The Patient's Wish to Die

The Patient's Wish to Die

Research, Ethics, and Palliative Care

Edited by

Christoph Rehmann-Sutter,

Heike Gudat,

and

Kathrin Ohnsorge

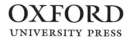

OXFORD

UNIVERSITY PRESS

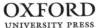
UNIVERSITY PRESS

Great Clarendon Street, Oxford, OX2 6DP,
United Kingdom

Oxford University Press is a department of the University of Oxford.
It furthers the University's objective of excellence in research, scholarship,
and education by publishing worldwide. Oxford is a registered trade mark of
Oxford University Press in the UK and in certain other countries

Published in the United States of America by Oxford University Press
198 Madison Avenue, New York, NY 10016, United States of America

British Library Cataloguing in Publication Data
Data available

Library of Congress Control Number: 2015930595

ISBN 978–0–19–871398–2

Printed in Great Britain by
Clays Ltd, St Ives plc

Acknowledgments

This book could not have been produced without the substantial contributions of numerous patients, family members, and healthcare professionals who were involved in the different studies on which the chapters report. As editors we thank Monica Buckland (all chapters except 2, 3, 4, 6, 7 and 12) and Ann Maloney (Chapters 19 and 20) for translating and revising the manuscripts written by authors whose first language is not English. We are grateful to Professor Jackie Leach Scully for her helpful questions on innumerable key details during the revision. We thank Judith Voellmy and Nadja Wilhelm for their patience and sharp eyes while putting the texts into the correct style and format. Special thanks to Professor Christina Schües for suggestions on earlier versions of Chapter 1 and Chapter 15, and to Professor Guy Widdershoven for his equally helpful comments to Chapter 8. We are grateful to Caroline Smith of Oxford University Press for her encouragement and support. Some parts of the book originated at a conference that the editors organized in June 2012 at the University of Basel in Switzerland. The production of the book was made possible thanks to research grants from Oncosuisse and the Swiss National Science Foundation.

Contents

Contributors

Albert Balaguer
Faculty of Medicine and Health Sciences,
Universitat Internacional de Catalunya,
Barcelona, Spain

Nessa Coyle
Ethics Committee and Clinical Ethics
Consultation Team,
Memorial Sloan-Kettering Cancer Center,
New York, USA

Luc Deliens
End-of-Life Care Research Group,
Vrije Universiteit Brussels and Ghent,
University Belgium,
Belgium

Heike Gudat
Hospiz im Park,
Arlesheim, Switzerland

Yasmin Gunaratnam
Department of Sociology,
Goldsmiths College,
University of London, UK

Christopher Lo
University Health Network,
University of Toronto, Canada

Lars Johan Materstvedt
Department of Philosophy
and Religious Studies,
Norwegian University of Science
and Technology (NTNU),
Trondheim, Norway

Alexandre Mauron
Institute for Ethics, History,
and the Humanities,
Faculty of Medicine,
University of Geneva,
Geneva, Switzerland

Bert Molewijk
Department of Medical Humanities,
EMGO+ Institute for Health and Care
Research,
VU University Medical Centre,
Amsterdam, The Netherlands

Cristina Monforte-Royo
Nursing Department,
Faculty of Medicine and Health Sciences,
Universitat Internacional de Catalunya,
Barcelona, Spain

Settimio Monteverde
Institute of Biomedical Ethics and
History of Medicine,
University of Zurich,
Zurich, Switzerland

H. Christof Müller-Busch
Consultant for Palliative Medicine
(now retired),
Pain Therapy and Anesthesiology,
Gemeinschaftskrankenhaus Havelhöhe,
Berlin, Germany

Rinat Nissim
Department of Psychiatry,
University of Toronto,
Canada

Kathrin Ohnsorge
Hospiz im Park,
Arlesheim, Switzerland

Bregje Onwuteaka-Philipsen
Department of Public and Occupational
Health,
EMGO Institute for Health and Care
Research,
VU University Medical Center,
Amsterdam, The Netherlands

Christoph Rehmann-Sutter
Institute for History of Medicine
and Science Studies,
University of Lübeck,
Lübeck, Germany

Gary Rodin
Department of Psychiatry,
University of Toronto,
Canada

Tracy Schroepfer
School of Social Work,
University of Wisconsin-Madison,
USA

Lois Sculco (1937–2012)
Radcliffe College, Harvard University,
Cambridge, USA

Tinne Smets
End-of-Life Care Research Group,
Vrije Universiteit Brussels
and Ghent University,
Belgium

Margreet Stolper
Department of Medical Humanities,
EMGO+ Institute for Health and Care
Research,
VU University Medical Centre,
Amsterdam, The Netherlands

Marian A. Verkerk
Faculty of Medical Sciences,
University of Groningen,
Groningen, The Netherlands

Christian Villavicencio-Chávez
Palliative Care Service, Institut Català
d'Oncologia,
Faculty of Medicine and Health
Sciences,
Universitat Internacional de Catalunya,
Barcelona, Spain

Guy Widdershoven
Department of Medical Humanities,
VU University Medical Center,
Amsterdam, The Netherlands

Part I

Introduction

Chapter 1

Why it is important to know about patients' wishes to die

Christoph Rehmann-Sutter, Heike Gudat, and Kathrin Ohnsorge

Die.
What a powerful word
Yet spoken so lightly.
Die.
[...]

Legion[1]

Wish to die: an introduction

Most people, even early on in their lives, have wishes about *how* they want to die: without pain, in dignity, surrounded by their loved ones, in private, and so on. Most people hope that relatives, healthcare professionals, and medical institutions will support them in these wishes. If, however, somebody knows that she or he is already terminally ill and the end seems to be coming inexorably, and soon, it is quite understandable that wishes about how one wants to die may also comprise another component: the wish *for death to come*. Some patients in similar situations may still want to continue living. This book is about wishes of this sort: the wishes of patients about their dying that do not just cover the circumstances of death but, most importantly, the wish for death itself to come. The chapters explore the agency of patients who hold and formulate such wishes, and the meanings these wishes may have for them.

For those involved in (palliative) care it can be troubling to be confronted with a patient's wish to die in this sense. It can pose a serious emotional and moral challenge. The ethical dilemmas require sensitive and empathetic understanding, and this again requires a particular respect for the patient's subjectivity. Palliative care specialists are aware of this challenge, even though opinions differ on how to respond to such wishes in practice, especially if they also involve a request for the ending of life-supporting treatments or even for assisted dying. How far should medical care go, and what can medical institutions endorse as being ethically appropriate and possible? Does respecting the patient's wish to die always mean fulfilling it or are other responses more appropriate? How can we distinguish between different kinds of wishes to die—which may also appear before illness has become terminal?

There are underlying issues that need to be clarified before we can reasonably discuss which responses are ethically acceptable and which are not. What might a patient actually be up to when she or he expresses a wish to die? What *is* a wish to die in the first place, as a psychological and social phenomenon of human intentionality? And what are the relevant contextual factors that may trigger it? How can healthcare professionals understand a wish to die? There is a widespread consensus today that wishes to die can have different meanings and that they are *not always* a symptom of less-than-optimal care or a sign that the patient has 'given up' or is suffering from depression. It has been acknowledged that in some patients a wish to die persists even with access to the best palliative care (Arnold et al. 2004).

Wishes to die: an emerging topic in end-of-life research

Two groundbreaking studies about dying appeared in the 1960s: Barney G. Glaser and Anselm L. Strauss's sociological report *Awareness of Dying* in 1965 (Glaser and Strauss 2005) and Elisabeth Kübler-Ross's psychological research *On Death and Dying* in 1969 (Kübler-Ross 2009). Glaser and Strauss investigated the secrecy or openness about the fact that a patient has a terminal illness, depending on whether the patient knows about her or his situation. Extensive qualitative data were collected in clinics in the Bay Area of San Francisco. If a patient knows that he will die soon and that medical care can no longer save his life, he might, as the authors wrote, actually develop a 'wish to die' (Glaser and Strauss 2005, p. 80). So the term 'wish to die' appears in the psychosocial literature. But the wish to die in Glaser and Strauss's book was not understood as a wish that death may come, or that it may come sooner, but rather as the wish to die in particular ways: without pain, with dignity, etc.

In Kübler-Ross's famous account of the five stages of coming to terms with one's own dying, the first stage is denial of death and isolation: not even being willing to *know* that one is going to die. The last stage, which might be closest to a wish to die, however, sees no alternative to an acceptance of approaching death. It is 'a stage during which he is neither depressed nor angry about his "fate" ' (Kübler-Ross 2009, p. 91). In Kübler-Ross's concept of acceptance, the possibility of a *wish* to die does not appear. The time was not yet ripe explicitly to investigate wishes to die at the end of life that contained a desire for that life to end. Other questions were still in the foreground at that time: the disclosure of the true facts to the patient and the effect of non-disclosure or disclosure on communication within the clinic and in the families (Glaser and Strauss), or the learning process and the personal transformations that a dying person undergoes (Kübler-Ross).

During the 1980s, however, psychosocial research in medicine acknowledged the possibility of potentially 'normal' (i.e. non-pathological) wishes to die in terminally ill patients (Brown et al. 1986). The existence of wishes and desires to die was of course known, but their significance then became less clear. Brown et al. (1986) asked, 'Is it normal for terminally ill patients to desire to die?' Should wishes to die be qualified as symptoms of a psychiatric disorder (depression) or always as a symptom of inadequate medical care (including untreated depression)? Or can they also be, as psychiatrist

Harvey Chochinov's group wrote, 'part of a normal adaptation to a life-threatening disease' (Chochinov et al. 1994, p. 537)? And where is the line between the 'normal' and the pathological? The answers to these questions also depend on philosophical assumptions about the normative significance of end-of-life care and of dying that transcend the medical sphere and therefore should not be discussed by medical professionals alone.

Studies of the factors leading to wish to die statements highlighted a multifactorial aetiology. Physical symptoms (if well controlled) are considered less influential than psychosocial and existential–spiritual distress, such as depression, demoralization, hopelessness, spiritual abandonment, fears about the future, fear of losing control, or fear of losing a sense of self. In a systematic meta-analysis of seven recent qualitative studies of patients' views, Monforte-Royo et al. (2010) found the wish to hasten death to be a response of the patient to multidimensional suffering. They developed a model of the factors that lead to the emergence of a wish to hasten death, which included 'total suffering, loss of self, and fear, which together produce an overwhelming emotional distress in relation to which the wish to hasten death is seen as a way out, i.e. the individual wishes to cease living in this way and to put an end to suffering while maintaining some control over the situation' (Monforte-Royo et al. 2010, p. 12). There is a certain amount of evidence for various aetiological factors, but there has been a lack of insight into the significance of the wish to die in the individual narrative context, as seen from the perspective of patients themselves. Adequately describing subjective matters is methodologically challenging, and requires a phenomenological–hermeneutic approach. One of the first studies of this type was published by Nessa Coyle and Lois Sculco (2004) and is reprinted in this volume. What patients *mean* when they say that they wish to die was the focus of that study. It became clear that these meanings are complex and can also be misinterpreted. More elaborate analytical tools needed to be developed to understand adequately what patients mean when they express a wish to die. For example, patients can mean different things by a fear of 'losing autonomy': is it a fear of becoming physically dependent on life-supporting technology, of finding themselves in a situation of social dependence, of losing the possibility of meaningful activity, or of being exposed to hospital routines? Or is the patient expressing a desire to preserve self-determination in planning what happens during the last moments of her or his life? Similarly nuanced meanings can be expected for other triggering factors, such as the fear of being a burden to others, a perceived loss of dignity, or a loss of meaning in life. This suggests that empirical findings, even if self-reported by patients in survey studies, have only a limited explanatory value if they are not complemented by a deeper understanding of the individual person's views on these items, which requires qualitative and narrative methodologies.

The idea of the book

In many countries there has been a public debate over several decades about the appropriate regulation of hastening death and other aspects of end-of-life care. The debates, however, often run in ideologically constrained circles and are not sensitive to the finer tuning of both the clinical reality and the subjective experiences and moral understandings of patients themselves as their lives draw to a close. This book brings together different research approaches to examine these phenomena, and makes them accessible to a broader audience than just the small, but international, 'wish to die' research community. Empirical research has been carried out for more than a decade on the phenomena of wishes to die and desires for a hastened death at the end of life. This book reflects the best currently available knowledge and research methodologies about patients' wishes at the end of life, together with a series of ethical views and a discussion of the clinical implications for palliative care.

When somebody says, 'I really want to die', 'I would prefer to be dead soon', 'Please, let me die more quickly'—or similar things—the underlying wish expressed may be very complex. In order to respond competently and compassionately, the healthcare professional needs to grasp the dimensions immanent in wishes to die, both in general and in regard to the concrete individually expressed concerns of the particular patient. This requires deeper knowledge of the structure, the meanings, and the dynamics of this phenomenon and of the interactions in which it is embedded. However, talking with patients in depth about wish to die statements is still seen as challenging, and is therefore often avoided by healthcare professionals (see Kohlwes et al. 2001). A superficial understanding of the statement risks taking it at face value (just fulfilling what is requested in the name of a superficially understood 'patient autonomy') without recognizing the patient fully as the person she or he is, who may be experiencing deeply ambivalent feelings at the end of life and who might express this as one element within a larger dialogue with healthcare professionals and relatives—and also in an inner dialogue with her- or himself. Another risk would be to 'medicalize' the expressed wish to die, i.e. to treat it as a sign or symptom of depression or anxiety in every single case which automatically demands treatment. Both reactions can lead to suboptimal palliative care, to shortcomings in the caring relationship, and, if things develop unhappily, even to an unnecessary abandonment of the patient.

The intended audience of this book is primarily healthcare practitioners involved in end-of-life care but also interdisciplinary scholars interested in palliative care and medical ethics, including its specific challenges in the last phases of life. The book attempts to contribute in an open manner to the medical, ethical, and public debates on this topic. It aims to be sensitive to the spiritual and existential dimensions of dying and to the different cultural views that provide meaning to the individual.

We have invited some of the best-known palliative care research specialists and ethics scholars from different countries to reflect on this sensitive issue based on an empirically informed and patient-centred view. Many, but not all, of the authors discuss the topic from a hermeneutical, phenomenological, or narrative perspective. The collection includes palliative care practitioners and end-of-life scholars from countries where different forms of assisted dying practices (such as assisted suicide or euthanasia) are legalized and from other countries where they are not.

A basic priority and its context

The topic of 'wishes to die' raises many deep philosophical questions. We can mention only one here: the assumption that life is better than death. This is a fundamental requisite for the continued existence of human societies—a basic priority for human life. Humans are expected to wish for life, not death. But on an individual level circumstances can be exceptional and the priority can switch. However, circumstances are not accountable for everything. There might also be—for some—the wish to maintain control over the situation when (or by) wishing to die, i.e. a decisional element, a sort of radical responsibility. The existentialist philosopher Albert Camus (1975, p. 11) wrote about this responsibility and considered the decision to live and *not* to stop living (i.e. not to commit suicide), while it remains a possible choice, as the most important of all questions: 'There is but one truly serious philosophical problem and that is suicide. Judging whether life is or is not worth living amounts to answering the fundamental question of philosophy.' Importantly, in Camus' thinking it is the decision *not* to wish for death that opens this question. Death wishes are not positively embraced, even though they are acknowledged as one *possible* element of the human condition.

It is a fact that, under difficult circumstances that render their situation hopeless, individuals can lose their desire to continue living; they may have an overriding reason to end their life, and may even kill themselves. This has been an important topic in literature since antiquity. We could mention King Saul's (heroic) suicide on the battlefield to avoid being captured by his enemies (1 Samuel 31: 3–6). Death was an act of *ultima ratio*, the ace up his sleeve, a way out; maybe the only way out. The will to die in such stories emerged from context, both physical and sociocultural.

Wishes to die in clinical contexts are in some way related to norms and moral attitudes concerning life and death (including suicide), however much they vary. The disease trajectory belongs to the situation, but is bound to the person. Patients' wishes to die also emerge from contextual considerations, and their meaning can only be understood within the local narratives. The special situation of a patient is to be in an unwanted state—to be terminally ill and to be extremely restricted as a consequence—and to wish for something that, according to social norms and moral attitudes, one should not wish. Most patients would want to live, but not under these circumstances. And in their despair they may even feel a need to justify this wish.

One narrative that has in recent decades underpinned many defences of autonomy at the end of life is the vision of being caught in a spider's web of medical technology. Philippe Ariès (1974) famously described the historical processes that made death a 'forbidden' event (to be prevented by all means) in the twentieth century and at the same time a communicative taboo. The typical new version of the frightening figure of death, he suggested, the image that replaced the Grim Reaper of earlier times, is the fear of being hooked up to life-support machines, of hanging on tubes, ending up in a state of complete dependence and inability to act. This version of fearful death is, however, not the fear of death arriving at the wrong time. Quite the contrary: it is the fear of *not* being able to die at the right time. It is the fear of being blocked from dying well, of being coerced to stay in a life that leaves no possibility for being oneself, that senselessly prolongs suffering, or that is no more than half-conscious organic functioning. The fear of being *over*treated by medicine animates much of the present discussion about wishes to die in hospital contexts. Here, a topic for ethical reflection has emerged: the 'good death' (Hagger and Woods 2013).

What is the wish in a 'wish to die'?

When we talk about wishes to die we also need to clarify what we mean when we address something in our minds as 'a wish'. Wishes are familiar experiences, but describing them analytically is not at all trivial. The discussion starts with looking for the correct overarching category to which the wishes belong. 'States of the mind' would be an obvious and frequently used category. We believe, however, that wishes cannot satisfactorily be categorized as 'states' of the mind. Wishes are not at all static but rather dynamic dispositions that play a role in interactive social processes and are sometimes conscious, sometimes hidden. A wish to die can appear in a moment as a state of the mind, but only if we do not pay attention to its motions. Why then suggest that it is static at all? A wish is a dynamic and interactive process. Always, when we say 'X has a wish' we mean that X is doing something: X is wishing. Wishing is a mental activity, not something one 'has' like one has a toothache. Strictly speaking, a wish is not an entity that could be identified by a noun.

Wishes to die deal with existential themes and therefore come from 'deep within'. How can this be explained? Wishes as such matter for the person. And wishes to die, especially, are not ideas that can easily be changed, like more casual wishes. Wishes emerge and may be overwhelming; they may suddenly present as the result of pondering about circumstances over a long period of time. But although such wishes are often not consciously formed, at least not entirely, people still grapple with them. They deal and fight with them; they develop them.

Traditionally, Western thought, and especially liberal thought, envisioned the act of willing (and wishing, although this is a distinct notion, which has sometimes been understood as part of forming a will) as a single moment of choice in which an autonomous individual asserts his or her own personal freedom, based on his or her independent cognitive capacities. Referring to the writings of Iris Murdoch, Cheryl Mattingly draws attention to the fact that in this concept of will as a moment of choice the 'notion of struggle is curiously absent' (Mattingly 2010, p. 56). Rather than conceptualizing willing as a single moment, or even a sequence of choices, it should be seen as 'a kind of practice, one that involves significant internal work', a kind of work that is about 'cultivating' moral ideas and emotions connected to one's self-understandings. Applying these to wishing, or more concretely to wishes to die, makes final wishes appear not just as expressions of decisive moments of choice but as internal work—most likely not without struggle—of coming to terms with what one wants for oneself (and for others with regard to oneself) at the end of life.

In this perspective, wishes to die are not single moments of decisions, neither are they entirely endured, but they do have an active side to them. Wishing to die is an active–passive dispositional practice. Humans can refocus the attention that is contained in it. Some wishes they themselves view as forbidden. And wishes do not come singly. We can have some wishes that contradict, and tend to cancel out, others. Wishing always develops in relation to all kind of things that matter to us in our lives. To arrive at what we wish, we evaluate and re-evaluate our moral understandings, self-images, convictions, and deepest commitments. And we do not usually do this in abstraction from our relation to others, but with respect or in contrast to what they wish and want. For this reason, Mattingly (2010, p. 68) speaks of willing as a process of 're-envisioning and re-orienting'. Continuing her line of thought, wishes to die might be seen as an inner work, a process of re-orienting or re-evaluating one's intentions about dying. Similarly, Margaret Archer (2003) has described internal conversations as personal reflexivity, which of course also includes conversation with others. Reflexively, individuals exert a form of agency that should be recognized as moral work on wishes.

Wishes in general are diverse, not just in content but also in kind. A closer look at them tells us that they populate a variable landscape of mountains and interconnected valleys. Like willing, wishing as a process is indeed moral work, since in wishing one usually evaluates what has significance for oneself against one's own moral understandings. But in contrast to a will, which represents an intention that is directed to an act, a wish is not necessarily directed towards acting. It is one of the essential characteristics of the wish that, in contrast to the will, it is possible to wish without performing the act for which one is wishing in physical reality. A wish is still a wish if it remains a hope for something. And it is not the realization of the wish that represents the sense of agency in wishing; it is the force of wishing itself that represents it. In a situation of fading vitality the wish to die may restore a kind of activity, sometimes without externally doing something, and to some degree help to re-appropriate the process of dying.

The psychologist and philosopher William James, writing in 1890, referred to common experience when beginning his chapter on 'will' in his *Principles of Psychology* with the following: 'Desire, wish, will, are states of the mind which everyone knows, and which no definition can make plainer' (James 1983, p. 1098). As the will must be distinguished from the act that follows, the wish can also be distinguished from willing and from acting. Anyone can wish impossible things, such as being able to fly like a bird, but still be unable act them out. The possibility of a wish, as we have said, does not depend on the possibility of its realization. But James goes on with a further important point: volition, he emphasizes, is a relation between an idea we have on the one hand and our Self on the other. This applies to the wish as well. An idea *stings* us in such a way that we say, *let it be* a reality (James 1983, pp. 1172ff.; cf. Garro 2010). A wish is therefore more than an idea; it is the relation to the Self that we may describe as *hope*: when I wish to fly, my idea ('me flying') is connected to myself in the sense that I would like to fly. A wish to die, accordingly, is more than imagining ceasing to exist, more than the idea or the certain knowledge that one will be dead at some time in the future. What it refers to is the relation to the Self, which is captured by James's word 'sting'. The idea of dying stings the person who is wishing to die: wishing to die is hoping that the idea of dying may come true. Hope can have many senses and intensities (see Bloch 1959).

With this in mind it is easier to draw out the distinctive characteristics of the wish in contrast to the will (Rehmann-Sutter 2013). Drawing on phenomenological literature— Bergson, Schutz, and Ricoeur—Jason Throop (2010) gives a helpful account of three constitutive dimensions of an act of willing: (1) own-ness—this is the sense that one is the author of one's own thoughts, ideas and actions; (2) anticipation/goal directedness— one anticipates an outcome as it unfolds into the future; (3) effortful-ness: one's intended act or behaviour requires effort or energy.

However, if somebody is wishing rather than willing, three dimensions can also be captured as being constitutive. The first, own-ness (1), is quite similar to willing.

In wishing one has the sense of being the author of one's own thoughts, ideas, and imaginings, but one can also wish that *others* act in certain ways (which is impossible in willing). There is also (2) an anticipatory dimension: in wishing one anticipates the content of the imagination to become or to be real. The intentional dimension, which in Throop's account of willing is effortful and directed towards a behaviour, is different in wishing: (3) the imaginative content of the wish is *hoped* to be or to become real. A wish does not necessarily aim for the act whose achievement needs energy. Wishing is more airy, but it still can require effort: both when wishes come into conflict with each other and need to be clarified, and when they need to be maintained under difficulties.

As we can see here, wishes are important parts of everybody's experience and of everybody's handling of reality. They are particularly important for those who are severely ill. It is therefore key to look into them more closely—which we will do in this book.

The structure of the book

The chapters illuminate the anatomy of the wishes to die of severely ill people. The diversity of possible points of view and possible practical conclusions shows us that we all (researchers as well) are imprinted by our own cultural context and by our own experiences. Taking this into account gives us an opportunity to reflect deeply on our own ideas and to proceed to new questions.

Part II (Research) looks at the state of empirical psychosocial research on wishes to die. Yasmin Gunaratnam (Chapter 2) introduces a narrative method for investigating the meaning contained in suffering, which is particularly relevant to uncovering the content of wishes to die. We then reprint as Chapter 3 the 2004 paper by Nessa Coyle and Lois Sculco, which was the first to provide an extensive and comparative insight into the meaningful construction of a wish to hasten death. It is followed by a new afterword by Nessa Coyle. A particularly interesting country for studying the impact of a changed, i.e. more liberal, legal framework on assisted dying, is Belgium, where a euthanasia law was introduced in 2002 and end-of-life research has been undertaken since then in a particularly intense way. In Chapter 5 Luc Deliens and Tinne Smets summarize the main highlights from this research so far. Tracy Schroepfer (Chapter 6) has developed a model for describing and understanding wishes to hasten death that includes psychosocial, spiritual, and physical motivating factors and temporal stability. In Chapter 7 Rinat Nissim, Chris Lo, and Gary Rodin report from their extended mixed methods study on the desire for hastened death in patients with advanced cancer undergoing outpatient treatment, and develop a three-factor model that includes multiple meanings of desires for hastened death. Then in Chapter 8 Kathrin Ohnsorge presents an analytical model resulting from a qualitative study that identifies three dimensions of wishes to die in patients in palliative care (intentions, motivations, and social interactions). That study was conducted in Switzerland, which is the only country where right-to-die organizations can legally offer assistance in suicide. Alexandre Mauron in Chapter 9 describes and explains the particulars of the Swiss situation. Another country where both euthanasia and (physician) assisted suicide are legal is the Netherlands, and in Chapter 10 Bregje Onwuteaka-Philipsen reports on extensive research that has been performed there to monitor the effects of the liberal governance. She describes five situations that can trigger a death wish in older people.

Part III (Ethics) offers four lenses or perspectives on the ethics of practically responding to wishes to die. The first is the Kantian approach to self-determination. In Chapter 12 Lars Johan Materstvedt undertakes a new reading of Kant's ethics and connects it with assisted dying in the context of palliative care. He arrives at a nuanced view of the idea that the patient is the best judge of her or his own interests. Then, in Chapter 13, Marian Verkerk introduces the perspective of 'responsive knowing' and epistemic justice. Speaking from Dutch experience, she applies these concepts to the moral conversation between doctor and patient. Conversations are also a topic of Chapter 14 by Guy Widdershoven, Margreet Stolper, and Bert Molewijk, although in a different sense: these authors discuss the application of an interactive and hermeneutic method of moral inquiry, 'moral case deliberation', to the moral dilemmas arising from requests for euthanasia. In Chapter 15 Christoph Rehmann-Sutter focuses on the perspective of patients' wishes and defends their own moral perspective as a space of moral deliberation, stressing that the topic of ethical debate should not be restricted to the dilemmas of healthcare professionals but should also include patients' own dilemmas in coping with their own wishes to die.

In Part IV (Practice), practical issues are discussed as they are encountered in palliative care for patients at the end of life who express wishes to die. The authors differ in what they consider an appropriate response to these wishes. Christof Müller-Busch begins in Chapter 17 by opening a value perspective on the intentions and principles of palliative medicine in the process of effective communication and thoughtful decision making when handling requests for hastening death. Then in Chapter 18 Settimio Monteverde introduces the spiritual dimension of living and dying, exploring a 'spiritual turn' within medicine. He also discusses the definition and assessment of spirituality in the context of patients' wishes to die. In Chapter 19, on issues of communication, Heike Gudat, Christoph Rehmann-Sutter, and Kathrin Ohnsorge address the relationship between healthcare professionals and patients as unequal dialogue partners. They stress the importance of narratives as communication tools. In Chapter 20 Heike Gudat analyses two examples of patients who explained their wishes to die and to live, how far they would go, and why they had their different wishes, some of them in tension with each other. The patient in palliative care is a social actor with a role to play in the social context of the hospital, and in Chapter 21 Cristina Monforte-Royo, Albert Balaguer, and Christian Villavicencio-Chàvez explore and discuss the different meanings of wishes to die in this clinical context.

The interactive pieces at the end of some parts of the book (Chapters 11, 16, and 22) were collated from an email conversation between the authors on a few selected questions that came up while preparing this volume.

Notes

1   Reproduced from Legion, *Die*, Copyright © 2013, Joe Stahl. Dated 9 July 2013. The poet Joe Stahl, writing under the name Legion, was born 1996 in Chicago. Courtesy of the author; originally published on: <http://www.hellopoetry.com>.

References

Archer, M. (2003). *Structure, Agency and the Internal Conversation*. Cambridge: Cambridge University Press.

Ariès, P. (1974). *Western Attitudes Toward Death. From the Middle Ages to the Present* (transl. P. M. Ranum). Baltimore: Johns Hopkins University Press.

Arnold, E. M., Artin, K. A., Person, J. L., and Griffith, D. L. (2004). Consideration of hastening death among hospice patients and their families. *Journal of Pain and Symptom Management*, **6**, 523–532.

Bloch, E. (1959). *Das Prinzip Hoffnung*, **3** vols. Frankfurt am Main: Suhrkamp.

Brown, J. H., Henteleff, P., Barakat, S., and Rowe, C. J. (1986). Is it normal for terminally ill patients to desire death? *American Journal of Psychiatry*, **143**, 208–211.

Camus, A. (1975). *The Myth of Sysiphus* (transl. J. O'Brien). Harmondsworth: Penguin (originally published 1942).

Chochinov, H. M., Wilson, K. G., Enns, M., and Lander, S. (1994). Prevalence of depression in the terminally ill: Effects of diagnostic criteria and symptom threshold judgments. *American Journal of Psychiatry*, **151**, 537–540.

Coyle, N. and Sculco, L. (2004). Expressed desire for hastened death in seven patients living with advanced cancer: a phenomenologic inquiry. *Oncology Nursing Forum*, **31**, 699–706.

Garro, L. C. (2010). By the will of others or by one's own action? In: K. M. Murphy and C. J. Throop (eds), *Toward and Anthropology of the Will*, pp. 69–100. Stanford: Stanford University Press.

Glaser, B. G. and Strauss, A. L. (2005). *Awareness of Dying*. New Brunswick: Aldine Transaction (originally published 1965).

Hagger, L. and Woods, S. (eds) (2013). *A Good Death? Law and Ethics in Practice*. Farnham: Ashgate.

James, W. (1983). *The Principles of Psychology*. Cambridge, MA: Harvard University Press (originally published 1890).

Kohlwes, R. J., Koepsell, T. D., Rhodes, L. A., and Pearlman, R. A. (2001). Physicians' responses to patients' requests for physician-assisted suicide. *Archives of Internal Medicine*, **161**, 657–663.

Kübler-Ross, E. (2009). *On Death and Dying. What the Dying Have to Teach Doctors, Nurses, Clergy and Their Own Families*, 40th anniversary edn. London: Routledge (originally published 1969).

Mattingly, C. (2010). Moral willing as narrative re-envisioning. In: K. M. Murphy and C. J. Throop (eds), *Toward an Anthropology of the Will*, pp. 50–68. Stanford: Stanford University Press.

Monforte-Royo, C., Villavicencio-Chavez, C., Tomas-Sabado, J., Mahatani-Chugani, V., and Balaguer, A. (2010). What lies behind the wish to hasten death? A systematic review and meta-ethnography from the perspective of patients. *PLoS One*, **7**(5), e37117, doi: 10.1371/journal.pone.0037117.

Rehmann-Sutter, C. (2013). Sterben als Teil des Lebens und als Handlungsraum. Ethische Überlegungen. In: H. Greif and M. G. Weiss (eds), *Ethics, Society, Politics. Proceedings of the 35th International Wittgenstein Symposium, Kirchberg am Wechsel, Austria, 2012*, pp. 483–518. Berlin: DeGruyter Ontos.

Throop, C. J. (2010). In the midst of action. In: K. M. Murphy and C. J. Throop (eds), *Toward an Anthropology of the Will*, 28–49. Stanford: Stanford University Press.

Part II

Research

Chapter 2

Illness narratives, meaning making, and epistemic injustice in research at the end of life

Yasmin Gunaratnam

Cultural contexts and personhood

In an ethnographic study of an English hospice, the anthropologist Julia Lawton (2000) came across people whose bodily boundaries were disintegrating because of their advanced disease. Though not always in physical pain, the patients' symptoms, which included the leaking of excreta and smells, were causing profound anguish and a loss of dignity. Selfhood was seeping out through their bodies, Lawton suggested, rendering them 'non-persons', physically present but subjectively absent. Recording what she observed, Lawton tells us about their end-of-life responses and wishes:

> Other patients, like Annie, made more explicit attempts to 'switch themselves off' by requesting heavy sedation. Kath for example, asked that she be moved to a side room and given a large dose of analgesics after commenting . . . 'you wouldn't put a dog through this' . . . Some patients, like Deborah, refused to eat or drink, thereby accelerating their own demise; others like Dolly, made direct requests for euthanasia. Stan, a patient with cancer of the prostate . . . repeatedly asked the staff to help him to die.

> Reproduced from Julia Lawton, *The Dying Process: Patients' Experiences of Palliative Care*, p. 132, Routledge, Oxford, Copyright © 2000, Routledge.

Requests for hastened death, among this group of dying people, were sometimes direct and explicit. In other cases, wishes were not so much spoken but were enacted in the refusal to eat or drink or in the withdrawal from human contact. Elsewhere in Lawton's study, we discover how last wishes are not atemporal but can change over time, for instance when symptoms are temporarily controlled and an individual no longer talks about wanting to die. For Lawton, suffering and the desire for a hastened death are connected to the Western idealization of personhood and dignity as self-contained. The most important cultural attributes of such ideals, as Lawton has identified them, are 'a bounded, physically sealed, enclosed body' and 'the bodily ability to act as the agent of one's embodied actions and intentions' (Lawton 2000, p. 7).

I begin my chapter by quoting these evocative ethnographic stories because they describe what it can be like to live with suffering, bodily decay, and fluctuating feelings at the most intimate of levels. These experiences can be missing from academic discussions, where Western perspectives of personhood, rational choice, and consistent and linear narrating are normative. Although I do not have the space to discuss the consequences of this normativity here, I want to keep these relationships in mind as I introduce narrative approaches and consider their relevance to research on end-of-life wishes and plans.

In what follows, I will first say something about the terms 'narrative' and 'story', before providing a general flavour of relevant themes from the literature on illness narratives. Next, I discuss speech act theory, as one approach to interpreting the meaning of last wishes that takes into account the impact of the social and cultural milieu on the creation and understanding of meaning. Finally, drawing from the palliative care concept of 'total pain', I offer thoughts on the limitations of narrative and empathic understanding when people are suffering. It is here that I will point to the ways in which narrative approaches can be valuable to care professionals and researchers in recognizing the challenges of being receptive to ambiguous, and discontinuous meanings.

Narratives and stories

It is important to acknowledge at the outset that for some writers, the process of defining, categorizing, and analysing the features of narrative and stories is less than fruitful, leading to decontextualized understanding and a distancing from the moral and relational demands of stories (Frank 2010). For others, knowledge of the distinctive features of a narrative and story can provide a deeper appreciation of the narrator's portrayal of themselves and how the structure of a narrative can work upon the listener (Greenhalgh and Hurwitz 1998, 1999; Paley and Eva 2005). This interest in the qualities of narrative is not wholly abstracted and theoretical. Sayantani DasGupta (2008), a physician and practitioner in the narrative medicine program at Columbia University, New York, believes that 'narrative humility' is a necessary and moral stance for care professionals. In DasGupta's words, narrative humility helps a practitioner 'to place herself in a position of receptivity, where she does not merely act upon others, but is in turn acted upon' (DasGupta 2008, p. 981).

Using concepts from literary criticism, Paley and Eva (2005) similarly believe that stories work upon those who receive them, but they take a different view. They argue that because the structuring of an account can affect us emotionally, we need to be attentive to the differences between a narrative and a story. Paley and Eva define a narrative as a sequence of events that are causally related, with one event leading on from another (Bal 1997). In this developmental framework, a story is a thickened and complicated narrative. In addition to related events, a story has a character(s), a problem, an explanation, and an underlying plot. A distinguishing feature of the 'narrative machinery' of a story is how it works to elicit an emotional response (Paley 2009). In light of the emotional magnetism of stories, Paley and Eva advise 'narrative vigilance', warning that we can be drawn to certain stories and persuaded by their surface meanings (as well as being repelled by others), because of their emotional resonance and our related judgements about how reliable a narrator is.

There are ethical as well as practical implications to this recognition of the differences between a narrative and a story. Using Miranda Fricker's (2007) idea of 'epistemic injustice', Carel and Kidd (2014) propose that illness narratives can be regarded with particular suspicion in health care, because patients are seen as being overly emotional and unstable as a result of their illness. For Carel and Kidd, the valuing of impersonal, third-person reports—that is, narratives rather than stories—disadvantages those who do not conform to these preferred styles of condensed, coherent and selective reporting. They remind us, furthermore, that the experience of illness and the emotional and bodily chaos that accompanies it, can be difficult, sometimes impossible, to make sense of and to narrate.

There are other aspects to epistemic injustice in end-of-life care that I would like to highlight. In my qualitative research with dying migrants to the United Kingdom, I have found that cultural and language differences can flatten patients' stories into narratives, lacking in emotional depth and nuance. In these situations, the stripped back narrative, alongside social and cultural differences, can get in the way of empathy and the ability to see an illness within the unique psychosocial tapestry of a life. The failure to imagine other lives, which perhaps have been more precarious and difficult than our own, can lead to what Fricker calls 'structural hermeneutical injustice'. That is: 'The injustice of having some significant area of one's social experience obscured from collective understanding owing to a structural identity prejudice in the collective hermeneutic resource' (Fricker 2007, p. 155).

In my research on social pain, defined by neuroscientists as the pain of social rejection and exclusion (Eisenberger 2012), I have begun to explore how past experiences of social pain and structural hermeneutical injustice can meld and gather over a person's lifetime. At the end of life, experiences of social inequality, together with cultural difference, can become further entangled with the symptoms of disease, blurring the boundaries between physical and social suffering, constraining meaningful exchanges (Gunaratnam 2014). Alongside the recognition of unreliable narrators, the predicament of the 'unreliable witness' is also apparent. Professionals can doubt whether they have fully understood a person's experience. For example, a hospice nurse, Gill, told me about a refugee from Uganda, with suspected dementia, who was dying of AIDs-related conditions. The woman, who was a mother, did not speak English and did not have friends or family in the United Kingdom. She appeared to be suspicious of care professionals, and Gill's efforts to communicate with her—to 'get alongside' her, as Gill put it—were unsuccessful. 'I suppose I view that as a failure of care in a way' Gill said. 'But then can you, can we ever, as somebody from a completely different culture . . . could I ever have done that you know, given more time?' (Gunaratnam 2013, p. 41).

Illness narratives

From this brief overview of discussions about the qualities of narratives and stories, it is possible to see how all kinds of narratives and stories—patient and professional accounts, diagnoses, medical histories, advanced care plans, case reviews, rumours, and hearsay—characterize the worlds of illness and dying. Indeed, from the very beginnings of modern hospice care in the 1960s, the value of building empathetic communication by listening to the stories of patients and those close to them has been advocated as good therapeutic practice (Saunders 1988).

Rita Charon (2006), a physician and leading exponent of contemporary narrative medicine, believes that narrative knowledge and 'competence' are vital in cultivating empathy and helping professionals to develop the hermeneutic resources to counter what Carel and Kidd have seen as the devaluing of patients' stories and points of view. Of her early experiences of learning about narrative knowledge in everyday care, Charon writes:

> I had to follow the patient's narrative thread, identify the metaphors or images used in the telling, tolerate ambiguity . . . identify the unspoken subtexts, and hear one story in light of others told by the teller . . . I also had to be aware of my own response to what I heard, allowing myself to be personally moved to action on behalf of the patient . . . pain, suffering, worry, anguish, and the sense of something not being right are conditions very difficult, if not impossible, to put into words.
>
> Reproduced from Rita Charon *Narrative Medicine: Honoring the Stories of Illness*, p. 4, Oxford University Press, New York, Copyright © 2006, Oxford University Press.

An underlying belief in such approaches, which can also inform the use of narrative interview methods with dying people (see Gunaratnam 2009), is that narrative and stories are relational *events* of meaning-making, conveying the phenomenological experience of illness that is much more than a medical or 'naturalistic' account (Carel 2008). As Arthur Kleinman (1988, p. xiii) has written, 'Illness narratives edify us about how life problems are created, controlled, made meaningful.' By telling stories, Bochner believes, we become a part of 'the project of self-understanding, an endeavour that may be unreachable but, for most of us, appears to be inescapable' (Bochner 2001, p. 154).

The sociologist Gareth Williams (1984) has argued that narrative provides a means to reconstruct continuity in the face of the 'biographical disruption' of illness (Bury 1982). In the narratology of Arthur Frank (2009), attending to a person's stories at the end of a life can help a dying person to regain a sense of agency and responsibility, a capacity all too often eroded by illness and institutional care. Frank believes that this restoring of agency happens when stories make connections in three different ways: when a story conveys the singular interconnectedness of experienced events; when it shares 'affiliations' with other stories (see also Charon 2006); and through the relationship between the narrator and listener. It is the offered presence of the listener as an 'empathetic witness' (Kleinman 1988) to another's suffering that is seen as constituting the unique moral and therapeutic qualities of a story.

Thinking of narratives and stories as relational *events* of meaning-making and as involving moral relationships marks a shift away from a mimetic or realist assumption: that narratives are a transparent reflection of a person's experience and rational choices, a view that has been called 'narrative fundamentalism'(Shapiro 2011, p. 68). Sometimes referred to as 'constructivist' (see Bruner 1987) or 'dialogic' (Frank 2010), what these latter approaches share is the belief that we continually create and refine our experience, and indeed our moral agency, through the stories that we tell (Schafer 1981). Related to what has been called a 'crisis of representation', constructivist/dialogic perspectives recognize the potential for the meaning of stories to be encoded and/or polysemic. They also question the presumption that researchers can be emotionally detached from the narratives we encounter.

That there can be a surplus or a withdrawal of meaning to what a person is able to narrate is a belief that is central to psychosocial approaches to narrative, which recognize how unconscious emotional defences against anxiety and threat, can affect what people are able to think and say. For the psychologists Wendy Hollway and Tony Jefferson, both the researcher and the research participant are 'defended subjects', who are motivated, often unconsciously, to protect their vulnerabilities through denial and avoidance (Hollway and Jefferson 2013). Such protective defensiveness is seen to lie behind the discontinuities of what people narrate, prompting some researchers to highlight the need for interpretation to preserve the 'disrupting and disorganising' qualities of a narrative as they are likely to lie closer to the narrator's perspective (Frosh 2007, p. 641). However, others, such as the writer John Berger (Berger and Mohr 1995, p. 285), believe that the recognition of 'unstated connections' in narratives and stories is culturally implicit and taken for granted in the West. 'No story is like a wheeled vehicle whose contact with the road is continuous', Berger writes. 'Stories walk, like animals or men' (p. 284).

To summarize, the ideas that I have examined so far problematize rationalist models of decision-making, subjectivity, and intersubjective communication. With regard to last wishes, these ideas serve to question assumptions that final wishes and plans can:

reflect unambiguous and rational desires and choices

be clearly communicated to another person who understands their meaning

remain unchanged as they are communicated

are stable over time.

By unsettling these beliefs, narrative approaches have the potential to add interpretive depth to what is also being found in quantitative and qualitative research—that the meaning of last wishes and care preferences can be ambiguous and can change over time (Johansen et al. 2005; Evans et al. 2012). This is not to promote practices of 'hermeneutical obstinacy' (see Chapter 9), where the recognition of complexities in meaning can be used to manage and suppress the choices of those who are dying. Rather, my aim is to contribute to the expansion of hermeneutic resources in end-of-life care.

Last wishes and narrative

A critical difficulty with interpreting last wishes and 'desire to die' statements is that of ambiguity and ambivalence in meaning (Van Loon 1999). As Hudson et al. (2006) have found, there is considerable uncertainty as to whether desire to die statements are a direct request for hastened death, an expression of suffering, or are a part of confronting the future that should not be taken literally. It is also the case that most end-of-life decisions are made by family members, as surrogate decision-makers. For example, a study of 26 end-of-life decision-making meetings between hospital staff and relatives found competing moral frameworks, where what was thought to be in the patient's 'best interests' took precedence over that person's own wishes (Karasz et al. 2010). In such circumstances, researchers and care professionals can be faced with various accounts and interpretations of last wishes—including from their colleagues (Seale 2009)—and the dying person's stated desires and choices will need to be considered both within and outside of the context in which they were originally given. In this sense, there are different orders of last wishes: first-order accounts from the dying person themselves and second-order accounts that come from the narratives of others.

If we think of last wishes from the perspective of narratives and stories, it is possible to see how they share something in common with stories in other areas of life. We tell stories about ourselves to ourselves and we tell stories about others. In turn, others tell our stories. And all the time these interrelating stories are shaped by our changing circumstances and by cultural meta-narratives and prescriptions (Skultans 2007), a phenomenon that Greenhalgh and Collard (2003, p. xiii) call 'stories-within-stories'.

Meanwhile, technological changes and online social networking platforms such as Facebook and Instagram are transforming the medium and cultural mores of narratives and storytelling, not least for those who are ill and dying. Researchers have found that the internet has led to a huge increase in the sharing of illness narratives (Bingley et al. 2008). These new modes of storytelling can further complicate the interpretation of end-of-life wishes because of the differences that can emerge between online and 'real world' selves (see Walter et al. 2011).

In a study of 'Identity construction on Facebook', Shanyang Zhao et al. (2008) found that online identities in the nonymous digital community expressed ideal-type selves (Yurchisin et al. 2005), or what the philosopher Stanley Cavell (1990) has called our 'next self'. In the social sciences, the 'impression management' of public selves and the desire to show oneself in the best possible light have been seen as vital parts of social relationships, particularly when negotiating cultural stigma and threat (Goffman 1971). How, then, might we begin to understand these different qualities of what people say and when? One approach, which is concerned with the impact of social and interpersonal contexts on the interpretation of meaning, is speech act theory.

End-of-life wishes as speech acts

In taking account of the differences, noted earlier, between narratives and stories, it is possible to see that last wishes might not always be stories and can sometimes be pared-down narratives, where the chain of related events emplotted in a last wish are implicit. A wish or request for palliative sedation or for assisted dying, such as those observed by Julia Lawton, are a genre of narrative (see Atkinson 2005) that the philosopher J. L. Austin (1975/1962) has called 'speech acts'. Speech act theory, a part of 'ordinary language philosophy', is concerned with how language works in day-to-day life, not only to convey meaning but also to achieve certain effects. For Austin, we cannot understand the meaning of words or 'utterances' (units of speech) in isolation, as a priori. We need to appreciate language within its contexts of use. In speech act theory there are three main features of speech acts that are important in the interpretation of meaning:

the literal meaning of words and their associations in the settings where they are usually found (the locution) what the words are intended to perform, such as requesting, suggesting, convincing, arguing, and so on (the illocution)

the consequences of words (the perlocution).

Because the context of language use is vital to the flow of communication and understanding, speech act theory recognizes that the meaning of the same words can change according to different situations (for example with varying emphasis, tone, and gestures, as well as in different cultural and social settings). This is not to say that words themselves are unimportant, but rather that words can have different meanings because we can each experience the world differently and because interactional and institutional situations are layered. Landa (1992), for instance, differentiates between *direct* speech acts, where there is no conflict between the literal meanings of words and what is intended, and *indirect* speech acts, such as when a wish for euthanasia might be formulated/intended as a request but expresses fears about the future (see Johansen et al. 2005).

In speech act theory, it is believed that indirect communication can be best understood when it is a part of shared perspectives, but in some cases it can require further 'translation'. It is these relationships between intention, shared understanding, and the 'decoding' of what could be indirect communication that are at the heart of many of the interpretive and clinical dilemmas that surround last wishes. For example, if a final wish is an indirect communication of existential suffering, how appropriate is a clinical response (Materstvedt and Bosshard 2009)? Or alternatively, how might our willingness to interpret last wishes as indirect communication, with ambiguous meaning, be an example of the workings of 'epistemic injustice' (Fricker 2007), undermining a dying person's capacity to speak from her own sensibilities? Two crucial ideas in speech act theory, that of 'uptake' and 'effect', are especially relevant to the interpretation of end-of-life wishes (Austin 1975/1962). Uptake refers to how an individual can get a listener to recognize both the force and the meaning of what they are saying, while for a speech act to take effect, it is argued, it must produce certain normative states. For last wishes, these normative states can be thought of as commitments or obligations.

We can better see some of the ethical implications of speech act theory in the practice of medicine in the next section.

Words, emotions, and meaning

The relationship between ordinary language use and end-of-life decision-making has been the subject of a study of family members by Barnato and Arnold (2013). The study—a randomized, controlled simulation experiment with 256 people who were surrogate decision-makers for a spouse or parent—used different words and terms to heighten or decrease emotion with regard to statements about cardiopulmonary resuscitation (CPR). During the simulation, an actor playing a doctor used different wording to ask the participants whether or not they wanted CPR for their loved one. One group of participants was asked whether they wanted their family member to receive CPR, which had a 10% chance of saving their life, or if they wanted a 'do not resuscitate'

(DNR) order. With this explanation about 60% chose the CPR option. When the term 'allow natural death' was used 49% chose CPR.

Barnato and Arnold (2013) argue that the term 'allow natural death' altered the emotionality (i.e. it lessened the threat) of the explanation, reducing feelings of guilt, anxiety, and stress that have been found among family members facing end-of-life decisions (see McAdam et al. 2010). An important ethical question here is the extent to which language should be manipulated to persuade family members to concur with the thinking of healthcare professionals, or indeed in research to encourage people to disclose difficult feelings or information.

From the perspective of speech act theory, 'allow natural death' may on the surface perform an explanation; nevertheless, its effect (the perlocution) is to persuade/convince/sway family decision-making away from the choice of CPR. This is not to suggest that persuasion is necessarily a 'bad' ethical practice. As those, such as Eva (2009) and Frank (2009) have pointed out, individuals can become attached, if not trapped, within certain stories, unable to see alternative possibilities and outcomes for themselves. This point is significant, because it speaks directly to the use and ethics of speech acts and narrative approaches as a part of care practices. 'The delicate balance of clinical work' Frank suggests, 'is how gently or how hard to push people off one story and towards another' (Frank 2009, p. 173).

Having outlined some of the ways in which narrative knowledge can help a researcher to make sense of the complexities of how meaning in produced in last wishes, I now want to turn to Cicely Saunders' concept of total pain to consider the importance of recognizing the emotional demands of narrative research in care at the end of life.

Narrative research with pain, suffering, and death—'being there'

In developing the palliative care philosophy of 'total pain' in the late 1950s and 1960s, Cicely Saunders, regarded as the founder of the modern hospice movement, provided some of the earliest examples of narrative-based research and medicine. Saunders collected over a thousand patient case studies, including transcripts of patient interviews, drawings, poems, and photographs, in developing her ideas about hospice care. Her archived documents give a flavour of how she approached the matters of attention, representation, and affiliation that Rita Charon (2006) has seen as the cornerstones of 'narrative competence' and that apply as much to narrative research as to care. Attention is the striving for empathic understanding. As Charon describes it, for the clinician, 'one wants to join, with the patient, as a whole presence, deploying all of one's human gifts of intuition, empathy, and ability to bear witness to each patient one sees' (Charon 2006, p. 133). Affiliation is the connection made between different stories, of illness; and struggles of *representation* refer to how we might describe, evoke, and interpret patient stories in ways that support epistemic justice.

What is unusual about Saunders' conceptualization of total pain is that she recognized the limits of narrative, empathy, and representation when someone is suffering, so that her ontology of pain acknowledges the non-relational (see Gunaratnam 2012). What I mean by the non-relational are modes of bodily existence and sensibility that are withdrawn from social life and relationships (Gunaratnam 2013). One example of the non-relational occurs in palliative sedation. Another is a 'psychic switching off' from the social world that can be a consequence of trauma and suffering, as Julia Lawton (2000) found in her hospice study, discussed at the beginning of this chapter.

Connected to these non-relational aspects of suffering, Saunders recognized the limitations of active care at the end of life. In the case of emotional distress, she wrote, 'a good deal of suffering has to be lived through' (Saunders 1988, p. 219; 2006). In such circumstances, Saunders envisaged the role of the care practitioner as largely passive, accompanying and 'being there' for patients in their suffering and tolerating ambiguity and not-knowing: 'We are not there to take away or explain, or even to understand but simply to "Watch with me"' she contended (Saunders 1988, p. 219; 2006). As Monica Greco has phrased it, this opening towards indeterminacy, gestures to both knowing and not knowing, 'knowing that you can give, without knowing the positive content of the aim of that giving' (Greco 2009, p. 26).

Drawing upon psychoanalytic ideas, the social work educator Margot Waddell (1989) has argued that the ability to provide a receptive presence to pain and distress, requires the capacity of 'standing by' and what the poet Keats, writing in 1817, called 'negative capability': the capacity to tolerate incomplete understanding and mystery (Keats 1958). In arguing for the value of negative capability and 'non-action' rather than 'inaction' in care, Waddell distinguishes between 'servicing' (implying action) and 'serving' (which may constitute not 'doing' anything). She writes:

> 'Servicing' urges itself as a substitute for 'serving' because the not-acting of serving brings us in contact with feelings: feelings which are very hard to bear . . .
>
> Reproduced from Margot Waddell, *Living in Two Worlds: Psychodynamic Theory and Social Work Practice*, p. 13, Copyright © 1989, The Author. Licensed under Creative Commons Attribution 3.0.

In Waddell's view, the imperative for professionals to be seen to be 'doing something' is accompanied by incessant attacks upon serving and 'emotional thinking' in caregiving that marginalize or make illicit the emotional demands of being receptive to another's suffering. Meier et al. (2001) have described some of the consequences for doctors of such unrecognized emotions, which include feelings of powerlessness, fear, and grief.

Although research is providing more evidence of caregivers' experiences and how the failure to acknowledge difficult feelings can adversely affect clinical practice (Wilson and Kirshbaum 2011; Granek et al. 2012), there has been comparatively little discussion of the emotions of researchers when undertaking narrative research with dying people.

Methodological practices that support the recognition and exploration of a researcher's feelings in narrative research include the writing of detailed fieldnotes that record interview dynamics and the researcher's emotions, regular fieldwork/clinical supervision, and panel initiated data analysis (see Wengraf 2001). In my research I have also developed techniques derived from narrative medicine that include reflective accounts of interview relationships and the writing of short stories and poems (see Gunaratnam 2013).

DasGupta et al. (2009) provide an example of the use of written narratives by professionals in the story of Ashley, a doctor who wrote about her experiences as a medical student some 2 years previously. Ashley described how she had been asked to help a patient—Mary, with acute respiratory distress syndrome—to relax, while other doctors worked to prevent her decline. Despite the care team's efforts, Mary died. 'I just wish I'd been able to do something for Mary, like everyone else' Ashley wrote, 'I felt so helpless. Just useless and in the way.' (DasGupta et al. 2009, p. 42). Through writing and discussing her story with others, Ashley began to see the importance of what Waddell (1989) calls 'serving'—an emotional standing-by and witnessing of another person's suffering. The story also provided a means of memorialization. 'Only in writing *about this* experience and through the discussion that followed, did Ashley discover the value in her actions', DasGupta and colleagues write, adding:

> In our work in Narrative Medicine, we find that writing, constructing a poem or short narrative, gives shape and context to experience, providing the writer access to experiences which—without a self-imposed form—could prove potentially overwhelming.
>
> Reproduced from Sayantani Das Gupta, Craig Irvine, and Maura Spiegel, 'The possibilities of narrative palliative care medicine: "Giving Sorrow Words" ', in *Narrative and Stories in Health Care: Illness, Dying and Bereavement.* p. 43, Oxford University Press, Copyright © 2009, Oxford University Press.

Conclusion

Narrative approaches complexify a mimetic interpretation of last wishes by recognizing how meaning is created through cultural and interpersonal relationships, not in isolation. Because last wishes are relational, it is important that we consider how cultural, interpersonal, and institutional settings can shape what is narrated and how certain forms of narrative can be valued or marginalized.

In addition to the challenges of interpreting the meaning of last wishes, especially when a person is in pain, research with death and dying places onerous demands upon the narrative researcher as a witness to suffering, sometimes over prolonged periods of time and with an intimacy that can be more intense than is found with other research methods. Yet narrative methods can also provide the researcher with valuable opportunities to document and interrogate feelings and the co-production of meaning, countering the alienating effects of certain scientific research paradigms that regard a researcher's emotions as irrelevant or at least antithetical to objectivity. As Riessman (2005, p. 473) has pointed out, 'The investigator's emotions are highly relevant to conversations about ethics because emotions do moral work: they embody judgments about value'. As well as enriching ethical discussions and practices of reflexivity, I believe that researcher stories can help us to commemorate losses and to remain open to the emotional consequences of being close to someone's last wishes.

References

Atkinson, P. (2005). Qualitative research—unity and diversity. *Forum Qualitative Sozialforschung/ Forum: Qualitative Social Research*, **6**(3). Available at: <http://www.qualitative-research.net/ index.php/fqs/article/view/4> (accessed 22 December 2013).

Austin, J. L. (1975/1962). *How to Do Things with Words*, 2nd edn. Oxford: Oxford University Press.

Bal, M. (1997). *Narratology: Introduction to the Theory of Narrative*. Toronto: University of Toronto Press.

Barnato, A. E. and Arnold, R. M. (2013). The effect of emotion and physician communication behaviors on surrogates' life-sustaining treatment decisions: a randomized simulation experiment. *Critical Care Medicine*, **41**, 1686–1691.

Berger, J. and Mohr, J. (1995). *Another Way of Telling*. New York: Vintage International.

Bingley, A. F., Thomas, C., Brown, J., et al. (2008). Developing narrative research in supportive and palliative care: the focus on illness narratives. *Palliative Medicine*, **22**, 653–658.

Bochner, A. P. (2001). Narrative's virtues. *Qualitative Inquiry*, **7**, 131–157.

Bruner, J. (1987). Life as narrative. *Social Research*, **54**, 11–32.

Bury, M. (1982). Chronic illness as biographical disruption. *Sociology of Health and Illness*, **4**, 167–182.

Carel, H. (2008). *Illness: The Cry of the Flesh*. Stocksfield: Acumen.

Carel, H. and Kidd, I. J. (2014). Epistemic injustice in healthcare: a philosophical injustice. *Medicine, Health Care and Philosophy*, **17**, 529–540.

Cavell, S. (1990). *Conditions Handsome and Unhandsome. The Constitution of Emersonian Perfectionism: the Carus Lectures (1988)*. Chicago: University of Chicago Press.

Charon, R. (2006). *Narrative Medicine: Honoring the Stories of Illness*, 1st edn. Oxford: Oxford University Press.

DasGupta, S. (2008). Narrative humility. *The Lancet*, **371**, 980–981.

DasGupta, S., Irvine, C., and Spiegel, M. (2009). The possibilities of narrative care medicine: 'Giving sorrow words'. In: Y. Gunaratnam and D. Oliviere (eds), *Narrative and Stories in Health Care: Illness, Dying and Bereavement*, pp. 33–46. Oxford: Oxford University Press.

Eisenberger, N. I. (2012). Broken hearts and broken bones: a neural perspective on the similarities between social and physical pain. *Current Directions in Psychological Science*, **21**, 42–47.

Evans, N., Pasman, H. R., Payne, S. A., et al. (2012). Older patients' attitudes towards and experiences of patient-physician end-of-life communication: a secondary analysis of interviews from British, Dutch and Belgian patients. *BMC Palliative Care*, **11**, 24.

Frank, A. W. (2009). The necessity and dangers of illness narratives, especially at the end of life. In: Y. Gunaratnam and D. Oliviere (eds), *Narrative and Stories in Health Care: Illness, Dying and Bereavement*, pp. 161–75. Oxford: Oxford University Press.

Frank, A. W. (2010). *Letting Stories Breathe: A Socio-Narratology*. Chicago: University of Chicago Press.

Fricker, M. (2007). *Epistemic Injustice: Power and the Ethics of Knowing*. Oxford: Oxford University Press.

Frosh, S. (2007). Disintegrating qualitative research. *Theory and Psychology*, **17**, 635–653.

Goffman, E. (1971). *The Presentation of Self in Everyday Life*, 1st edn. Harmondsworth: Penguin Books.

Granek, L., Tozer, R., Mazzotta, P., et al. (2012). Nature and impact of grief over patient loss on oncologists' personal and professional lives. *Archives of Internal Medicine*, **172**, 964–966.

Greco, M. (2009). On the art of life: a vitalist reading medical humanities. *The Sociological Review*, **56**(Suppl. 2), 22–45.

Greenhalgh, T. and Collard, A. (2003). *Narrative Based Healthcare: Sharing Stories—a Multiprofessional Workbook*, 1st edn. London: BMJ Books.

Greenhalgh, T. and Hurwitz, B. (1998). *Narrative Based Medicine: Dialogue and Discourse in Clinical Practice*. London: BMJ Books.

Greenhalgh, T. and Hurwitz, B. (1999). Why study narrative? *British Medical Journal*, **318**, 48–50.

Gunaratnam, Y. (2009). Narrative interviews and research. In: Y. Gunaratnam and D. Oliviere (eds), *Narrative and Stories in Health Care: Illness, Dying and Bereavement*, pp. 47–61. Oxford: Oxford University Press.

Gunaratnam, Y. (2012). Learning to be affected: social suffering and total pain at life's borders. *The Sociological Review*, **60**(Suppl. 1), 108–123.

Gunaratnam, Y. (2013). *Death and the Migrant: Bodies, Borders, Care*. London: Bloomsbury Academic.

Gunaratnam, Y. (2014). Morbid mixtures: hybridity, pain and transnational dying. *Subjectivity*, **7**, 74–91.

Hollway, W. and Jefferson, T. (2013). *Doing Qualitative Research Differently: A Psychosocial Approach*. London: SAGE.

Hudson, P. L., Schofield, P., Kelly, B., et al. (2006). Responding to desire to die statements from patients with advanced disease: recommendations for health professionals. *Palliative Medicine*, **20**, 703–710.

Johansen, S., Hølen, J. C., Kaasa, S., et al. (2005). Attitudes towards, and wishes for, euthanasia in advanced cancer patients at a palliative medicine unit. *Palliative Medicine*, **19**, 454–460.

Karasz, A., Sacajiu, G., Kogan, M., et al. (2010). The rational choice model in family decision making at the end of life. *Journal of Clinical Ethics*, 21, 189–200.

Keats, J. (1958). Letter to George and Tom Keats, 21 December, 1817. In: H. E. Rollins (ed.), *The Letters of J. Keats: 1814–1821*, p. 193. Cambridge: Cambridge University Press.

Kleinman, A. (1988). *The Illness Narratives: Suffering, Healing, and the Human Condition*. New York: Basic Books.

Landa, J. (1992). Speech act theory and the concept of intention in literary criticism. *Review of English Studies Canaria*, **24**, 89–104.

Lawton, J. (2000). *The Dying Process: Patients' Experiences of Palliative Care*. London: Routledge.

McAdam, J. L., Dracup, K. A., White, D. B., et al. (2010). Symptom experiences of family members of intensive care unit patients at high risk for dying. *Critical Care Medicine*, **38**, 1078–1085.

Materstvedt, L. J. and Bosshard, G. (2009). Deep and continuous palliative sedation (terminal sedation): clinical-ethical and philosophical aspects. *The Lancet Oncology*, **10**, 622–627.

Meier, D., Back, A., and Morrison, R. (2001). The inner life of physicians and care of the seriously ill. *Journal of the American Medical Association*, **286**, 3007–3014.

Paley, J. (2009). Narrative machinery. In: Y. Gunaratnam and D. Oliviere (eds), *Narrative and Stories in Health Care: Illness, Dying and Bereavement*, pp. 17–32. Oxford: Oxford University Press.

Paley, J. and Eva, G. (2005). Narrative vigilance: the analysis of stories in health care. *Nursing Philosophy: An International Journal for Healthcare Professionals*, **6**, 83–97.

Riessman, C. (2005). Exporting ethics: a narrative about narrative research in South India. *Health*, **9**, 473–490.

Saunders, C. M. (1988). The evolution of the hospices. In: R. Mann (ed.), *The History of the Management of Pain: From Early Principles to Present Practice. The Proceedings of a Conference Organised by the Section of the History of Medicine of the Royal Society of Medicine, London*, pp. 167–178. Carnforth: Parthenon Publishing Group Ltd.

Saunders, C. M. (2006). *Cicely Saunders: Selected Writing 1958–2004*. Oxford: Oxford University Press.

Schafer, R. (1981). Narration on psychoanalytic dialogue. In: W. J. T. Mitchell (ed.), *On Narrative*, pp. 25–49. Chicago: University of Chicago Press.

Seale, C. (2009). End-of-life decisions in the UK involving medical practitioners. *Palliative Medicine*, **23**, 198–204.

Shapiro, J. (2011). Illness narratives: reliability, authenticity and the empathic witness. *Medical Humanities*, **37**, 68–72.

Skultans, V. (2007). *Empathy and Healing: Essays in Medical and Narrative Anthropology*. New York: Berghahn Books.

Van Loon, R. A. (1999). Desire to die in terminally ill people: a framework for assessment and intervention. *Health and Social Work*, **24**, 260–268.

Waddell, M. (1989). Living in two worlds: psychodynamic theory and social work practice. *Free Associations*, **15**, 11–35.

Walter, T., Hourizi, R., Moncur, W., et al. (2011). Does the internet change how we die and mourn? Overview and analysis. *Omega (Westport)*, **64**, 275–302.

Wengraf, T. (2001). *Qualitative Research Interviewing: Biographic Narrative and Semi-Structured Methods*. London: Sage Publications.

Williams, G. (1984). The genesis of chronic illness: narrative re-construction. *Sociology of Health and Illness*, **6**, 175–200.

Wilson, J. and Kirshbaum, M. (2011). Effects of patient death on nursing staff: a literature review. *British Journal of Nursing*, **20**, 559–563.

Yurchisin, J., Watchravesringkan, K., and Brown Mccabe, D. (2005). An exploration of identity re-creation in the context of internet dating. *Social Behavior and Personality*, **33**, 735–750.

Zhao, S., Grasmuck, S., and Martin, J. (2008). Identity construction on Facebook: digital empowerment in anchored relationships. *Computers in Human Behavior*, **24**, 1816–1836.

Chapter 3

Expressed desire for hastened death in seven patients living with advanced cancer: a phenomenologic inquiry

Nessa Coyle and Lois Sculco

Introduction to expressed desire for hastened death

Individuals living with advanced cancer sometimes express desire for hastened death (Brown et al. 1986; Coyle et al. 1990; Seale and Addington-Hall 1994 Chochinov et al. 1995; Breitbart et al. 2000; Emanuel et al. 2000; Rosenfeld et al. 2000). The need to have a clear understanding of what such an expression means and what the individual is asking for is present at clinical and societal levels. Clinically, nurses and physicians need to understand such an expression so that they can respond appropriately to the individual's needs. At a societal level, understanding also is needed so that rational social policies can be formulated regarding how to respond as a society when a terminally ill patient with cancer expresses desire for hastened death. For this study, the researcher postulated that gaining insight into the lived experience of a cohort of patients with advanced cancer who had expressed, at least once, desire for hastened death would provide insight into the meanings and uses of such an expression. This is one in a series of articles arising from that study (Coyle 2002).

Literature review

Research to explore why terminally ill patients with cancer express desire for hastened death has focused in large part on the relationship between depression or psychological distress and the desire for death (Chochinov et al. 1995; Breitbart and Rosenfeld 1999; Breitbart et al. 2000; Chochinov 2002; Ganzini et al. 2002). Psychological and social factors typically have appeared to have more influence than physical symptoms such as pain. Overall, the studies have attempted to understand patients' experiences through preselected domains of study. Little in-depth research could be found that examined individual meanings and uses of an expressed desire for hastened death derived directly from narratives of terminally ill patients with cancer (Mak and Elwyn 2003).

A body of literature does exist on euthanasia, clinician-assisted suicide, and suicide in the terminally ill, all of which are potential outcomes of an expressed desire for hastened death, and therefore was appropriate to review for the study. This literature reflects various perspectives, including caregivers' perspectives of dying patients' desire for death (Seale and Addington-Hall 1994; Jacobson et al. 1995; Emanuel et al. 2000; Matzo and Schwarz 2001;), dying patients who acknowledge desire for death (Brown et al. 1986; Chochinov et al. 1995; Suarez-Almazor et al. 1997; Breitbart et al. 2000; Mak and Elwyn 2003), and patients whose behaviour suggests that they might be considering hastening death sometime in the future (Owen et al 1992; Emanuel et al. 1996), as well as suicide, one outcome of desire for death (Breitbart 1987; Quill 1991; Grzybowska and Finlay 1997; Ferrell et al. 2000; Filiberti et al. 2001; Matzo and Schwarz 2001; Ganzini et al. 2002). The current study was designed using a different methodological approach from those used in the previously described studies. The design was selected as one that would provide added insight into the lived experience of a patient with advanced cancer who had expressed, at least once, desire for hastened death. Through this insight, the researcher hoped that a clearer understanding of the meanings and uses of an expressed desire for hastened death in this population could be gained. No assumptions were made in the current study as to whether an expressed desire for hastened death was or was not a literal request.

Methods

Phenomenology (from the Greek word phenomenon, which means to show itself) was the methodological basis for this qualitative study. This approach is one of discovery and description and emphasizes meaning and understanding in the study of the lived experience of individuals (van Manen 1990; Creswell 1998). Phenomenologic research requires active involvement from the researcher, study participants, and audience who eventually will read and evaluate the research report. Reinharz (1983) described this process as one of 'transformation' of private experience into public knowledge and has outlined specific steps to explain it. These steps include self-revelation by the study participant; listening, interpreting, and producing a coherent and meaningful written account of the phenomenon by the researcher; and creation of a personal understanding by the reader of the final report. A good phenomenologic description is 'something that we can nod to, recognizing it as an experience that we have had or could have had' (van Manen 1990, p. 27). Van Manen also wrote that 'a phenomenologic description is always one interpretation, and no single interpretation of human experience will ever exhaust the possibility of yet another complementary, or even potentially richer or deeper transcription' (van Manen 1990, p. 31). The study findings report one interpretation of the meanings and uses of an expressed desire for hastened death in a select group of patients living with advanced cancer.

Setting and sample

The sample was limited to English-speaking adults with advanced cancer who were followed by the pain and palliative care service at an urban cancer research centre either as inpatients or outpatients who were not known to the researcher from her clinical practice and who had expressed, at least once, a desire for hastened death. This expression could be either verbal or nonverbal, that is, expressed by an action that was interpreted by the physician as reflecting such a desire. Patients who fulfilled these criteria were eligible for the study.

Attending palliative care physicians were asked to approach patients who met the study criteria to determine whether they were interested in participating in the study. Patients who expressed interest in participating were given the option either to contact the researcher directly or have their attending physicians ask the researcher to initiate the contact. Once the researcher had been informed about an interested potential study participant, she contacted that individual either that day or the following day in person or by telephone. After a brief explanation of the purpose of the study, if the individual remained interested, the researcher set up a convenient time to explain the study protocol in full, to ask whether the individual would like the researcher to speak with a family member, and to leave a copy of the study protocol and informed consent for the individual to review. The rationale for these steps was that, in the researcher's experience, terminally ill individuals often like to include family members or friends in the decision-making process. The researcher recontacted the individual within 2 days to see whether he or she was interested in participating in the study. If interested, a time was set for the researcher to obtain a signed consent and conduct the first interview. In addition to the signed informed consent, process consent was used throughout the study, that is, the researcher obtained consent verbally prior to each interview. New participants continued to be recruited until no further themes of the lived experience of advanced cancer emerged (known as reaching 'theoretical saturation'). No more than two interview series were ongoing at any one time.

Protection of participants

The study was approved by the Memorial Sloan-Kettering Cancer Center and New York University institutional review boards. Pseudonyms were used for all identifying information about the participants to protect confidentiality.

Interview process

One researcher conducted all of the interviews. A series of two to six in-depth interviews was conducted with each participant for a duration of 30–60 minutes each at intervals ranging from 1 day to 6 months apart. The basis for deciding on the number of interviews per participant was that each interview series would continue until no new information was forthcoming from the participant (saturation) or until circumstances intervened that prevented further interviews from being conducted with the participant. The initial study protocol specified a time interval of 3 to 4 weeks between interviews. However, when the interview process began, the researcher noted that some participants were very eager to continue the interview process within a much shorter time frame and, on occasion, to extend the interval between interviews to a longer period. The protocol was amended with institutional review board approval to accommodate the participants' wishes. These flexible time frames and interview lengths reflecting individual patients' needs are consistent with the research method.

The interviews were held at a place that was convenient to each patient, either at home or in the hospital, outpatient clinic, or long-term care facility. Each interview was audiotaped, transcribed, and reviewed before the next interview. At the beginning of each interview series, the researcher explained to participants that she was

- ◆ The entire set of interviews was examined as a whole to get an overall understanding of the text.
- ◆ The text of each interview and then all interviews for each participant were summarized (into narrative summaries and individual portraits).
- ◆ Themes were identified from the codes. Excerpts from the interviews were organized to support interpretations resulting in thematic consensus.
- ◆ A second person reviewed the coding and themes. Where necessary, clarification was achieved through data review and discussion.
- ◆ Themes that cut across all participants were identified as supported from the data.
- ◆ Finally, an interpretive narrative using the identified themes was written. Sufficient data were organized to support the interpretive analysis and allow for validation of the findings by the reader.

Fig. 3.1 Steps in data analysis.

there to learn from them about their experience of living with a serious illness and how that experience had affected their attitudes toward life and death. The follow-up question asked participants to describe their lives before they were sick and their lives at the present time. Follow-up probe questions were flexible and dependent on an individual's responses. Each patient's interview series continued until no new information was forthcoming, the patient developed cognitive impairment, the patient became too weak or fatigued to continue, or death intervened.

Data analysis

During the interview series with each participant, the researcher conducted ongoing initial content analysis of the data. Each line of text was the unit of analysis. The researcher coded for meaning, clustered codes into conceptual categories, and identified the need for further data collection for clarification or expansion of categories. Consistent with the philosophical underpinnings of the study, data analysis was an interactive process with the researcher reading and rereading the transcripts and interacting with and interpreting the data (van Manen 1990; Creswell 1998). This ongoing analysis between interviews allowed the researcher to explore and verify with the participant themes that had been uncovered and to 'member check' that her interpretation of what had been said was valid. Data were analysed at the completion of all of the interviews according to the steps in Fig. 3.1.

A solid data trail, documenting each step of the research process and open to scrutiny, was maintained. Two master's of art-prepared individuals (one in philosophy and one in anthropology) provided an external check that the coding and themes were grounded in the narratives. In addition, an auditor ensured that the researcher adhered to the planned process and that the coding and derivation of themes adequately represented the raw data (Lincoln and Guba 1985; van Manen 1990; Ely 1991).

Findings and interpretative analysis

Sample

Eight patients were approached for the study. Seven agreed to participate, and one patient declined because of deep fatigue. Participant demographics can be found in

Table 3.1 Participant Demographics (*n* = 7)

Characteristic	*n*
Age (years)	
40–49	1
50–59	2
60–69	2
70–79	2
Gender	
Male	4
Female	3
Cancer diagnosis	
Endometrial	1
Lymphoma/HIV	1
Lymphoma	1
Lung	1
Prostate	1
Rectal	1
Sarcoma	1
Ethnicity	
White	6
Hispanic/Latino	1
Religion	
Jewish	3
Catholic	2
Protestant	2
Occupation	
Professional	5
White collar	1
Blue collar	1

Table 3.1. The number of interviews per participant ranged from two to six, and time period for the interviews varied from 2 days to 6 months. The reasons for terminating an interview series were cognitive impairment (*n* = 2), information saturation (*n* = 2), and death (*n* = 2), and a participant believed that she had completed her contribution to this research (*n* = 1) (see Table 3.2). Although information saturation was reached in only two participants, theoretical saturation across all participants was reached after recruitment of the seven participants. That is, no new themes were forthcoming across participants. Six of the seven participants had died by the time the study was completed.

Table 3.2 Interview characteristics

Participant	Number of interviews	Time period for interviews	Location of Interviews	Reason interview series halted	Patient status
1	6	3 weeks	Cancer centre (4) Terminal care hospital (2)	Cognitive impairment	Died 7 days after last interview
2	3	3 months	Participant's home (1) Cancer centre (1) Outpatient clinic (1)	Information saturation	Alive at time of study completion
3	2	2 days	Terminal care hospital (2)	Cognitive impairment	Died 1 month after last interview
4	3	4 weeks	Participant's home (1) Cancer centre (2)	Death	Died 7 days after last interview
5	4	2 months	Cancer centre (1) Rehabilitation centre (2) Student residence (1)	Participant believed that she had completed her contribution to this research	Died 4 months after last interview
6	3	4 weeks	Participant's home (3)	Death	Died 1 month after last interview
7	6	6 months	Researcher's office (5) Cancer centre (1)	Information saturation	Died 1 year after last interview

Antecedents and trigger events preceding expression of desire for hastened death

Chronic antecedents or triggers that preceded expression of desire for hastened death in these participants included debilitating progression of disease; perception of chronic and progressive loss of social supports, dignity, autonomy, and sense of worth; loss of sense of purpose (place) in the world; and perception of being a burden on self or others in the present or future. Acute events included uncontrolled pain, shortness of breath, and medical information that produced fear, hopelessness, and a sense of dread. Antecedents and trigger events for the expressed desire for hastened death in these participants were chronic, acute, or acute superimposed on chronic.

Forms of expression of desire for hastened death

Although most of the expressions of desire for hastened death by these participants were in verbal form, two were expressed by action. One participant refused surgery that had the potential to lengthen her life by several years without significant morbidity, and a second acquiesced to transfer from an acute care cancer hospital to a terminal care facility, an action perceived by him as helping to realize his goal of a hastened death. Examples of circumstances under which each participant expressed a desire for hastened death and forms this expression took are seen in Table 3.3.

Meaning and uses of an expression of desire for hastened death

The seven participants illustrated the complexity of the meanings and uses of an expressed desire for hastened death. Sometimes the meanings and uses were explicit and directly stated, and other times they were more indirect and inferred or interpreted by the researcher within the context of what each participant described. The expression of a desire for hastened death was, in all instances, a tool of communication, and the examples evidenced in the individual narratives are explicated in the following paragraphs. The researcher found that the meanings and uses of this expression of desire for hastened death could be different from patient to patient and from intent to intent. For example, one patient might wish to call attention to him- or herself and also to signal an urgent need for help. In another instance, the expression might be used to affect a participant's support systems and/or to express despair. The meanings and uses often were intertwined and overlapping—the same and yet different for each expression and each patient. Nine distinct and yet sometimes intertwined and overlapping meanings and uses of an expressed desire for hastened death were extrapolated from the narratives.

A manifestation of the will to live

The researcher named this the 'primary paradox', that is, the participant's behaviour evidenced the will to live despite having expressed at least once a desire for hastened death. 'The goal is now to die. . . . I'm using my flexibility not to devote my time toward how I am going to die and praying, etc. . . . I'm using my flexibility in time management to do things that the living do, not the dying.' The paradox and struggle also were

Table 3.3 Participants' desire for hastened death

Participant	Circumstances	Forms of expression
1	When first diagnosed with cancer to prevent his family having to 'go through' his terminal illness Later in response to an increasingly debilitated state and loss of bowel and bladder control Later still in the setting of severe pain	In written form, in a personal diary and shared with no one until shown to researcher; no plan outlined In verbal form, shared with his wife; various plans such as blowing air into his central line discussed In verbal form, shared with his wife and palliative care physician; no plan outlined
2	In response to decreased ability to walk, chronic pain, and loss of sense of self-worth	In verbal form, a constant rumination to staff; no plan outlined
3	In response to feeling a burden on his family and not wanting them to remember him as a debilitated and dependent person	In form of action, accepting transfer to a terminal care hospital that he stated was an act that would hasten his death because he would no longer be in a mode of life-prolonging care
4	In response to fear of a suffocating death after experiencing an acute episode of dyspnoea	In verbal form to palliative care physician and nurse, discussed various plans: taking an overdose of morphine available to him for pain, jumping in front of a train, selecting an institution for terminal care that would not interfere with self-administration of medication
5	As the only way to get staff to 'really hear' her	In verbal form to the inpatient staff which triggered a palliative care referral; later in thoughts of the future if she became 'sicker' or pain increased; no plan outlined
6	In response to lack of mobility, chronic neuropathic pain, and inability to live in a personally meaningful way	In verbal form to her palliative care physician; no plan outlined: 'How does one do it? I don't know.'
7	In response to fear of living for a prolonged time in a dependent state and using her financial resources to the detriment of her family	In form of action, refusing treatment that might have prolonged her life for several years without significant morbidity

evidenced in the following statement: 'See, there's a problem while planning or pursuing your death. . . . On the one hand, I am saying all these things, and, on the other hand, I am going down for radiation.'

The ability to live a full and normal life shrunk with the progression of the disease and sometimes led to the expression of desire for hastened death. Yet the participants frequently found a way to value aspects of their life that remained, such as being with their family, and to affirm the urge for continued existence.

I think passively sitting in my own garden, sitting on my own deck, would still be preferable to, to, to death. Quality of life, the concept of quality of life is shifted. I can live with an inactive life . . . and I'd still fight a bit to gain incrementally.

This response shift was a sign of the will to live despite having expressed desire for hastened death.

The dying process itself was so difficult that an early death was preferred

This was named by the researcher as the 'secondary paradox'. In these situations, the expression of desire for hastened death reflected that the dying process itself was so difficult that death was better than going through it. The secondary paradox also could be characterized as, 'I can't bear the dying process so I'll short circuit it by dying', or 'I don't want to go through the dying process so I'll kill myself'. Thus, expressed desire for hastened death could reflect a desire to end a dying process that had become too overwhelming and burdensome for a participant. 'I don't want to undergo that [expletive] feeling of helplessness, that there's not a [expletive] thing that I or anyone else can do', or 'Sometimes I start yelling at my shrink that this is horrible, that why don't I die right now? . . . Why do I have to live through this?'

In these situations, the reasons triggering the expression of a desire for hastened death were multiple and often overlapping, including uncontrolled symptoms, perceived loss of dignity, a feeling of having no place in the world, and the fear of leaving a damaged legacy. 'After a while, your family, who you love so dearly, will remember you as a washed-out role model. . . . It will remind them of what they have to go through, the lack of strength, the weakness, and so forth.' The desire was to end the process before further destruction of self occurred. These participants did not wish to cease existing, but they saw no point in going through the process and wanted it to end.

The immediate situation was unendurable and required instant action

An expressed desire for hastened death in these situations was an urgent request for help that the immediate situation was unendurable and required instant action. 'There were many times when I was in such pain and such misery. I said, let me go . . . finished . . . no more of this torture.' This called attention to any variety of problems arising from the lived experience of advanced cancer: physical, psychological, social, spiritual, and existential. The message sent was, 'You don't know how much I am suffering. Come and deal with me; I need your attention and help.' One participant gave this signal through nonverbal communication by refusing surgery that could have prolonged her life for several years without significant morbidity. Others expressed their suffering verbally. 'I feel, deep inside, I don't want to feel hurtin [sic] . . . that I want to end this. . . . I ask God why he don't take me, why I suffer so much.' The urgent need for help was indicative of a layer of suffering experienced by a participant that was so confusing and overwhelming that he or she was unable to specifically indicate what was causing the suffering and what was required. On the other hand, when a participant was focused on a specific experience or event that he or she knew would be intolerable, the expression of desire for hastened death took another form, the 'if–then' proposition.

A hastened death was an option to extract oneself from an unendurable situation

The option to extract oneself from an untenable situation through a hastened death sometimes was expressed as an 'if–then' proposition; for example, 'If the pain gets worse, then I want to be dead.' 'Pain is my biggest fear. It puts me in a darkness and a lack of will to go forward and a desire to die. . . . The pain wants me to have a vehicle to just, just stop my life.' Severe pain or acute, severe shortness of breath were the two symptoms that overwhelmed the participants and were identified as being incompatible with life. 'If I had to go through [an acute episode of shortness of breath] again, I would throw myself in front of a subway train. I am not going through that again.'

A manifestation of the last control the dying person can exert

The expression of desire for hastened death was sometimes an assertion of ultimate control over an untenable situation as reflected in many of the previously described situations. Loss of control so frequently was a source of suffering for these participants that it warranted a category in and of itself. An example was the participant who said that he would throw himself under a train if he was in a situation of uncontrolled shortness of breath again. 'If I had to go through [an episode of acute shortness of breath] again, I would throw myself in front of a subway train. I am not going through that again.' The 'if–then' situation and a manifestation of the last control a dying person can exert are intertwined concepts, but separating them conveys a broader understanding of the human struggles and thoughts behind the expression of desire for hastened death.

A way of drawing attention to 'me as a unique individual'

The demand from the participants that they be understood and heard as individuals with a life and valued outside of their role as patients was another use of the expression of desire for hastened death. Patients sometimes have difficulty making themselves visible as persons in the hospital environment. Attention is focused on the disease process, disease management pathways, and protocols. One participant reported using an expressed desire for hastened death specifically as a tool to draw attention to self and be heard, listened to, and understood in the depth of her experiences, her losses, and her suffering. No other form of communication had worked for her.

A gesture of altruism

In some cases, the desire for hastened death was to relieve the family of the burden of care and of witnessing the participant's progressive deterioration. In some instances, this use of expressed desire for hastened death occurred early in the disease process when disease progression was anticipated: 'There have been times I've felt so much a burden on my family that maybe it is best for me to die just to relieve them of going through the terminal phase of my disease.' Another participant stated that he did not want his family to witness what 'they would have to go through themselves' at some point (their own dying). He accepted transfer to a terminal care facility to spare his family the burden and responsibility of his physical care and the daily witnessing of his physical deterioration. In another instance, when a participant acknowledged that no tumour-directed therapy options were possible for him:

> All of a sudden, it dawned on me that there was no solution, and if there was no solution to my cancer, then why was I hanging around? I got thinking about death as a practical matter. Why hang around and cause a lot of people a lot of grief?

An attempt at manipulation of the family to avoid abandonment

The expressed desire for hastened death can be a message to those around an individual as to how dependent he or she is upon them. One participant described involving his family in every decision that was made regarding his care, including his thoughts about a hastened death:

> I shared that I wouldn't do it until we discussed it together. . . . She didn't have to worry about me taking the pills. . . . It wasn't fair to them. . . . It would leave them wondering, did they do, you know, contribute to it, did they do all they could. . . . And I want them to feel comfortable that they've done everything.

Could any family really say, 'Yes, we are burdened by your care, and yes, both you and I would be better off if you were dead'? Involving the family in this way almost certainly reinforced to his family how vulnerable he was to their presence, their care, and his desperate need for them. Shifting the responsibility for decision making onto the family might be interpreted as a way of ensuring that they stayed by his side. This appeared to be the case with this participant: He was never left alone, and his family constantly reinforced to him the benefit they were deriving from his care and his presence.

A despairing cry depicting the misery of the current situation

Finally, the expression of desire for hastened death sometimes took on the form of a lament—a despairing cry to the universe about the misery of the current situation. Sometimes the cry was directed to the ear of a compassionate and trusted healthcare professional; at other times, the lament was voiced to heaven. A sense of abandonment by God was expressed by two of the participants. This lament, which was given voice from time to time, was the visible part of a deep-seated well of grief. 'Why do I have to go through this? Why can't I just die right now?' and, 'When I pray, I use [sic] to feel the power of God on me. . . . Now I sometimes feel as though I am talking to the air.'

Discussion

The topic explored in this study was the expression of desire for hastened death by individuals living with advanced cancer. The researcher postulated that an exploration of the lived experience of these individuals through a series of face-to-face interviews would shed light on the meanings and uses of this expression. The intent of this qualitative study was to explore the human dimensions of living with advanced cancer, the impact of that experience on the individual, and how that impact led to an expression of a desire for hastened death. A paradox was seen: on one side, the expressed desire for hastened death represents the desire for cessation of life; on the other side, the evidence for the desire for life and continued existence is strong.

Parse (1981, 1992), a nursing theorist, has recognized the paradoxical nature of people's experiences as living human beings. Parse's (1992) theory of Human Becoming (formerly Man-Living-Health; Parse 1981) is what 'is embedded in meanings patterns in relationships, and in hopes and dreams' (Parse 1992, p. 37). She described paradox as 'apparent opposites' but emphasized that these are not opposites but rather two sides of the same coin.

The expression of a desire for hastened death seems consistent with the paradoxical pattern of Human Becoming described by Parse (1992). In this conceptual model, the present participle is used to express continuous process. Parse suggested that development (becoming) is a combination of affirmation and negation: a paradoxical process. The expression of a desire for hastened death—a movement from being to non-being— is consistent with Parse's definition of 'powering', which is the continuous affirming of self in the light of non-being. As demonstrated in the current study and other studies (e.g. Chochinov et al. 1995), an expressed desire for hastened death is not always continuous. It can be understood as a transformation or the struggle toward what is not yet. According to Parse (1998), 'These rhythmical patterns are not opposites, they are both sides of the same rhythm that coexist as a whole, and both sides of the rhythm are present simultaneously' (Parse 1998, p. 42). Through the expression of a desire for hastened death, the transformation that is sought—the regaining of dignity, autonomy, and wholeness—may occur.

When a patient with advanced cancer expresses a desire for hastened death, the process described by Parse (1992) is very apparent. The reality of 'becoming' pushes and pulls patients with advanced cancer in a quest to guide and control the becoming. 'Revealing–concealing' in the expressed desire for hastened death is illustrative of how little we know about the lives of the patients for whom we care. The person we see, the present revealed, conceals the past and the becoming. 'Enabling–limiting' in the expression of desire for hastened death attempts to control the future and, through that control, may cut off the future. Ambivalence is common. 'Connecting–separating' in the expression of desire for hastened death often draws the individual closer to the family as they plan to separate. The individual's sense of the imminence of nonexistence can intensify the separating and connecting. Parse (1992) saw paradox as a model for human experience and identifies opposing forces in human behaviour and understanding. The findings from the current study support this view. The particular applicability of this insight to the understanding of the end-of-life experience of the patient with advanced cancer is striking. The parallels between palliative nursing and Parse's (1992) theory of Human Becoming have been described previously (Hutchings 2002). Leaving aside the complexities of her theory, the insight that Parse (1992) described in the paradoxical nature of human experiences and human feelings elicits the 'phenomenologic nod' (van Manen 1990) from the researcher. For the person living with advanced cancer, the paradox is poignantly present in the urge to live and the inevitability of death. The experience of belonging to both the world of the living and the world of the dying can be bewildering and confusing. Similar findings were shown by Benzein et al. (2001), when exploring the experience of hope in 11 patients followed in palliative home care. The participants were described as being torn between a will to live and the awareness of a final capitulation to death. The prominence of one domain over the other varied with the individual's changing physical and emotional circumstances.

The findings from the current study suggest that the expression of a desire for hastened death is a complex language and may not be generated by suicidal ideation but rather by the lived experience of the individual with advanced cancer. Although some of the expressions of desire for hastened death may be associated with depression and hopelessness, this study has illuminated several factors pervading the experience of the dying patient that may underlie or trigger the expression of desire for hastened death, providing a broader basis to understand this language.

Limitations

The number of participants was small, and the participant pool was limited by recruiting them only from the pain and palliative care service of an urban cancer research centre. Most were white professionals older than 50. The implication of these small numbers and the limited participant pool is that the study findings are not traditionally generalizable. However, the aim of qualitative research is not to find significant numbers but rather themes that emerge from the narratives that are indicative of common human experiences.

Nursing implications

Practice

Listening to patients' stories through the narrative interview and giving them an opportunity to describe their lived experience of advanced cancer may help nurses and others to understand what actually is being asked for when a patient expresses desire for hastened death. This is extraordinarily important because many patients living with advanced cancer are not able to identify or articulate the particulars of what is causing them such overwhelming distress and may indicate their distress globally through the expression of desire for hastened death. This expression is a communication tool in all instances and has many meanings and uses that appear to be common to patients with advanced cancer and unique to individual patients. Their uniqueness to the particular person can be understood best within the context of that person's current situation, life history, and experiences. The findings of the current study help to provide a framework or matrix of categories for nurses to listen to and address the needs of a patient with advanced cancer who expresses a desire for hastened death. Time for the narrative interview needs to be built into palliative nursing practice.

Education

The research findings suggest that the vulnerability of patients with advanced cancer cared for in an urban research cancer centre is profound. They also suggest that nurses can educate patients to reduce that vulnerability. The research suggests that patients can be empowered by learning how to communicate with their doctors and nurses, to address their pain issues, and to understand their treatment options. The research findings also underscore the importance of nurses being prepared to provide patients with answers to questions about how they might die and what their options are for care at the end of life. Empowerment through education can help to provide those living in the face of death with a systematic way of dealing with their sense of vulnerability.

Research

This is a small exploratory study that raises many questions and areas for future research. The methodology used in the study included an interpretive analysis in determining the uses and meanings conveyed by each participant when expressing desire for hastened death. The researcher did not in all instances ask the participants if that interpretation was the one that was intended. Future research on the uses and meanings of an expressed desire for hastened death could use the categories delineated through the research as a guide to see if they hold true in other populations in a similar environment or in a different environment such as a hospice setting. Only patients were included in the current study. Research is needed on how staff interpret and respond to the expression of desire for hastened death by patients and the impact of that expression on their attitudes and behaviour toward patients following such an expression. Research also is needed regarding how families interpret and respond to the expression of desire for hastened death and the impact of that expression on their attitudes and behaviour toward the patient following such an expression. Finally, researchers should ask the following questions. Can 'vulnerability markers' be identified in patients who express desire for hastened death? What are these markers? If identified early would interventions decrease future suffering?

Acknowledgement

This article has originally appeared as N. Coyle and L. Sculco, Expressed desire for hastened death in seven patients living with advanced cancer: a phenomenologic inquiry, in: *Oncology Nursing Forum* 31(4), pp. 699–706. Copyright © 2004, Oncology Nursing Society, courtesy of the Oncology Nursing Society (ONS). All rights reserved.

The primary author gratefully acknowledges the following people for making this work possible: first, the participants of the study who gave the researcher hours of their time when time was what they did not have and second, numerous colleagues who devoted many hours to reading and critiquing selected parts of the broad research. Special mention goes to Doris Aach, MA, William Breitbart, MD, Kathleen Foley, MD, Russell Portenoy, MD, Bruce Rapkin, MD, and Richard Payne, MD, for his ongoing support.

References

Benzein, E., Norberg, A., and Saveman, B. I. (2001). The meaning of the lived experience of hope in patients with cancer in palliative home care. *Palliative Medicine*, **15**, 117–126.

Breitbart, W. (1987). Suicide in cancer patients. *Oncology (Huntington)*, **1**(2),49–54.

Breitbart, W. and Rosenfeld, B. D. (1999). Physician-assisted suicide: the in- fluence of psychologic issues. *Cancer Control*, **6**, 146–161.

Breitbart, W., Rosenfeld, B., Pessin, H., et al. (2000). Depression, hopelessness, and desire for hastened death in terminally ill patients with cancer. *Journal of the American Medical Association*, **284**, 2907–2911.

Brown, J. H., Henteleff, P., Barakat, S., and Rowe, C. J. (1986). Is it normal for terminally ill patients to desire death? *American Journal of Psychiatry*, **143**, 208–211.

Chochinov, H. M. (2002). Dignity-conserving care—a new model for palliative care: helping the patient feel valued. *Journal of the American Medical Association*, **287**, 2253–2260.

Chochinov, H. M., Wilson, K. G., Enns, M., et al. (1995). Desire for death in the terminally ill. *American Journal of Psychiatry*, **152**, 1185–1191.

Coyle, N. (2002). Expressed desire for hastened death in a select group of people living with advanced cancer: a phenomenologic inquiry. *Dissertation Abstracts International*, **63**-11B, 5156.

Coyle, N., Adelhardt, J., Foley, K. M., and Portenoy, R.K. (1990). Character of terminal illness in the advanced cancer patient: pain and other symptoms in the last four weeks of life. *Journal of Pain and Symptom Management*, **5**, 83–93.

Creswell, J. W. (1998). *Qualitative Inquiry and Research Design: Choosing Among Five Traditions*. Thousand Oaks, CA: Sage.

Ely, M. (1991). *Doing Qualitative Research: Circles Within Circles*. Washington, DC: Falmer Press.

Emanuel, E. J., Fairclough, D. L., Daniels, E. R., and Clarridge, B.R. (1996). Euthanasia and physician-assisted suicide: attitudes and experiences of oncology patients, oncologists, and the public. *Lancet*, **347**, 1805–1810.

Emanuel, E. J., Fairclough, D. L., and Emanuel, L. L. (2000). Attitudes and desires related to euthanasia and physician-assisted suicide among terminally ill patients and their caregivers. *Journal of the American Medical Association*, **284**, 2460–2468.

Ferrell, B., Virani, R., Grant, M., Coyne, P., and Uman, G. (2000). Beyond the Supreme Court decision: Nursing perspectives on end-of-life care. *Oncology Nursing Forum*, **27**, 445–455.

Filiberti, A., Ripamonti, C., Totis, A., et al. (2001). Characteristics of terminal cancer patients who committed suicide during a home palliative care program. *Journal of Pain and Symptom Management*, **22**, 544–553.

Ganzini, L., Harvath, T. A., Jackson, A., Goy, E. R., Miller, L. L., and Delorit, M. A. (2002). Experiences of Oregon nurses and social workers with hospice patients who requested assistance with suicide. *New England Journal of Medicine*, **347**, 582–588.

Grzybowska, P. and Finlay, I. (1997). The incidence of suicide in palliative care patients. *Palliative Medicine*, **11**, 313–316.

Hutchings, D. (2002). Parallels in practice: palliative nursing practice and Parse's theory of Human Becoming. *American Journal of Hospice and Palliative Care*, **19**, 408–414.

Jacobson, J. A., Kasworm, E. M., Battin, M. P., Botkin, J. R., Francis, L. P., and Green, D. (1995). Decedents' reported preferences for physician-assisted death: a survey of informants listed on death certificates in Utah. *Journal of Clinical Ethics*, **6**, 149–157.

Lincoln, Y. and Guba, E. (1985). *Naturalistic Inquiry*. Beverly Hills, CA: Sage.

Mak, Y. and Elwyn, G. (2003). Use of hermeneutic research in understanding the meaning of desire for euthanasia. *Palliative Medicine*, **17**, 395–402.

van Manen, M. (1990). *Researching Lived Experience: Human Science for an Action Sensitive Pedagogy*. Albany, NY: State University of New York.

Matzo, M.L. and Schwarz, J.K. (2001). In their own words: oncology nurses respond to patient requests for assisted suicide and euthanasia. *Applied Nursing Research*, **14**(2), 64–71.

Owen, C., Tennant, C., and Jones, M. (1992). Suicide and euthanasia: patients attitudes in the context of cancer. *Psycho-Oncology*, **1**(2), 79–88.

Parse, R .R. (1981). *Man-Living-Health: A Theory of Nursing*. New York: John Wiley and Sons.

Parse, R. R. (1992). Human Becoming: Parse's theory of nursing. *Nursing Science Quarterly*, **5**, 35–42.

Parse, R. R. (1998). *The Human Becoming School of Thought: A Perspective for Nurses and Other Professionals*. Thousand Oaks, CA: Sage.

Quill, T. (1991). Death and dignity—a case of individualized decision making. *New England Journal of Medicine*, **324**, 691–694.

Reinharz, S. (1983). Phenomenology as a dynamic process. *Phenomenology and Pedagogy*, **1**(1), 77–79.

Rosenfeld, B., Breitbart, W., Galietta, M., et al. (2000). The schedule of attitudes toward hastened death: measuring desire for death in terminally ill cancer patients. *Cancer*, **88**, 2868–2875.

Seale, C. and Addington-Hall, J. (1994). Euthanasia: why people want to die earlier. *Social Science and Medicine*, **39**, 647–654.

Suarez-Almazor, M. E., Belzile, M., and Bruera, E. (1997). Euthanasia and physician-assisted suicide: a comparative survey of physicians, terminally ill cancer patients, and the general population. *Journal of Clinical Oncology*, **15**, 418–427.

Chapter 4

Comment on 'Expressed desire for hastened death: a phenomenologic inquiry' 10 years later

Nessa Coyle

A nursing perspective

In reviewing the study 'Expressed desire for hastened death: a phenomenologic inquiry' (reprinted as Chapter 3) 10 years later as a palliative care nurse working with advanced cancer patients and their families, I am struck by how things are both the same and yet different. The conclusion of that study—that the expression of a desire for hastened death (DHD) has many meanings and uses and is a tool of communication—is still valid in my experience. Vulnerability, the multidimensional nature of suffering, a need to be heard, fear of abandonment, concern about burdening the family, and the importance both of kindness and 'presence' all appear to influence the meanings and uses of an expression of the DHD. The need for vigilance in managing pain, dyspnoea, and other forms of suffering, as well as the impact of uncontrolled symptoms on the desire for death also remain important factors. The fact that words really matter and the importance of how information is given remain unchanged. In addition it remains the case that, for a small number of people, controlling the time and manner of their death is important even when symptoms and suffering are well managed. Whether it is the place of medicine to provide the tools for assisting a hastened death in this population remains controversial.

The various dimensions outlined in the study reflect the importance of the terminally ill patient being seen as a person, a unique individual and not just a case—'I am more than my chart' as one patient told me. That the DHD fluctuates, and may be an expression of suffering rather than a literal request, is also unchanged. A paradox remains—on the one hand a DHD and on the other a desire for continued existence. The patient is simultaneously travelling on two different paths, that of the living and that of the dying.

One major difference, perhaps, since the 2004 study was conducted is that in those caring for the terminally ill there is a greater awareness of the multidimensional and interrelated factors experienced by the dying, and their influence on demoralization, hopelessness, and in turn the DHD. There is also a more conscious willingness and understanding of the imperative to be present, to suspend judgement, to listen to the patient, and to being open to what is being said without necessarily agreeing with the patient's conclusion. We may know what is best for ourselves but we can't provide guidance for patients unless we hear their voices. There has also developed a greater acknowledgment of how little we know about the patients we care for, and yet we seem to make assumptions about how the end of their lives should unfold. With awareness comes humility. Practitioners have observed that spirituality in its broadest terms and search for meaning come to the fore as life draws to a close. Meaning-centred psycho-therapy (Chochinov et al. 1995) is just one approach that has been developed to address this need.

There is an increased focus on interdisciplinary teams as well as the development of communication skill training. The rapidly growing hospital-based palliative care pro-grammes and home hospice programmes focus on presence, listening, symptom con-trol, and meaning-making as the team works to facilitate the best possible quality of life for the patient given their clinical reality. A caveat is that this focus may involve facili-tating the process of acquiring a lethal dose of medication for the patient to use if he or she chooses. Although that step is currently legal in five US states, many practitioners feel that this is not the role of medicine or nursing and is not part of palliative care. Alternatively there exists a growing literature about the option of voluntarily stopping eating and drinking. This option is generally accepted as the patient's right.

There is overall more discussion than 10 years ago about 'patient-controlled dying'— that is controlling the circumstances of dying if not the precise timing of one's death. In this regard there is increased information for the public and greater discussion in the lay press about self-determination and planning for the end of life through, for example, completing advanced directives, discontinuing unwanted life-prolonging in-terventions, and voluntarily stopping eating and drinking. Whether in fact increasing numbers of people are choosing to hasten their death is not known, but there is gen-erally more acceptance among clinicians, patients, and families about the benefits of having open discussions about end-of-life values and wishes.

Reference

Chochinov, H. M., Wilson, K.G., Enns, M., *et al.* (1995). Desire for death in the terminally ill. *American Journal of Psychiatry*, **152**, 1185–1191.

Chapter 5

Euthanasia (requests) after the implementation of the euthanasia law in Belgium in 2002. Results of empirical studies in Flanders, Belgium

Luc Deliens and Tinne Smets

Introduction to euthanasia

Following several years of intense ethical and political debate, euthanasia was legalized in Belgium in 2002, making it one of the few countries, together with the Netherlands and Luxembourg, where euthanasia is currently possible by law, albeit under strict conditions (Belgisch Staatsblad 2002a). Among other things, the patient requesting euthanasia must be of age (minimum age 18 years) and consciously aware at the time of the request, and be in a continuing situation of constant and unbearable physical or psychological suffering without relief as a result of an incurable condition caused by an illness or accident. The physician has to consult a second, independent, physician. Furthermore, under the euthanasia law the physician is obliged to report every case of euthanasia to the Federal Control and Evaluation Commission (Belgisch Staatsblad 2002a; Nijs and Deckers 2003; Distelmans 2004; Smets et al. 2009).

At almost the same time as the euthanasia law, there was a vote on a law on palliative care and a patient rights law. The palliative care law stipulates that each patient has a right to specialized palliative care and decides measures for the expansion and organization of palliative care provision (Belgisch Staatsblad 2002b). According to the law on patient rights, every patient has the right to be informed of his or her diagnosis and become involved in all treatment decisions (Belgisch Staatsblad 2002c). In general we can state that these laws show the increasing importance of patient autonomy and a high quality of life at the end of life.

In the light of this new legal context it is important to consider any possible effects these laws have had on the occurrence, decision-making, carrying out, and reporting of euthanasia. In the framework of the evaluation of the euthanasia law in Belgium by the MELC project (monitoring the quality of end-of-life care in Flanders) a number of studies have been carried out to map and evaluate the implementation of the euthanasia law and the practice of euthanasia in Belgium (MELC Consortium 2011). This chapter presents and discusses the main results of these studies.

Incidence of euthanasia

Before the euthanasia law came into force, the incidence and characteristics of end-of-life decisions had already been researched using a survey of death certificates signed by physicians in 1998 and 2001—the retrospective post-mortem surveys (Deliens et al. 2000; Van der Heide et al. 2003). These are large-scale surveys performed in Flanders, Belgium, based on a representative random sample of death certificates. Each death in Belgium must be registered by the physician using a death certificate; these certificates are handled by the Flemish Agency for Care and Health. For the surveys, the Flemish Agency for Care and Heath drew a large, stratified sample from the death certificates of people aged 1 year or older who died within a particular period. The sample was proportionately stratified according to province and month of death, but also disproportionately stratified according to the underlying cause of death. The likelihood of an end-of-life practice with a possible or certain life-shortening effect varies according to the underlying cause of death. Sampling fractions in the strata therefore rise correspondingly with higher likelihood of an end-of-life practice. A short questionnaire was mailed to the certifying physician of all sampled deaths. Further details on the methodology of the survey can be found elsewhere (Chambaere et al. 2008). The retrospective post-mortem survey was repeated in 2007; this enabled us to study the trends after the laws mentioned in the Introduction came into force (Chambaere et al. 2008). In 1998, a random sample of 3999 deaths was selected and 1925 deaths were described (the response rate was 52%) (Deliens et al. 2000). In 2007, 6927 deaths were sampled, and questionnaires were returned for 3623 deaths. Non-eligible cases were removed from the sample. The response rate for this survey was 58.4% (Bilsen et al. 2009).

In describing trends in the incidence and characteristics of euthanasia, we are mainly comparing the figures for 2007 with those for 1998. The 2001 figures might give a somewhat misleading picture, as a strong ethical and political debate was raging at that time about legalizing euthanasia. In addition, during this period legal proceedings were started against a number of physicians who were suspected of having carried out euthanasia, which resulted in a greater reluctance on the part of physicians to carry out euthanasia or to report it in a survey. Euthanasia was defined in this study as 'the administration of drugs with the sole purpose of hastening the death of the patient, at his or her explicit request'.

Trends in incidence of euthanasia

In 1998, 1.1% of all deaths in Flanders involved euthanasia (Deliens et al. 2000). In 2007 the incidence rose to 1.9%, i.e. slightly more than a thousand cases of euthanasia a year (Bilsen et al. 2009). The new legal context has therefore resulted in an increased incidence of euthanasia. It is likely that the atmosphere of openness and an emphasis on patient autonomy since the changes in the law have made the increase in euthanasia possible.

Changes within patient groups

No increase in the incidence of euthanasia was found in patients in residential homes. We mainly saw an increase in euthanasia in cancer patients and in younger patients up to the age of 64, the group in which euthanasia occurs most frequently. Euthanasia is, as expected, more frequently carried out at the patient's home (Chambaere et al. 2010a).

The fact that euthanasia occurs more frequently among cancer patients can be explained as the course of the illness is more predictable than for patients with different chronic conditions. In addition, the actual phase of dying is often more easily recognizable (Murray et al. 2005). Cancer patients also fear that their end of life will come with pain and other symptoms such as exhaustion and breathing difficulties. Knowledge or fear of what lies ahead can prompt patients and carers to speak about end-of-life options, and therefore euthanasia is preferred by some patients.

Euthanasia is most often carried out in the patient's home, as many patients would prefer to die at home surrounded by their family and friends. The fact that it can be carried out by their own GP, with whom the patient has often built a long-term and personal relationship, can for some people be an additional reason to want euthanasia to be carried out at home.

The fact that younger patients, too, more often ask for euthanasia may be linked to their greater awareness than older patients that they will die from their condition, and it may be easier for them to discuss end-of-life options with their physician. This age group is better educated on the whole than the elderly. Statistically, younger patients also die of cancer more often than patients in older age groups.

Euthanasia requests

In 2009, a large-scale countrywide research project was carried out using a questionnaire posted to a random sample of 3006 Belgian physicians whose clinical work gave them a greater chance of having to care for end-of-life patients. This survey examined attitudes towards and experiences of euthanasia. Nine hundred and fourteen questionnaires were returned, a response rate of 34%.

The results showed that 48% of the physicians who responded had received a euthanasia request (Van Wesemael et al. 2011). Physicians in Wallonia and the Brussels area received significantly fewer requests than those in the Flemish area (43% and 46% versus 51%, respectively). Of the physicians questioned, 39% had received a request *since the introduction of the euthanasia law*.

The recipients with the most requests were radiotherapists (100%), neurologists (73%), lung specialists (61%), and surgeons (50%). Physicians training in palliative care or who were part of a palliative care team received a request more often than physicians who were not training or who were not a member of a palliative care team (49% versus 30%) (MELC Consortium 2011).

When we looked at the influence of several variables at the same time, we found that physicians who are non-believers, physicians treating terminally ill patients, physicians training in palliative care, and physicians between the ages of 25 and 65 are more likely to receive a request for euthanasia than other physicians. Their attitude towards euthanasia is not a predictable factor in whether they receive a euthanasia request or not (Van Wesemael et al. 2011).

Physicians who had received a request since the law's introduction were asked to describe their latest euthanasia request. Three hundred and sixty-three requests were described. The request descriptions showed that 64% of the patients requesting euthanasia had cancer and 54% of requests were from patients between the ages of 60 and 79 years. The most apparent reasons for the requests were suffering without prospects of improvement (72%), loss of dignity (44%), and pain (34%) (Van Wesemael et al. 2011).

Of the 363 requests described, 171 resulted in euthanasia; in 18 cases the request was refused by the physician; 37 patients decided not to have euthanasia; in 82 cases the patient died before euthanasia could be carried out; and in 47 cases, the patient was still alive at the time the physician filled in the questionnaire. However, these results should be interpreted with caution considering that the response rate was only 34% (Van Wesemael et al. 2011).

Decision-making and clinical practice of euthanasia

Consultation of a second physician

According to the euthanasia law, prior to carrying out euthanasia a physician is obliged to consult another physician about the patient's serious and incurable condition, and to advise him or her of the reasons for this consultation. The second physician must be independent of the physician treating the patient as well as of the patient him- or herself, and must read the medical dossier, examine the patient, ascertain the continuous and unbearable physical suffering which cannot be relieved, and write a report on his or her findings. The second physician then gives a recommendation, although the treating physician is not obliged to follow this advice. The law does not give a precise definition of the second physician's independence with regard to the treating physician and the patient (Belgisch Staatsblad 2002a).

The study carried out by Chambaere et al. (2010b) showed that there was more discussion between physicians and their colleagues after the euthanasia law came into force than before. In 2007, discussion with colleagues took place in 78% of the euthanasia cases carried out in Flanders, while in 1998 this figure was only 50%. The increase can be explained by the regulation in the euthanasia law that a second physician (and a third in the case of a patient who is not terminally ill) has to be consulted during the euthanasia procedure. Despite these legal requirements, no second physician was consulted in 22% of euthanasia cases.

In addition, the physician survey gave information about consulting a second physician. This survey asked physicians to describe their last euthanasia request. In 65% of the 363 described euthanasia requests, the physician consulted a second physician (Van Wesemael et al. 2011). In 43% of the consultations the second physician was a GP, and in the remaining cases, a specialist. In 78% of the euthanasia requests where a second physician was consulted, the latter gave positive advice. Euthanasia was ultimately carried out on 78% of the patients who had received positive advice from the second physician.

We found significant differences between physicians in three different districts concerning the consultation of a second physician. In the Flemish and Brussels districts a majority of 73% and 68%, respectively, of physicians did consult, whereas in Wallonia only 49% of physicians consulted a second physician (Van Wesemael et al. 2011).

In terms of the physicians' work, our study showed that 96% of consultations between the physician treating the patient and the second physician were conducted orally. In 96% of consultations the second physician examined the dossier, 92% talked to the patient, and 66% carried out a physical examination of the patient. Furthermore, in 72% of cases the second physician talked to the family, 57% of them had discussions with the care team, and in 33% of cases the consultant had a conversation with another physician treating the patient. Thirty-two per cent of consulted physicians were present at the euthanasia itself, and the same number offered practical help in carrying it out. Of the second physicians consulted, 65% wrote a report and 30% assisted the physician treating the patient to fill in the registration form for the Review Commission (Van Wesemael et al. 2011).

Consultation of next of kin and other caregivers

In the mortality study we found that patients' next of kin, nursing staff, and carers specializing in palliative care had been increasingly involved in discussions surrounding decisions on euthanasia over the years (Chambaere et al. 2010b).

When the law legalizing euthanasia was drafted, there was a suggestion from some quarters that a procedure of 'palliative filter' should be included. This means that patients asking for euthanasia are first made aware of the possibilities that palliative care can offer them. The expectation was that provision of adequate palliative care would in many cases lead to the request for euthanasia being withdrawn. Although the palliative care filter was ultimately not included in the law, our research shows that carers specializing in palliative care are consulted in half of all euthanasia cases, and that this option is indeed explored but is often not enough to replace the request for euthanasia.

Reasons for euthanasia

The main reason physicians gave in the mortality study for carrying out euthanasia is a request or wish expressed by the patient (93%) (Chambaere et al. 2010a). Other important reasons were the patient's future expectations of their quality of life and suffering, i.e. 'no prospect of improvement' (84%), 'limited expected quality of life' (56%), and 'expectation of further suffering' (54%). A final important reason for carrying out euthanasia was the loss of patient dignity (51%). The wish of the next of kin (26%) and their unbearable situation (17%) were less often stated as important reasons for carrying out euthanasia.

Use of medication

In two-thirds of all cases, a combination of medicines was used, mostly barbiturates with muscle relaxants (29%) (Chambaere et al. 2010a). Barbiturates and muscle relaxants are the recommended medication for good practice in euthanasia, as described in various guidelines and recommendations. According to these guidelines, a barbiturate should be administered first, rendering the patient unconscious, after which (if the patient has not died by then) a muscle relaxant is administered to stop the heart (Battin and Lipman 1996; KNMP 2007). In 10% of cases a muscle relaxant was unnecessary after administering barbiturates (Chambaere et al. 2010a). In 22% of euthanasia cases, opiates alone were administered. The use of opiates for carrying out euthanasia is discouraged because of their uncertain life-shortening effect and because of possible undesirable side effects (Battin and Lipman 1996).

Since the euthanasia law came into force, a clear improvement in medication used in euthanasia has been noticeable (Chambaere et al. 2010a). An analysis of medication used in 1998 shows that opiates in particular were used to carry out euthanasia, whereas barbiturates and muscle relaxants are now the preferred medication. This is probably as a result of the legalization of euthanasia. Before, physicians were less sure of the medication available, but with the euthanasia law they have been able to search openly for the information on which medication to use. Despite this, euthanasia is still often carried out with opiates, which shows that many physicians remain uncertain about the appropriate medication.

Since euthanasia became lawful in Belgium, no clear guidelines regarding the administration of euthanasia have been set, although such guidelines could benefit the practice of euthanasia (MELC Consortium 2011). It is possible that physicians who administer opiates with the sole intention of ending a patient's life at their explicit request do not consider their action to be euthanasia (Chambaere et al. 2010a). These cases are not usually reported to the Federal Review Commission. It is also possible that, in some circumstances, physicians do not want to follow the procedures by using the recommended medication because their patient does not satisfy all the legal safeguarding conditions for euthanasia, or because they find the legal procedures too cumbersome (Smets et al. 2010a).

In 70% of the euthanasia cases studied, the physician alone administered the euthanasia medication (Chambaere et al. 2010a); in a few cases (8%) it was administered jointly with a nurse. It is problematic, however, that in 20% of euthanasia cases a nurse administered the medication alone. In the majority of these cases, the drugs administered were opiates. Legally, euthanasia needs to be done by a physician, who alone has the necessary expertise. Patient care and care in administering a drug are ultimately also the physician's responsibility. If the medication is administered by a nurse, especially in the absence of the treating physician, this can compromise the proper euthanasia procedure and is punishable by law. Despite this, we were able to establish that the involvement of nurses in the administering of euthanasia has diminished considerably compared with the situation in 1998. Before the euthanasia law, nurses were involved in 40% of the administration of all euthanasia cases. The legal rulings on euthanasia have to a certain extent produced the apparent behaviour change, but explicit guidelines on the possible role of carers involved in the euthanasia process are still lacking (Chambaere et al. 2010b; MELC Consortium 2011).

Reporting of euthanasia

Euthanasia is an exceptional medical practice and demands a kind of social control in order to avoid abuse. The law therefore makes it obligatory for the physician to report every case of euthanasia to the Federal Review Commission (Belgisch Staatsblad 2002a). One of this Commission's tasks is to examine the registration documents submitted by the physician to check whether all the legal rules on safeguards and procedures have been followed (Distelmans 2004; Smets et al. 2009). Once the members of the Review Commission are satisfied that all legal conditions have been met, the case is closed. If, however, they consider the law has been broken, the members of the Commission can then decide whether to send the dossier to the Public Prosecutor, who can prosecute the physician (Distelmans 2004; Smets et al. 2009). The Commission issues its ruling within 2 months. If everything has been carried out according to the law, the physician will not be informed. Only if the Review Commission requires additional information or wants to make comments will the physician be contacted to hear their verdict.

Reporting percentage and reasons for not reporting

The post-mortem survey also allowed us to estimate the extent to which physicians in Flanders did report their euthanasia cases (Smets et al. 2010b). In the survey, end-of-life practices were classified based on four key questions. These questions assessed: (1) whether the physician had withheld or withdrawn medical treatment while taking into account the possible hastening of death; (2) whether they had intensified measures to alleviate pain or other symptoms while taking into account or partly intending the possible hastening of death; (3) whether they had withheld or withdrawn medical treatment with the explicit intention of hastening death; or (4) whether they had administered drugs with the explicit intention of hastening death, resulting in the patient's death. If more than one of the four questions was answered affirmatively, the act that involved the most explicit intention was used to classify the case. If the intention was similar, the administration of drugs prevailed over the withholding or withdrawing of treatment. If question 4 was answered affirmatively, and if the act was done in response to an explicit request by the patient, the act was classified as euthanasia, regardless of how the physician labelled the act themselves. In 53% of all euthanasia administered by physicians in 2007, the physician indicated that they had reported it at the time. Both GPs and specialists reported their euthanasia cases at the same rate. As this is the first time the reporting percentage has been estimated, and no identity estimates are available for the other years since the euthanasia law came into force, we do not know whether this signifies an increase or decrease in the reporting percentage.

In all cases where the physician did not report the death, the reasons for not doing so were requested (Smets et al. 2010b). The main reason physicians gave for not reporting a euthanasia death was that they themselves did not consider the death as euthanasia (in 77% of non-reported euthanasia cases). Other reasons were also given, such as 're-porting is too much of an administrative hassle' (18%), 'possible non-compliance with all legal conditions and procedures' (12%), 'euthanasia is a matter between doctor and patient' (9%), and 'fear of possible legal consequences' (2%) (multiple answers were possible).

We did not ask for the reason why some physicians did not perceive the end-of-life practice as euthanasia. However, the discrepancy between the legal definition of euthanasia and the perception of the physician of what they had done might be explained by the following possible hypotheses.

The first is the 'grey zone' hypothesis. When a patient requests that their life be ended and the physician disproportionally increases the dose of opioids or sedatives instead of administering neuromuscular relaxants, the distinction between euthanasia and normal intensification of symptom treatment may become blurred. Because of the confusion that may arise in these situations, physicians may not perceive the act as euthanasia. A second hypothesis is that some physicians may feel reluctant to perform euthanasia although they do want to help the patient who is requesting it. In these situations physicians may choose to use opioids or sedatives because these drugs are not normally associated with euthanasia. By disguising the act as normal medical practice, whether deliberately or not, they feel they have granted their patient's wish without, in their perception, having actually performed euthanasia.

How a physician describes the action is evidently crucial in the decision on whether to report euthanasia or not. It also shows that Flemish physicians are more inclined to report euthanasia cases than physicians from Wallonia or Brussels. In addition, physicians who consider they are well enough informed about the euthanasia law are more likely to report euthanasia than those who are less well informed. Finally, it is not surprising that physicians who feel positive towards social control over the practice of euthanasia are more likely to report euthanasia cases than those with a negative attitude towards control (Smets et al. 2012).

Characteristics of the reported cases of euthanasia

An analysis of registered reported euthanasia cases requested by the Commission shows that in Belgium between 22 September 2002 and 31 December 2009 a total of 3443 cases of euthanasia had been reported by physicians (Smet et al. 2010a; Smets and Deliens 2011). The number of reported euthanasia cases had also risen each year from 235 in 2003 to 822 in 2009. Of all reported euthanasia cases, 82% were reported by Dutch-speaking physicians and only 17.8% by French-speaking ones. [For a better understanding of these findings note that 53.4% of all physicians (specialists and GPs) are located in Flanders, 33.3% in Wallonia, and 13.3% in Brussels Capital Region. About 60% of the population of Belgium live in the northern part, Flanders, and about 40% in the southern part, Wallonia.] Whether these findings indicate differing medical end-of-life practices between the Flemish and Walloon communities, and/or whether this reflects a difference in willingness to report among physicians of both communities, is unclear.

The annual rise in the number of reported euthanasia cases may be for various reasons. First, it is likely that physicians have become more aware over the years of the legal reporting regulations, together with the fact that physicians' acceptance of euthanasia has also increased, possibly due to the many debates on euthanasia in the media and other public forums. Physicians no longer have to act in secret and are therefore more inclined to be transparent. Finally, it has become clear that the risk of legal action resulting from reporting is effectively zero. Since the Commission came into being, not a single case of euthanasia has been referred to the Public Prosecutor, which will have given physicians more confidence in the reporting procedure.

Of all reported euthanasia cases, 51.8% of patients were male and 48.2% female. Most patients who received euthanasia were between the ages of 40 and 79 (76.5%). Euthanasia does not occur as often with patients aged 80 or older; only 21% of cases studied involved people older than 80, although this number has increased considerably since 2008 and 2009 compared with previous years (from an average of 17% of all reported cases between 2002 and 2007 to an average of 24% in 2008 and 2009). Nearly half of euthanasias administered (48.8%) took place in hospital, and 43.2% at home. In care homes, it is only sporadically administered (5.8%). Most of the euthanasia patients had cancer (82%); a minority had been diagnosed with a neuromuscular or cardiovascular disease. In nearly every case reported (97.5%) the physician indicated that the patient was experiencing physical suffering. Psychological suffering was also indicated in 8 out of 10 reported cases. According to the reporting physician, the majority of patients were terminally ill (93%), and only 7% of all reported cases were non-terminal. These patients mainly suffered diseases other than cancer, such as progressive or non-progressive neuromuscular disease (52%) or cardiovascular disease (9%). Over the years, their numbers have not increased significantly (Smets et al. 2010a).

In practically all cases physicians had consulted a second independent physician, as stated in the euthanasia law. For patients who, according to their physician, are not (yet) terminally ill, the law requires a third independent physician to be consulted. In most cases, this was a psychiatrist (64.5%). In more than a third of reported euthanasia cases, the physician had consulted more than the obligatory number of physicians.

In all cases reported between 2002 and 2009, the Commission judged that all legal requirements for euthanasia had been adhered to and not a single dossier was referred to the Public Prosecutor (Smets et al. 2010a).

Application of the legal requirements of due care in euthanasia

The mortality study enabled us to compare reported and non-reported euthanasia cases, and the meticulous care taken with them (Smets et al. 2010b). This analysis showed that euthanasia cases that were not being reported were also treated with less care by the physician than euthanasia cases that were reported. An oral and written request, as stipulated in the euthanasia law, was present in 73% of the reported cases, though these were generally absent for the non-reported cases (88% had an oral request only and 9% an oral as well as a written request). In non-reported cases of euthanasia there was often much less consultation with others. In only 55% of the non-reported cases were other physicians consulted, compared with 72% of the reported cases where consultation had taken place. There is also less consultation with palliative care specialists and nursing staff in non-reported euthanasia cases. Dutch research also shows a strong relationship between the consultation of a second independent physician and the reporting of euthanasia: the main reason quoted in the research for not consulting a second physician was that the physician was not intending to report the euthanasia (Onwuteaka-Philipsen et al. 2000; Jansen-van der Weide et al. 2004).

Physicians who reported their case of euthanasia generally used barbiturates and muscle relaxants to carry it out. Physicians who did not report their case of euthanasia more often used medicines not specified for use in euthanasia, such as opiates and sedatives. Although in reported euthanasia cases the life-ending medicine was always administered by a physician, as stipulated by the euthanasia law, this did not happen with the non-reported euthanasia cases. Often (41% of all cases) the administration was carried out by nursing staff (Smets et al. 2010b).

Attitudes of physicians

The physicians' survey gauged their attitude towards euthanasia and the euthanasia law (Smets et al. 2011). The survey showed that the vast majority of physicians (90%) identify euthanasia for terminally ill patients with extreme uncontrollable pain or other suffering. This shows a very high acceptance level, which has also risen since the euthanasia law. The euthanasia law, the law on palliative care, and the patient rights law, together with debates prior to these laws, may have led to an increased awareness of the rights of terminally ill patients and increased support for patient self-determination about medical decisions at the end of life. Although the level of acceptance of euthanasia is high, the level of preparedness by physicians to administer euthanasia themselves is lower (63%). This makes sense, as it is easier to support a practice than to take responsibility for carrying it out personally.

Physicians accept not just euthanasia but also the use of life-ending medication *without* a request from terminally ill incompetent patients, to a fairly high degree, although this practice is illegal in Belgium. Over half the physicians considered that they, together with the care team, should be able to make a decision to administer life-ending medication if a terminally ill patient is suffering unbearably and is incapable of making their own decisions. It was notable that physicians who had more experience in the care of dying patients were more likely to end life without a request than less experienced physicians. In the first instance this may appear contradictory because we might expect that these physicians in particular are well aware that this treatment is illegal. However, it might be explained as being precisely because of their experience in caring for dying patients. The constant and personal experience of human suffering might make these physicians see the use of life-ending medication without a request as a justified choice for incompetent patients whose suffering cannot be relieved in any other way (Smets et al. 2011).

In Belgium, the opinion that euthanasia can form part of good care at the end of life is supported by 75% of physicians involved with end-of-life care; 10% consider that euthanasia hinders the further development of palliative care. It is also noticeable that physicians who had trained in palliative care did not have a negative attitude towards euthanasia any more often than physicians who had not. In fact, physicians with palliative care training considered that the euthanasia law had less of a negative effect on the development of palliative care, and had themselves administered euthanasia more frequently than other physicians (Smets et al. 2011).

The statement that consultation with a second physician was meaningful for every case of a euthanasia request was agreed by 81% of the respondents, and 46% of physicians agreed that they would have had to have specialist training to give advice as second physician. A third of physicians disagreed with the statement. Furthermore, 82% of those who responded considered that the consultation with a second physician contributes to how careful and thorough physicians' medical behaviour is at the end of life (Van Wesemael et al. 2012).

The vast majority of physicians consulted also supported the need for social control over the practice of euthanasia (68%). Nevertheless, 25% of physicians considered that euthanasia is a private matter and should not be under the control of the Commission. Physicians from Wallonia and Brussels, in particular, expressed this opinion. According to 66% of physicians, the euthanasia law should supplement medical treatment and care at the end of life (Smets et al. 2011).

A majority of the physicians (nearly 80%) support the extension of the euthanasia law to minors, whereas slightly less than half support the extending of the law to mentally incapable patients, such as those with dementia, who are in possession of a legal written declaration requesting euthanasia.

Conclusions

Since the introduction of the euthanasia law, the incidence of euthanasia in Flanders has risen from 1.1% in 1998 to 1.9% in 2007. The higher incidence is particularly noticeable among cancer patients and younger patients up to the age of 64. These are also the patients who most frequently request euthanasia. Among reported euthanasia cases, these patient groups are also clearly over-represented compared with patients with a different diagnosis and older patients.

Compared with 1998, we determined that in 2007 a request for euthanasia was more frequently discussed with the patient's next of kin, other physicians, nursing staff, and carers specializing in palliative care. There was an especially large increase in consultation with other physicians, which is clearly connected to the legal obligation to consult a second independent physician in a case of euthanasia. Despite these legal obligations, a second physician had not been consulted in nearly 25% of the administered euthanasia cases.

However, although compared with 1998 there has been a noticeable improvement in the choices of drugs administered in euthanasia, opiates are used far too often (and frequently on their own), showing that many physicians remain unclear about which substances to use. In addition, the involvement of nursing staff in euthanasia is still problematic. When the euthanasia law came into force in Belgium, clear guidelines for performing euthanasia were omitted. The publication of such guidelines would benefit the practice of euthanasia.

In Flanders in 2007, 53% of all euthanasia cases carried out were reported by physicians to the Federal Review Commission. Euthanasia cases not reported are often not considered euthanasia by the physicians who carry them out. Non-reported euthanasia cases are in general carried out with less care than reported ones.

Most physicians have a positive attitude towards euthanasia for terminally ill patients who are experiencing extreme suffering. The majority are also positive about consulting a second physician, as well as about social control of the practice of euthanasia. Nevertheless, our research found that one in four physicians considered euthanasia to be a matter between physician and patient that does not require societal control by a Review Commission. This is certainly problematic as far as social control of the practice of euthanasia is concerned.

We conclude that having a euthanasia law on its own is not sufficient to achieve a caring and transparent medical system for the implementation of euthanasia. There will probably need to be additional measures. Physicians need to receive enough information about the euthanasia law and the interpretation of the legal conditions for due care. Intensive training for those physicians caring for patients at the end of life, the availability of support for physicians who are faced with patients' requests for euthanasia, and the development of guidelines for a safe procedure are needed.

References

Battin, M. P. and Lipman, A. G. (eds) (1996). *Drug Use in Assisted-Suicide and Euthanasia*. New York: Haworth Press.

Belgisch Staatsblad (2002a). Wet betreffende euthanasie, 22 June 2002.

Belgisch Staatsblad (2002b). Wet betreffende palliatieve zorg, 26 October 2002.

Belgisch Staatsblad (2002c). Wet op de patiëntenrechten, 22 August 2002.

Bilsen, J., Cohen, J., Chambaere, K., et al. (2009). Medical end-of-life practices under the euthanasia law in Belgium. A nationwide post-mortem survey. *New England Journal of Medicine*, **361**, 1119–1121.

Chambaere, K., Bilsen, J., Cohen, J., et al. (2008). A post-mortem survey on end-of-life decisions using a representative sample of death certificates in Flanders, Belgium: research protocol. *BMC Public Health*, **8**, 299.

Chambaere, K., Bilsen, J., Cohen, J., Onwuteaka-Philipsen, B. D., Mortier, F., and Deliens, L. (2010a). Physician-assisted deaths under the euthanasia law in Belgium: a population-based survey. *Canadian Medical Association Journal*, **182**, 895–901.

Chambaere, K., Bilsen, J., Cohen, J., et al. (2010b). Trends in medical end-of-life decision making in Flanders, Belgium 1998–2001–2007. *Medical Decision Making*, **31**, 500–510.

Deliens, L., Mortier, F., Bilsen, J., et al. (2000). End-of-life decisions in medical practice in Flanders, Belgium: a nationwide survey. *Lancet*, **356**, 1806–1811.

Distelmans, W. (2004). De Federale Controle- en Evaluatiecommissie inzake de toepassing van de wet van 28 mei 2002 betreffende de euthanasie. *Tijdschrift voor Geneeskunde*, **60**, 232–234.

Jansen-van der Weide, M. C., Onwuteaka-Philipsen, B. D., and van der Wal, G. (2004). Implementation of the project support and consultation for general practitioners of the project support and consultation for general practitioners concerning euthanasia in the Netherlands. *Health Policy*, **69**, 365–373.

KNMP (Koninklije Nederlandse Maatschappijter Bevordering der Pharmacie) (2007). *Standaard Euthanatica*, 4th edn. The Hague: KNMP.

MELC Consortium (2011). *Palliatieve Zorg en Euthanasie in België. Evaluatie van de Praktijk en de Wetten*. Brussels: Academic and Scientific Publishers.

Murray, S. A., Kendall, M., Boyd, K., and Sheikh, A. (2005). Illness trajectories and palliative care. *British Medical Journal*, **330**, 1007–1011.

Nijs, H. and Deckers, E. (2003). *Nieuwe Wetgeving Inzake Euthanasie*. Mechelen: Kluwer.

Onwuteaka-Philipsen, B. D., van der Wal, G., Kostense, P. J., and van der Maas, P. J. (2000). Consultation with another physician on euthanasia and assisted suicide in the Netherlands. *Social Science and Medicine*, **51**, 429–438.

Smets, T. and Deliens, L. (2011). Euthanasie in België: recente resultaten van studies naar praktijken en attitudes van artsen. *Onco-Hemato*, **5**, 226–230.

Smets, T., Bilsen, J., Cohen, J., Rurup, M. L., De Keyser, E., and Deliens, L. (2009). The medical practice of euthanasia in Belgium and the Netherlands: legal notification, control and evaluation procedures. *Health Policy*, **90**, 181–187.

Smets, T., Bilsen, J., Cohen, J., Rurup, M. L., and Deliens, L. (2010a). Legal euthanasia in Belgium: characteristics of all reported euthanasia cases. *Medical Care*, **48**, 187–192.

Smets, T., Bilsen, J., Cohen, J., Rurup, M. L., Mortier, F., and Deliens, L. (2010b). Reporting of euthanasia in medical practice in Flanders, Belgium: cross sectional analysis of reported and unreported cases. *British Medical Journal*, **341**, c5174.

Smets, T., Cohen, J., Bilsen, J., van Wesemael, Y., Rurup, M. L., and Deliens, L. (2011). Attitudes and experiences of Belgian physicians regarding euthanasia practice and the euthanasia law. *Journal of Pain and Symptom Management*, **41**, 580–593.

Smets, T., Cohen, J., Bilsen, J., van Wesemael, Y., Rurup, M. L., and Deliens, L. (2012). The labeling and reporting of euthanasia by Belgian physicians: a study of hypothetical cases. *European Journal of Public Health*, **22**, 19–26.

Van der Heide, A., Deliens, L., Faisst, K., et al., on behalf of the EURELD Consortium (2003). End-of-life decision-making in six European countries: descriptive study. *Lancet*, **362**, 345–350.

Van Wesemael, Y., Cohen, J., Bilsen, J., Smets, T., Onwuteaka-Philipsen, B. D., and Deliens, L. (2011). Process and outcomes of euthanasia requests under the Belgian Act on Euthanasia: a nationwide survey. *Journal of Pain and Symptom Management*, **42**, 721–733.

Van Wesemael, Y., Cohen, J., Bilsen, J., Smets, T., Onwuteaka-Philipsen, B. D., and Deliens, L. (2012). Implementation of a service for physicians' consultation and information in euthanasia requests in Belgium. *Health Policy*, **104**, 272–278.

Chapter 6

The journey to understanding the wish to hasten death

Tracy Schroepfer

Introduction to 'wish to hasten death'

Legal or not, terminally ill patients across the world have continued to voice the wish to hasten death (WTHD); however, that voice is often quickly silenced due to the ethical struggles of healthcare professionals, the fear of what is not legal where the patient resides, or the desire by a loved one for the patient to fight for life. Another key reason, though, is a lack of understanding regarding what it means when an individual vocalizes such a wish. This lack of understanding has served as an impetus to numerous studies of the potential physical and psychosocial factors motivating the WTHD (Chochinov et al. 1995; Breitbart et al. 1996; Emanuel et al. 1996, 2000; Kelly et al. 2003; Arnold et al. 2004; Albert et al. 2005; Schroepfer 2006, 2007, 2008; Villavicencio-Chavez et al. 2014), a conceptual framework that would capture the nuances of the WTHD (Monforte-Royo et al. 2011; Ohnsorge et al. 2014), the temporal stability of the WTHD (O'Mahony et al. 2005; Monforte-Royo et al. 2011; Ohnsorge et al. 2014), and instruments to measure effectively the WTHD (Monforte-Royo et al. 2011; Villavicencio-Chavez et al. 2014). As well as providing evidence that a WTHD can offer a deeper understanding of an individual's unmet emotional, physical, spiritual, and social needs, these and other studies also afford insight into the complexity of a WTHD. Expressing the WTHD may be less about an actual desire to actively end one's life than an expression of feelings about the current situation, a way to communicate psychosocial, spiritual, or physical suffering (Hudson et al. 2006), or a way to attract attention when no one is listening (Coyle and Sculco 2004). By silencing patients, the opportunity for their expression of feelings or suffering is lost, as is the opportunity for the healthcare professional to gain insight into the patient's needs so they can be effectively addressed. That said, it is understandable that without a deeper knowledge of the WTHD that seeks to reassure and inform the professional and loved one, hesitancy about having such conversations will continue to exist. It was my concern about the lack of these conversations that led me to focus my research on the WTHD.

When I began my research on the WTHD in 2001, I did so for a variety of reasons, one of which was that I had witnessed patients being silenced when they voiced a wish for their death to come sooner. At the time I resided in Michigan, and Jack Kevorkian, also known as Dr Death, lived in Detroit. Since 1990, Dr Kevorkian had assisted with the suicide of numerous individuals with a terminal illness (Nicol et al. 2006).

He created a suicide machine that allowed for patients to press a button to administer a lethal dose to stop their heart. He videotaped each assisted suicide and required the patient to verbally express their WTHD. In 1998, he was arrested for administering a lethal injection to a man in the final stages of Lou Gehrig's disease (amyotrophic lateral sclerosis). Kevorkian deemed the administration of a lethal injection to be an act of voluntary euthanasia, but the state of Michigan viewed it as second-degree murder, for which he was convicted and imprisoned (Nicol et al. 2006). Over the next year, I sought out and met with individuals who had been close to Kevorkian and/or had continued with his work of assisted suicide. I valued these discussions because I wanted to study the WTHD in order to gain a deeper understanding of the factors motivating such a wish, with the ultimate goal of developing an assessment instrument to be used by healthcare professionals. The insight I gained from these discussions served to inform my first study.

Factors motivating the WTHD and emerging frameworks

Over the years, researchers have adopted a retrospective or prospective method for studying the factors that motivate an individual's consideration to hasten his or her own death, but neither method is without its limitations. In the early studies on this topic, the retrospective approach was mostly adopted by researchers who interviewed physicians whose patients chose to hasten their death, as well as the patient's family and friends. Retrospective studies have led to the realization that psychosocial and spiritual factors appear to be more commonly reported as motivating the consideration of a hastened death than physical factors. This finding is reflected in the data reported by Oregon and Washington State where the Death with Dignity Act legalizing physician-assisted suicide (PAS) was passed in 1998 and 2009, respectively. Without exception, loss of autonomy, a decreased ability to participate in activities that make life enjoyable, and loss of dignity have been reported as the top three end-of-life concerns for the past 13 years in Oregon and the past 4 in Washington (Washington State Department of Health 2012; Oregon Department of Human Services 2014). Other factors found to play a role include feeling that one is a burden (Back et al. 1996; Meier et al. 1998; Washington State Department of Health 2012; Oregon Department of Human Services 2014), loss of control over the manner of death (Oregon Department of Human Services 2000; Volker 2001), and loss of meaning in life (Meirer et al. 1998). Two physical factors motivating the consideration to hasten death also surfaced. The first factor was the loss of control over bodily functions (Back et al. 1996; Washington State Department of Health 2012; Oregon Department of Human Services 2014) and the second was pain, which has been found to be more complex in nature. Two studies reported the role of *current* pain as a motivator for hastening death (Back et al. 1996; Meier et al. 1998); however, it is the *fear* of uncontrollable symptoms (Meier et al. 1998) or inadequate pain control at the end of life (Volker, 2001; Washington State Department of Health 2012; Oregon Department of Human Services 2014) that has been more often reported.

A recognized limitation of the retrospective approach has been the potential for recall bias, and so to address this bias researchers, including myself, have adopted a prospective approach. This approach involves interviewing individuals with a terminal illness (an illness likely to result in death) or individuals who have been defined as terminally ill (i.e. those with less than 6 months to live) about their WTHD and the factors motivating such a wish. As with retrospective studies, this method also possesses a limitation, which is that the individuals being interviewed are often not the ones who prior to the interview actually stated a WTHD. I knew this would not be a limitation for my research, as I felt it was also important to gain insight into the factors that led to patients not having a WTHD.

At the time of my first study in 2001, a thorough search of the literature revealed two gaps that I sought to address. The first gap was that I could not locate a study in which only terminally ill individuals had been interviewed about their WTHD; instead, terminally ill individuals and individuals with a terminal illness were often included in the same sample. I felt that such a mixed sample could prove problematic in that the views on dying and experiences of someone who has 6 months or less to live were likely to be very different from those of people who may live for years with a terminal illness. The second gap was in regard to the use of qualitative methodology; I could only find one qualitative study (Lavery et al. 2001) that addressed the WTHD. I felt strongly that it was too early in the research on the WTHD to be taking a quantitative approach since it meant working on an assumption that researchers knew which factors to measure. To address these gaps in the literature, I designed a mixed-methods study wherein respondents were elders who had been given a prognosis of 6 months or less to live. Quantitative measurements were made of depression, pain, education, and religiosity, all factors presumed at the time by healthcare professionals and researchers to motivate a WTHD. In addition, I asked open-ended questions to allow elders to discuss what *they* felt were factors behind the WTHD.

I conducted 96 interviews with terminally ill elders from all over Michigan, asking respondents if they had ever given serious consideration to hastening their death, as well as why they had or had not considered doing so. At that time, studies had focused on the dichotomy of either considering or not considering a hastened death, and so I had planned to report my findings based on this dichotomy. The qualitative analysis, however, revealed that respondents reported a more nuanced view of their dying process, the result of which was the emergence of six mind frames towards dying (Schroepfer 2006). I chose the term 'mind frames' because I felt 'stages' implied that elders moved through each or that there was a certain direction to that movement, neither of which my study was designed to test.

The six mind frames differed in terms of the consideration of a hastened death. The first three mind frames did not involve such a consideration; rather, these mind frames were focused on the respondent's acceptance of and readiness for dying. These three mind frames included neither ready nor accepting of dying, not ready but accepting of dying, and ready and accepting of dying. The other three mind frames involved a wish for death to come, a consideration of a hastened death with no specific plan, and a consideration of a hastened death that involved a specific plan. The three elders who wished death would come were resolute about not considering a hastened death; they found life difficult and wished for death, which they viewed as a 'better place' (Schroepfer 2006, p. S134). Their emotional pain was evident in the deep sadness and tearfulness that they exhibited. They spoke of not enjoying life, feeling useless, being exhausted, and experiencing daily pain. Family and their belief that it was God's decision when death will come were the two factors they reported as preventing them from actually taking steps to hasten their death. Nine of the 18 respondents considering a hastened death had not developed a specific plan and reported not enjoying life, being a burden, and feeling lonely, useless, and hopeless. Two of these nine respondents were currently in pain and two were fearful of experiencing pain in the future, which is yet another top reason for physician-assisted suicide requests in both Oregon and Washington State. None of the nine respondents had a plan, though, because they were struggling to balance their psychosocial and/or physical misery with their loved ones' desire for them to stay alive as long as possible. The other nine respondents did have a specific plan and talked about how having a plan gave them a sense of control in being able to die should life become unbearable in the future. They talked about their plan being motivated by feelings of uselessness, not enjoying life, and fearing future pain. All 21 respondents who wished for or were considering a hastened death reported that they were not actively looking to end their life at the time of their interview (Schroepfer 2006).

In addition to my prospective study, numerous others have not only provided support for the motivating factors described in retrospective studies, they have also uncovered a number of new factors. Reported psychological factors have included a higher level of anxiety (Kelly et al. 2003; Arnold et al. 2004), hopelessness (Albert et al. 2005; Schroepfer 2006), less optimism (Albert et al. 2005), emotional distress (Villavicencio-Chavez et al. 2014), and depression (Chochinov et al. 1995; Breitbart et al. 1996; Emanuel et al. 1996, 2000; Kelly et al. 2002, 2003; Arnold et al. 2004; Villavicencio-Chavez et al. 2014) for individuals considering a hastened death as opposed to those not doing so. With regard to social factors, patients reported few social supports (Breitbart et al. 1996; Kelly et al. 2003), a low quality of social support (Arnold et al. 2004; Chochinov et al. 1995; Breitbart et al. 1996; Kelly et al. 2002; Schroepfer 2007, 2008), conflictual social support (Schroepfer 2008), low family cohesion (Kelly et al. 2003), and low satisfaction with their social support (Kelly et al. 2003). As was found in the retrospective studies, the reported physical factors were more complex. In four studies pain was not found to be a significant predictor (Chochinov et al. 1995; Breitbart et al. 1996; Emanuel et al. 1996; Schroepfer 2008), but it was found to be significant in two other studies (Emanuel et al. 2000; Arnold et al. 2004). In addition, Kelly et al. (2002) found that respondents with a high WTHD reported as factors physical symptoms and lack of confidence concerning symptom control. Villavicencio-Chavez et al. (2014) found greater functional impairment and dependence, as well as loss of autonomy, which retrospective studies show as the number one reason for physician-assisted suicide requests in both Oregon and Washington State.

One benefit of prospective studies is that researchers can talk with patients about the role of social relationships in their WTHD. I used logistic regression to analyse quantitatively whether the relational content of social relationships significantly predicted the consideration of a hastened death (Schroepfer 2008). The four relational content variables were marital status, parental status, direct social control (how often someone told, reminded, or encouraged them to continue with their medical treatment or care), and social support (positive versus poor or conflictual social support); education, religiosity, depression, and pain intensity were included as control variables. I could not use the six mind frames as the dependent variable due to the small sample size ($n = 96$) and the number of predictor and control variables; therefore, I chose to dichotomize the mind frames into considering or not considering a hastened death. The results revealed that only one of the four relational content variables was significant. Those who reported receiving poor or conflictual social support, particularly those with a higher education, had greater odds of considering a hastened death regardless of depression, pain intensity, or religious beliefs. What was not clear from my results and those of other prospective studies was the type of support that respondents valued and from whom they would want to receive it. Clearly, social support, and its role in a WTHD, requires more research.

Temporal stability and assessment

Despite the limitations of retrospective and prospective methods, the results have afforded a deeper understanding of the factors motivating the WTHD, as well as an insight into possible frameworks that may prove useful in future research. What is not necessarily gleaned from the studies, however, is whether the WTHD fluctuates over time or dissipates when needs are addressed. Furthermore, the development of instruments that would assess both the WTHD and the factors motivating such a wish remains in its infancy. Gaining an understanding of the temporal stability of a WTHD, as well as developing an assessment tool, are necessary steps for ensuring that patients who have a WTHD are provided the opportunity for an open and uncensored discussion.

Temporal stability

In addition to the emergence of the mind frames in my first study, I also found evidence of the temporal nature of the WTHD (Schroepfer 2007). Fifteen (16%) of the 96 respondents spoke of four particular events that led them to wish for or consider a hastened death, as well as the end-of-life care practices that led to their no longer doing so. The four events were the perception of receiving insensitive and uncaring communication of a terminal diagnosis, dying in a distressing environment, unacknowledged feelings regarding undergoing chemotherapy or radiation treatment, and experiencing unbearable pain. For each of these events, respondents reported that the lack of acknowledgement for or listening to their concerns led to a wish for or consideration of a hastened death. They also reported that this desire passed when healthcare professionals or loved ones listened to their concerns and sought to address them. For example, a respondent was receiving radiation treatment to reduce her brain tumour and spoke about her intensive depression and ceaseless crying. She spoke with her brain surgeon, but he felt strongly that she should continue the radiation. The radiation oncologist, however, listened, acknowledged her feelings, and agreed to stop treatment. Her plan to hasten her death via an overdose of pills dissipated (Schroepfer 2007). Implications from this study centred on the importance of communication in order to ensure that when these and other events happen healthcare professionals have the communication skills necessary to provide patients with the information they need and an opportunity to voice their emotions and concerns. One could also argue that communication is only effective when the healthcare professional knows that the patient has a WTHD. Such knowledge could be gathered at the time of potential challenging events via assessment.

Assessment of the WTHD

In order to assess effectively the WTHD, as well as the factors often associated with such a wish, it is important that researchers have a deep enough understanding of those factors such that they can be measured. In 2006, I took another step towards my goal of developing an assessment instrument. Working with a psychometrician, I constructed a survey that sought to accomplish four goals. The first was to gain a more explicit comprehension of what terminally ill elders meant when they reported 'loss of control' as a factor motivating the WTHD. What was it that elders once had control over that they no longer did? What control did they wish to exercise during their dying process? How did they wish to exercise that control? Secondly, as previously noted, support has been found numerous times to serve as a motivating factor for the WTHD; however, the type of support that respondents value and from whom they would want to receive that support remain unclear. Thirdly, using the six mind frames, I created questions that I hoped would be a step toward assessing a patient's mind frame. Fourthly, I sought available valid and reliable scales to measure the motivating factors that respondents had reported in numerous studies. When I could not find a scale or question, I developed my own. Using this instrument, face-to-face interviews were conducted with a purposive sample of 102 terminally ill elders from hospices throughout southern Wisconsin. The findings were illuminating, and I will discuss some related to control and social support.

Of the 102 terminally ill elders interviewed, 84 responded to questions regarding over what aspects of the dying process they sought control, the strategies they used to exercise that control, and whether they desired more control. A direct content approach based on Schulz and Heckhausen's (1996) control strategies was used in analysing the data. These researchers theorize that individuals strive to exercise control over their lives to attain goals and proposed three control strategies they use in doing so. The first strategy is selective primary control, which requires the use of one's own abilities and efforts to attain a goal. The second strategy is compensatory primary control, which is when one's own abilities and efforts are no longer sufficient and assistance from others is necessary. The third strategy, compensatory secondary control, involves using cognitive strategies that devalue former goals, enhance the value of a new goal, require letting go of prior goals, and comparison of one's situation with another's that is deemed to be worse.

The results provided a great deal of insight into the role that control played in the dying process of these elders (Schroepfer et al. 2009). All 84 respondents reported using at least one primary control strategy, and 83 spoke of using an additional one, either compensatory primary control and/or compensatory secondary control. The results of a one-way ANOVA test found that using more than one control strategy was associated with a higher reported quality of life during the dying process. In regard to the areas of the dying process over which the respondents sought control, they reported decision-making, independence, mental attitude, activities of daily living, instrumental activities of daily living, and personal relationships. Over 50% of the respondents wanted to exercise more control but reported that their illness did not allow them to do so. These highlighted findings belie the richness of the data collected, and more details can be found in the article itself (Schroepfer et al. 2009). As reported by other researchers, control is clearly a crucial factor with regard to the WTHD; hence, the study results will be used to guide the development of control questions to be included in my assessment instrument.

As previously noted, another critical factor that has been reported as playing a role in the WTHD is social support. In my study, open-ended questions were asked of the terminally ill respondents to determine the role that social support played in their dying process. Although a number of findings surfaced, one unexpected finding was the anticipation of social support (Schroepfer and Noh 2010). Without prompting, 85 respondents discussed their anticipation of receiving support in the future and even after death. They talked about basing their anticipation on the past and/or current experiences they were having with received support, expectations based on who provided the support, and the feelings associated with the anticipation. For example, they noted that when support was timely and consistent, and when the caregiver was responsive and willing, they could feel positive in their anticipation of future support. Respondents also noted, however, that if they felt their caregivers were overburdened then they anticipated unhelpful support. Some respondents also reported feelings of guilt for anticipating that caregivers would have to provide more support in the future. Additional analyses have been run on all the support data and will be used to construct questions for the proposed assessment instrument.

Next steps

Although my research has been in hiatus for the past 4 years due to administrative responsibilities, having completed them I will now be resuming my work on the assessment of the WTHD and related factors. I plan to conduct a national survey of hospice and palliative care nurses and social workers regarding their assessment tools and what factors they feel should be included. I will then finalize a draft of my assessment tool and test it in hospice agencies and palliative care units. In addition, I have begun work on understanding the role played by culture in the dying process and plan to extend that work to the WTHD. Little research has been conducted in this area; yet, it makes sense to assume that a quality dying process would include attention to the beliefs, values, and traditions that are essential to terminally ill individuals.

Conclusion

From 1988 to 2003 I worked in the field with elders and, after earning my doctorate in 2003, my research and teaching has focused on them, particularly those who are terminally ill. I have been at the bedside of many elders during their dying process and with some at the time of their death. Before earning my doctorate, I remember how elders would tell healthcare professionals that they were dying and the professionals would quickly shush them and say that they were just fine. The elder's face would fill with sadness and their eyes with tears; they needed to talk about their dying process and they needed someone to listen. I also remember painful dying processes when elders would look beseechingly at me and vocalize their WTHD. I wanted to find a venue for their voices to be heard regarding why they wished for a hastened death and why it was important to them that such a vocalization not be shushed; my research is that venue. It is my hope that the research conducted on the WTHD will continue, and will be read and disseminated such that healthcare professionals to whom patients may vocalize a WTHD will listen. After all, the responsibility for safeguarding a patient's right to voice a WTHD without fear of being silenced lies with these professionals in whom patients have placed their trust for a quality dying process.

References

Albert, S. M., Rabkin, J. G., Del Bene, M. L., et al. (2005). Wish to die in end-stage ALS. *Neurology*, **65**, 68–74.

Arnold, E. M., Artin, K. A., Person, J. L., and Griffith, D. L. (2004). Consideration of hastening death among hospice patients and their families. *Journal of Pain and Symptom Management*, **27**, 523–532.

Back, A., Wallace, J., Starks, H., and Pearlman, R. (1996). Physician-assisted suicide and euthanasia in Washington state: Patient requests and physician responses. *Journal of the American Medical Association*, **275**, 919–925.

Breitbart, W., Rosenfeld, B., and Passik, S. (1996). Interest in physician-assisted suicide among ambulatory HIV-infected patients. *American Journal of Psychiatry*, **153**, 238–242.

Chochinov, H., Wilson, K. G., Enns, M., et al. (1995). Desire for death in the terminally ill. *American Journal of Psychiatry*, **152**(8), 1185–1191.

Coyle, N. and Sculco, L. (2004). Expressed desire for hastened death in seven patients living with advanced cancer: a phenomenologic inquiry. *Oncology Nursing Forum*, **31**, 699–709.

Emanuel, E., Fairclough, D., Daniels, E., and Clarridge, B. (1996). Euthanasia and physician-assisted suicide: Attitudes and experiences of oncology patients, oncologists, and the public. *Lancet*, **347**, 1805–1810.

Emanuel, E., Fairclough, D., and Emanuel, L. (2000). Attitudes and desires related to euthanasia and physician-assisted suicide among terminally ill patients and their caregivers. *Journal of the American Medical Association*, **284**, 2460–2468.

Hudson, P. L., Kristjanson, L. J., Ashby, M., et al. (2006). Desire for hastened death in patients with advanced disease and the evidence base of clinical guidelines: a systematic review. *Palliative Medicine*, **20**, 693–701.

Kelly, B., Burnett, P., Pelusi, D., Badger, S., Varghese, F., and Robertson, M. (2002). Terminally ill cancer patients' wish to hasten death. *Palliative Medicine*, **16**, 339–345.

Kelly, B., Burnett, P., Pelusi, D., Badger, S., Varghese, F., and Robertson, M. (2003). Factors associated with the wish to hasten death: a study of patients with terminal illness. *Psychological Medicine*, **33**, 75–81.

Lavery, J., Boyle, J., Dickens, B., Maclean, H., and Singer, P. (2001). Origins of the desire for euthanasia and assisted suicide in people with HIV-1 or AIDS: a qualitative study. *Lancet*, **358**, 362–367.

Meier, E., Emmons, C., Wallenstein, S., Quill, T., Morrison, R., and Cassel, C. (1998). A national survey of physician-assisted suicide and euthanasia in the United States. *New England Journal of Medicine*, **338**, 1193–1201.

Monforte-Royo, C., Villavicencio-Chavez, C., Tomas-Sabado, J., and Balaguer, A. (2011). The wish to hasten death: a review of clinical studies. *Psycho-Oncology*, **20**, 795–804.

Nicol, N., Wylie, H., and Rao, C. (2006). *Between the Dying and the Dead: Dr. Jack Kevorkian, the Assisted Suicide Machine and the Battle to Legalise Euthanasia*. London: Vision.

Ohnsorge, K., Gudat, H., and Rehmann-Sutter, C. (2014). Intentions in wishes to die: analysis and a typology—a report of 30 qualitative case studies of terminally ill cancer patients in palliative care. *Psycho-Oncology*, **23**, 1021–1026.

O'Mahony, S., Goulet, J., Kornblith, A., et al. (2005). Desire for hastened death, cancer pain and depression: report of a longitudinal observational study. *Journal of Pain and Symptom Management*, **29**, 446–457.

Oregon Department of Human Services (2000). *Oregon's Death with Dignity Act: The Second Year's Experience*. Portland: Oregon Health Division.

Oregon Department of Human Services (2014). *Thirteenth Annual Report on Oregon's Death with Dignity Act*. Portland: Oregon Health Division.

Schroepfer, T. (2006). Mind frames towards dying and factors motivating their adoption by terminally ill elders. *Journal of Gerontology: Social Sciences*, **61B**, S129–S139.

Schroepfer, T. (2007). Critical events in the dying process: the potential for physical and psychosocial suffering. *Journal of Palliative Medicine*, **10**, 136–147.

Schroepfer, T. (2008). Social relationships and their role in the consideration to hasten death. *The Gerontologist*, **48**, 612–621.

Schroepfer, T. A. and Noh, H. (2010). Terminally ill elders' anticipation of support in dying and death. *Journal of Social Work in End-of-Life and Palliative Care*, **6**, 73–90.

Schroepfer, T. A., Noh, H., and Kavanaugh, M. (2009). The myriad strategies for seeking control in the dying process. *The Gerontologist*, **49**, 755–766.

Schulz, R. and Heckhausen, J. (1996). A life span model of successful aging. *American Psychologist*, **31**, 702–714.

Villavicencio-Chavez, C., Monforte-Royo, C., Tomas-Sabado, J., Maier, M., Porta-Sales, J., and Balaguer, A. (2014). Physical and psychological factors and the wish to hasten death in advanced care patients. *Psycho-Oncology*, **23**, 1125–1132.

Volker, D. (2001). Oncology nurses' experiences with requests for assisted dying from terminally ill patients with cancer. *Oncology Nursing Forum*, **28**, 39–49.

Washington State Department of Health (2012). *Washington State Department of Health 2012 Death with Dignity Act Report. Executive Summary*, DOH 422-109. URL: <http://www.doh.wa.gov/portals/1/Documents/Pubs/422-109-DeathWithDignityAct2012.pdf>

Chapter 7

The desire for hastened death in patients in palliative care

Rinat Nissim, Christopher Lo, and Gary Rodin

The desire for hastened death: an introduction

The desire for hastened death (DHD), when expressed in the context of a life-threatening illness, poses complicated legal and ethical questions. Research on the prevalence of the DHD and on the factors that motivate it has important implications for the improvement of the quality of life of individuals near the end of life and for the growing public debate about the legalization of physician-assisted suicide (PAS) and euthanasia. Much of the research to date on the DHD in the context of a life-threatening medical illness has focused on individuals with cancer, especially in advanced stages, utilizing either quantitative or qualitative methods (Hudson et al. 2006).

The prevalence of the DHD has traditionally been estimated by the rates of suicidal behaviours and the seeking of PAS or euthanasia. Epidemiological studies have consistently demonstrated that the rate of suicide in cancer patients is higher than in the general population, although less than 1% of individuals with cancer take this course of action (Björkenstam et al. 2005). Similarly, the reported incidence of cancer-related PAS and euthanasia in countries in which these practices are legalized is relatively low, ranging from 0.1–2.9% of all deaths (van der Heide et al. 2007; Steck et al. 2013). However, a more subtle approach to the assessment of the DHD in advanced cancer has been to examine it in individuals who have not necessarily expressed the wish to act on this desire.

The study of passive wishes to die or to hasten death has been aided by the development of self-report rating scales of the DHD, the most widely used one being that developed by Rosenfeld et al. (1999). This scale, the Schedule of Attitudes Toward Hastened Death (SAHD), is a 20-item self-report instrument designed to assess the continuum of the DHD, ranging from a passive desire for death to plans to facilitate one's own death. The SAHD was shown to have good psychometric properties, with factor analysis supporting a single-factor structure when used with hospitalized palliative care cancer patients (Breitbart et al. 2000). Administering the SAHD, Breitbart et al. (2000) reported that of 92 patients in an American palliative care unit, 17% could be classified as having a high DHD based on a cut-off score of 10 out of 20 on this measure. In other studies involving the SAHD or similar scales, the reported prevalence of a high DHD in patients in palliative care units ranged from 8 to 22% (Chochinov et al. 1995; Tiernan et al. 2002; Mystakidou et al. 2005).

While the quantitative assessment of the DHD provides valuable information about its prevalence in palliative care settings, important information about the dimensionality of the DHD can be gleaned from studies utilizing qualitative interview-based methods. For example, Coyle and Sculco (2004) conducted a phenomenological study with seven cancer patients in palliative care who expressed a desire for hastened death. Based on their findings, the researchers interpreted the expression of the DHD as a communication tool used by these patients to communicate at least one of nine different messages. While such qualitative studies of the DHD suggest that the DHD in the context of advanced cancer is a multidimensional construct, quantitative studies tend to assess the incidence or degree of the DHD as if it were a one-dimensional construct. In order to better understand the relationship between the qualitative and quantitative dimensions, we designed a mixed-methods study, assessing the incidence and correlates of the DHD in a large sample of ambulatory patients with advanced cancer, with qualitative interviews in a small subset of participants selected based on purposeful sampling (Rodin et al. 2007, 2009; Nissim et al. 2009). Here we will elucidate the process and outcome of this unique study to illustrate what can be learned about the DHD from qualitative and quantitative methodologies.

The research process

Using Tashakkori and Teddlie's (2003) typology of mixed-methods research designs, we employed a concurrent nested design, which included the simultaneous use of quantitative and qualitative methods each attempting to answer different research questions regarding the DHD. The quantitative method was used to assess the frequency of the DHD and its correlates, such as depression, hopelessness, and pain. The qualitative method was used to understand the meaning and clinical significance of the DHD.

Sampling procedures were designed separately for the quantitative and qualitative components of our study, dictated by their respective methodological considerations. Sampling for the quantitative component was consecutive, leading to a total of 406 patients who completed the study questionnaire package. All participants had been diagnosed with stage III or IV lung cancer or stage IV gastrointestinal cancer, and were approached in outpatient and inpatient units at a comprehensive cancer centre in Toronto, Ontario, Canada. Participants' ages ranged from 21 to 88, with a mean age of 61, and 234 (57%) of them were men. Participants completed a package of self-report instruments, providing ratings of psychosocial and physical distress, including the SAHD. Medical and demographic data were extracted from the medical record of each patient (Rodin et al. 2007, 2009).

Sampling and data collection procedures for the qualitative component were developed according to the grounded theory method (Glaser and Strauss 1967), as modified for psychological inquiry by Rennie et al. (1988). Sampling involved the ongoing screening of the questionnaire packages of the 406 participants in the quantitative component to identify those who met recruitment criteria for the qualitative interviews. Recruitment criteria evolved throughout the study. Initially, participants with elevated scores on the SAHD or on measures of hopelessness or depression were sought. Selection of additional participants was theory-based, directed to enhance and to check the understanding achieved from the ongoing qualitative analyses. Using these evolving criteria, 27 participants were interviewed, 12 (44%) of whom were men, ranging in age from 45 to 82, with a mean age of 61 (Nissim et al. 2009). Interviews were designed to explore the experience of living with advanced cancer in a discovery-oriented manner. All interviews were audiotaped and transcribed verbatim and analysed using the grounded theory method (Nissim et al. 2009).

Findings and integration

The qualitative study generated a theoretical model regarding the global experience of living with advanced cancer, which subsumed the experience of the DHD in this context (Nissim et al. 2009, 2012a). This model accounts for the DHD as a multidimensional construct, represented under three distinct categories: (1) the DHD as a hypothetical exit plan; (2) the DHD as an expression of despair; and (3) the DHD as a manifestation of letting go. These categories are described in this section.

The DHD as a hypothetical exit plan represents the most common form of the DHD. It involves the contemplation of suicide as a future 'exit plan' to be executed if one's situation becomes unbearable. This hypothetical 'exit plan' is understood as a response to the multiple fears of participants regarding their future. These fears were sometimes fed by dreadful memories of the dying process of family members or friends, as well as by cultural and media stereotypes of dying of cancer. Participants typically stated that if these fears were to become a reality, life would no longer be worth living and that suicide would be their best option. This sentiment is illustrated by a quote from one of the participants:

> I never thought about giving up, but my fear was that I didn't know much about cancer. There are so many people that linger, and I was afraid that I could not cope. I know I will die, but I don't want to be lingering and suffering and people around me to suffer with me. . . . It's the only thing that makes me feel a little bit emotional. I don't want to deal with it so I think I would speed up things myself. I don't want to be lingering here in palliative care, lying day by day, slowly dying. Oh no, I don't want to do that . . . So, suicide is a way of exiting. I don't want to talk about that, because I like life and I have lots to live for, but if I come to the point when I am too weak to do anything, then I don't want to stay.

The formulation of this hypothetical 'exit plan' allowed participants to tolerate their fears regarding their future and provided them with a sense of having a safety net. In this context, some participants spoke in favour of the legislation of PAS and euthanasia. They viewed euthanasia as essential because they realized that when they reach a stage when life is no longer worth living they may be too incapacitated, mentally or physically, to end their lives themselves. In addition, even if they were able at that stage to commit suicide, they viewed the option of PAS as more dignified than that of suicide:

> I think that anybody with a terminal illness should have the right to assisted suicide . . .
> I think that should be a fundamental right people have . . . I wouldn't like to be like that sick poor man who was in the news recently, who put a plastic bag on his head. I mean, he must have felt really bad to be able to do that, and I'm sorry that he had to do that because he should have had a more dignified option, and he shouldn't have had to do it by himself.

The idea of suicide at an anticipated time in the future when life would no longer seem worth living was contemplated by most participants through most of the course of their illness, but it was typically not discussed with others. Asking the oncologist about this future exit plan was perceived as a waste of the oncologist's valuable time and as pointless for the patient because it was understood that it is illegal where they lived for others to assist in this. As one participant remarked, 'If we lived in the Netherlands then, yeah, I can discuss my thoughts because you have an option, but here you don't have an option, so why discuss it with your doctor? Why discuss future thoughts when the doctor can't do anything anyway?'

DHD as an expression of despair represents a short-lived and less common form of the DHD. It involves the contemplation of hastening death as the best, or even only, action that one can take in the present, to escape from overwhelming feelings of despair, meaninglessness, helplessness, and panic:

> I'm just saying to myself when I go to sleep, 'Just let me die.' I don't want to have to wake up and face this . . . I honestly I just pray that I would just die in my sleep. I have nothing to live for, absolutely nothing. There's nothing coming up in my life that I am living towards, and if there was it would be so terrible because it probably wouldn't happen.

The thought of death as a means to escape from despair was contemplated at different points on the illness trajectory. Indeed, despair may be a common, although transient, response to the communication of 'bad news', and to the experience of suffering and loss. In particular, despair, and subsequent contemplation of hastening death as a way to flee this state, was noted following interactions with physicians in which participants felt emotionally abandoned or during periods of severe physical pain. Participants reported that severe pain deprived them of the ability to focus on anything else, or to hope for a more tolerable future, and that death in this circumstance was perceived as 'preferable' to this state:

> I've experienced such incredible pain over the last little while and more in the last week. Such incredible pain that it made me think that death is preferable to this . . . I'll sit there for two hours in terrible pain. Such pain where I can't yawn even, and I get only half a yawn and my whole insides turn and waiting for the medication to start to work . . . I'd love to have forty-eight hours let's say, I'd love to have this weekend where I could plan to have a nice weekend and have no pain. I'd love to do that and it doesn't happen, and the pain affects everything. It makes you tired. It affects how you can eat. It affects your mood. It affects other people, and the fact is that even if you try to hide it, you can't . . . So that's hard . . . and I know it's gonna get worse, so that's hard too. It's great to be alive, and pain takes that life out of you, and to sit there for two hours with a blanket around you just shivering, with no solution, is really hard.

The emotional tone of this form of the DHD was very different from that of the DHD as a hypothetical exit plan. While hastening death as a future 'exit plan' was considered calmly and rationally, the contemplation of death out of despair emerged in a state of anguish, confusion, and panic. Moreover, the contemplation of hastening death in this context did not provide any sense of relief, but rather increased the state of havoc.

Importantly, three participants in our study denied desiring death at any point on their illness trajectory, either at times of despair or as a future 'exit plan'. What was unique about them was their strong religious conviction. For them, death was considered to be in God's hands, and their 'job', as one participant described it, was to follow God's will until the very end:

> What I do believe is, as the scripture said, 'He knew me before He formed me.' So He knew the day when I come in this world and He knows the day He's gonna take me out. So until then I just have to say 'Lord, you just keep me strong till you take me home. Keep me strong. Draw me closer to you. Let me have a closer walk with you.'

DHD as a manifestation of letting go represents a form of the DHD which was most common in the final weeks of life. It involves the embodied knowing that, as one participant noted, 'my time has come', and that now it was time to let nature run its course. Thus, while the previous two forms of the DHD involve the contemplation of hastening death, this form of the DHD does not involve an active wish to hasten death but rather a recognition that death is imminent, and that one can no longer resist it. This is both a mental and physical experience, as stated in the excerpt below, of reaching one's 'limit' in terms of one's ability to delay the dying process:

> In a sense it's artificial that I'm still alive. Even a few years ago, that would not have been the case for me to survive that long, but there are limits to what any organism will take or can do, and I have reached my limit.

Our qualitative findings informed our quantitative analysis. Similarly to other studies of the DHD with ambulatory populations of advanced cancer (e.g. Ransom et al. 2006), the DHD scores in our sample were extremely low, with a mean SAHD total score of 1.7 (standard deviation = 2.2). Positive statistically significant correlations were identified between the scores on the SAHD and on measures of hopelessness, depression, and physical distress; statistically significant negative correlations were identified with physical functioning, spiritual well-being, social support, and self-esteem (for a complete description of the results see Rodin et al. 2007, 2009).

The qualitative findings regarding the multidimensionality of the DHD called for a careful inspection to determine whether the same multidimensionality could be identified in the quantitative data. First, the SAHD response patterns of the 27 participants who took part in the qualitative interviews were examined. A clear trend emerged, in which participants whose qualitative data revealed the first category of the DHD (DHD as a hypothetical exit plan) tended to endorse specific items on the SAHD, such as item 18 ('I plan to end my own life when my illness becomes too much to bear'); participants whose interviews matched the second category of the DHD (DHD as an expression of despair) tended to endorse items such as item 3 ('My illness has drained me so much that I do not want to go on living'); and participants whose interviews matched the third category of the DHD (DHD as a manifestation of letting go) tended to endorse items such as item 16 ('Because of my illness, the idea of dying seems comforting'). This relationship that was found between the qualitative categories and the response patterns of the SAHD led us to a subsequent step, namely, a factor analysis of the SAHD in the large quantitative sample.

The factor structure of the SAHD was conducted using an exploratory factor analysis, with an unweighted least-squares estimator, and an orthogonal (Varimax) rotation method. Items were considered to load substantially on a factor if the loading was greater than or equal to 0.30. Cross-loadings were not allowed. The decision regarding the number of factors to extract was theory-based (Preacher et al. 2013). Thus, in keeping with the qualitative categorical model, three factors were chosen for extraction. A clear fit between the resulting three-factor solution and the qualitative categories of the DHD was identified, allowing the qualitative interpretation of the DHD to inform the labelling process of the three factors. The first factor was labelled: [DHD as a hypothetical] 'exit plan'; the second factor was named [DHD as an expression of] 'despair'; and the third was labelled [DHD as a manifestation of] 'letting go' (see Box 7.1).

Box 7.1 Item composition of the three-factor model

First factor: the DHD as a hypothetical exit plan

1 I feel confident that I will be able to cope with the emotional stress of my illness.

2 I expect to suffer a great deal from emotional problems in the future because of my illness.

17 I expect to suffer a great deal from physical problems in the future because of my illness.

18 I plan to end my own life when my illness becomes too much to bear.

20 I am able to cope with the symptoms of my illness, and have no thoughts of ending my life.

Second factor: the DHD as an expression of despair

3 My illness has drained me so much that I do not want to go on living.

5 Unless my illness improves, I will consider taking steps to end my life.

7 Despite my illness, my life still has purpose and meaning.

8 I am careless about my treatment because I want to let the disease run its course.

12 I enjoy my present life, even with my illness, and would not consider ending it.

Third factor: the DHD as a manifestation of letting go

6 Dying seems like the best way to relieve the emotional suffering my illness causes.

10 I hope that my disease will progress rapidly because I would prefer to die rather than continue living with this illness.

13 Because my illness cannot be cured, I would prefer to die sooner, rather than later.

15 Dying seems like the best way to relieve the pain and discomfort my illness causes.

16 Because of my illness, the idea of dying seems comforting.

Furthermore, to provide a preliminary investigation of the criterion validity of this factor structure, correlational analyses were conducted, examining the associations between the summed score of each factor and concurrent variables of physical and psychological distress. The resulting differences between the three factors in terms of their pattern of statistically significant ($p < 0.05$) correlations were as follows:

◆ Age was positively correlated with the 'letting go' factor and negatively correlated with the 'exit plan' factor, and no statistically significant correlation was identified between age and the 'despair' factor.

◆ Scores on both the Rosenberg Self Esteem Scale (Rosenberg 1989) and the Faith subscale of the Functional Assessment of Chronic Illness Therapy-Spiritual Well-Being Scale (Cella et al. 1993), which measures the extent to which participants find comfort and strength in their religious beliefs, were negatively correlated with the 'exit plan' and the 'despair' factors, but not with the 'letting go' factor.

◆ Of the three factors, only the 'despair' factor was correlated with ratings of pain intensity as measured by the Brief Pain Inventory (Cleeland 1989).

Conclusions

Our mixed-methods study suggests that the DHD in ambulatory patients with advanced cancer is a multidimensional construct that has multiple meanings unrelated to the literal intention to take one's life. Our qualitative analysis identified three distinct categories of the DHD: (1) the DHD as a hypothetical exit plan; (2) the DHD as an expression of despair; and (3) the DHD as a manifestation of letting go. These qualitative findings informed the interpretation of the quantitative assessments of the DHD. The exploratory factor analysis of the SAHD in our sample of ambulatory patients with advanced cancer suggested a three-factor model that is consistent with the three dimensions identified qualitatively. This contrasts with reports that the SAHD measure had a single-factor structure, when it was used with hospitalized palliative care cancer patients (Breitbart et al. 2000). Lastly, examining the statistical relationships between the factor sum scores and other outcome variables provided preliminary evidence for the utility of the three-factor structure.

The first category of the DHD, the DHD as an expression of a *hypothetical 'exit plan'*, was the most common experience, expressed by the majority of participants in the qualitative study. In the quantitative analysis, the corresponding factor had a unique association with younger age, lower self-esteem, and lower spiritual faith. This category can be understood as a response to fears regarding the dying process, as illuminated in the qualitative interviews, as well as through the item composition of the quantitative three-factor solution (for example, the item with the highest loading on this factor was item 2, 'I expect to suffer a great deal from emotional problems in the future because of my illness').

In this context, the DHD serves to relieve and manage anticipatory fears. In this spirit, participants in our study also supported the legalization of PAS and euthanasia. Importantly, the contemplation of hastening death as a hypothetical 'exit plan', although common, was rarely discussed with others because they were perceived as legally unable to assist. Healthcare providers need to be aware of this potentially silenced issue and address patients' fears and concerns (Hudson et al. 2006). This conclusion is further supported by preliminary evidence of the high prevalence of death-related anxiety in patients with advanced cancer, as measured by the recently developed Death and Dying Distress Scale (Lo et al. 2011a; Neel et al. 2013). In addition, our pilot study of a brief, manualized, psychosocial intervention for individuals with advanced cancer indicated that participants reported benefit from having a safe place to discuss their fears about death and dying (Nissim et al. 2012b), which reduced death-related anxiety (Lo et al. 2014).

The second category of the DHD, the DHD as an *expression of despair*, was typically a short-lived experience. It was experienced during moments in the illness trajectory in which participants felt overwhelmed by feelings of meaninglessness, helplessness, and panic. This experience fits with what others have described as a demoralization syndrome (Kissane et al. 2001), a syndrome characterized by hopelessness, helplessness, loss of meaning, and existential distress brought about by the physical, mental, and social challenges of a medical illness. It may also fit with the construct of existential suffering at the end of life (Lo et al. 2011b).

The quantitative analysis suggested that the factor representing the experience of DHD as an expression of despair is associated with lower self-esteem and spiritual faith, and is uniquely correlated with pain intensity. This is consistent with our qualitative analysis, which demonstrated that the contemplation of death out of despair was most profound during periods of severe physical pain. Similarly, Wilson et al. (2007) indicated that almost 10% of their sample of patients in palliative care believed that they would have asked for PAS in the past, had it been legally available, and, most commonly, that the previous wish for PAS was related to experiences of uncontrolled pain. Correspondingly, this wish subsided once pain was resolved.

Lastly, the present study suggested that the DHD in the final weeks of life may be an expression of a general *experience of 'letting go'* at this stage, in which one disengages from life and welcomes death. This finding fits with Kubler-Ross's (1969) description of the final terminal phase of a prolonged medical illness as a stage of inward withdrawal. The state of letting go in the final weeks of life may account for the relatively high rates of the DHD that have been reported in patients in palliative care units (Breitbart et al. 2000) compared with the much lower rate in our sample of ambulatory patients with a longer expected survival (Rodin et al. 2007, 2009). Our quantitative analysis further suggests a unique association between the experience of 'letting go' and older age, which may be accounted for by a greater capacity to reflect on death (Lo et al. 2011b).

This study demonstrates that the integration of quantitative and qualitative methodologies can produce results that are richer than those from either method alone, and may minimize, or compensate for, the potential errors and biases that are inherent in any single methodology. A mixed-methods approach is more demanding in terms of funding and skills, and may not be justifiable in many cases. However, it may often be well suited to study the complex personal realities of a medical illness, and complex constructs such as the DHD.

In our mixed-methods study, the interplay between the contextualized qualitative knowledge and the quantitative knowledge allowed us to refine our understanding of the multidimensional nature of the DHD in individuals with advanced cancer. These findings highlight that DHD is at various times an adaptive strategy, a less organized expression of distress, and a form of passive resignation. Proposed interventions need to take into account the meaning of the DHD in particular individuals at particular stages of disease.

References

Björkenstam, C., Edberg, A., Ayoubi, S., and Rosén, M. (2005). Are cancer patients at higher suicide risk than the general population? A nation wide register study in Sweden from 1965–1999. *Scandinavian Journal of Public Health*, **33**, 208–214.

Breitbart, W., Rosenfeld, B., Pessin, H., et al. (2000). Depression, hopelessness, and desire for death in terminally ill cancer patients. *Journal of the American Medical Association*, **284**, 2907–2911.

Cella, D. F., Tulsky, D. S., Gray, G., et al. (1993). The functional assessment of cancer therapy scale: development and validation of the general measure. *Journal of Clinical Oncology*, **11**, 570–579.

Chochinov, H. M., Wilson, K. G., Enns, M., et al. (1995). Desire for death in the terminally ill. *American Journal of Psychiatry*, **152**, 1185–1191.

Cleeland, C. S. (1989). Measurement of pain by subjective report. In: C. R. Chapman and J. D. Loeser (eds), *Advances in Pain Research and Therapy*, 12th edn, pp. 391–403. New York: Raven.

Coyle, N. and Sculco, L. (2004). Expressed desire for hastened death in seven patients living with advanced cancer: a phenomenologic inquiry. *Oncology Nursing Forum*, **31**, 699–709.

Glaser, B. G. and Strauss, A. L. (1967). *The Discovery of Grounded Theory: Strategies for Qualitative Research*. Chicago: Aldine.

van der Heide, A., Onwuteaka-Philipsen, B. D., Rurup, M. L., et al. (2007). End-of-life practices in the Netherlands under the Euthanasia Act. *New England Journal of Medicine*, **356**, 1957–1965.

Hudson, P. L., Kristjanson, L. J., Ashby, M., et al. (2006). Desire for hastened death in patients with advanced disease and the evidence base on clinical guidelines: a systematic review. *Palliative Medicine*, **20**, 693–701.

Kissane, D. W., Clarke, D. M., and Street, A. F. (2001). Demoralization syndrome: a relevant psychiatric diagnosis for palliative care. *Journal of Palliative Care*, **17**, 12–21.

Kübler-Ross, E. (1969). *On Death and Dying*. London: Tavistock.

Lo, C., Hales, S., Jung, J., et al. (2014). Managing Cancer And Living Meaningfully (CALM): Phase 2 trial of a brief individual psychotherapy for patients with advanced cancer. *Palliative Medicine*, **28**, 234–242.

Lo, C., Hales, S., Zimmermann, C., Gagliese, L., Rydall, A., and Rodin, G. (2011a). Measuring death-related anxiety in advanced cancer: preliminary psychometrics of the Death and Dying Distress Scale. *Journal of Pediatric Hematology and Oncology*, **33**(Suppl. 2), S140–S145.

Lo, C., Zimmermann, C., Gagliese, L., Li, M., and Rodin, G. (2011b). Sources of spiritual well-being in advanced cancer. *BMJ Supportive and Palliative Care*, **1**, 149–153.

Mystakidou, K., Rosenfeld, B., Parpa, E., et al. (2005). Desire for death near the end of life: The role of depression, anxiety and pain. *General Hospital Psychiatry*, **27**, 258–262.

Neel, C., Lo, C., Rydall, A., Hales, S., and Rodin, G. (2013). Determinants of death anxiety in patients with advanced cancer. *BMJ Supportive and Palliative Care*, doi:10.1136/bmjspcare-2012-000420.

Nissim, R., Gagliese, L., and Rodin, G. (2009). The desire for hastened death in individuals with advanced cancer: a longitudinal qualitative study. *Social Science and Medicine*, **69**, 165–171.

Nissim, R., Rennie, D., Fleming, S., et al. (2012a). Goals at the end of life: findings from a qualitative longitudinal study with individuals with fatal cancer. *Death Studies*, **36**, 360–390.

Nissim, R., Freeman, E., Lo, C., et al. (2012b). Managing Cancer and Living Meaningfully (CALM): a qualitative study of a brief individual psychotherapy for individuals with advanced cancer. *Palliative Medicine*, **26**, 713–721.

Preacher, K. J., Zhang, G., Kim, C., and Mels, G. (2013). Choosing the optimal number of factors in exploratory factor analysis: a model selection perspective. *Multivariate Behavioral Research*, **48**, 28–56.

Ransom, S., Sacco, W. P., Weitzner, M. A., Azzarello, L. M., and McMillan, S. C. (2006). Interpersonal factors predict increased desire for hastened death in late-stage cancer patients. *Annals of Behavioral Medicine*, **31**, 63–69.

Rennie, D. L., Phillips, J. R., and Quartaro, G. K. (1988). Grounded theory: A promising approach to conceptualization in psychology? *Canadian Psychology*, **29**, 139–150.

Rodin, G., Lo, C., Mikulincer, M., Donner, A., Gagliese, L., and Zimmermann, C. (2009). Pathways to distress: the multiple determinants of depression, hopelessness, and desire for hastened death in metastatic cancer patients. *Social Science and Medicine*, **68**, 562–569.

Rodin, G., Zimmermann, C., Rydall, A., et al. (2007). The desire for hastened death in patients with metastatic cancer. *Journal of Pain and Symptom Management*, **33**, 661–675.

Rosenberg, M. (1989). *Society and the Adolescent Self-image*, revised edn. Middletown, CT: Wesleyan University.

Rosenfeld, B., Breitbart, W., Stein, K., et al. (1999). Measuring desire for death among patients with HIV/AIDS: The schedule of attitudes toward hastened death. *American Journal of Psychiatry*, **156**, 94–100.

Steck, N., Egger, M., Maessen, M., Reisch, T., and Zwahlen, M. (2013). Euthanasia and assisted suicide in selected European countries and US states: systematic literature review. *Medical Care*, **51**, 938–944.

Tashakkori, A. and Teddlie, C. (2003). *Handbook of Mixed Methods in Social and Behavioral Research*. Thousand Oaks: Sage.

Tiernan, E., Casey, P., O'Boyle, C., et al. (2002). Relations between desire for early death, depressive symptoms and antidepressant prescribing in terminally ill patients with cancer. *Journal of the Royal Society of Medicine*, **95**, 386–390.

Wilson, K. G., Chochinov, H. W., McPherson, C. J., et al. (2007). Desire for euthanasia or physician-assisted suicide in palliative cancer care. *Health Psychology*, **26**, 314–323.

Chapter 8

Intentions, motivations, and social interactions regarding a wish to die

Kathrin Ohnsorge

Walter

As part of a qualitative study, We interviewed 30 patients, their relatives, and associated healthcare professionals about their wishes around the end of life. Of all the interviews in the study, the first was one of the most difficult. The patient that my colleague and I interviewed—let us call him Walter—did not have what one would call an 'outspoken' personality. He preferred to deal with his thoughts on his own. Half Swiss, half Brazilian, he grew up in a rural corner of Brazil with an authoritarian father who 'expected him to obey, to do what has to be done, not to talk about it, and not to argue' [a nurse speaking about Walter]. Walter's wife said that this continued also to be his philosophy throughout their marriage. When he was 18, his father sent him to Switzerland 'to find a wife', which he did. But, contrary to his father's expectations, he did not return to Brazil. He lived with his wife and son in the Swiss countryside, working as a mechanic. His wife discovered only by chance that Walter had been diagnosed with prostate cancer several years previously, without having said a word to her. As Walter continued to refuse to talk to her about his illness, she had to ask their GP for more information. After several treatments and a longer hospitalization, Walter came to the hospice, where we interviewed him.

Now, Walter had consented to take part in an interview in which he knew that, as a severely ill person, he would be asked to tell us his ideas about living and dying. His opioid therapy made him tired, and talking with him for long periods was virtually impossible. The interview proceeded haltingly. His answers were monosyllabic, often with lengthy pauses. More than once he did not answer at all. His silence and apparent reluctance to talk placed me as the interviewer in some difficulty. Was his reluctance to speak due to the opioid therapy or was he experiencing difficulty in talking about himself? On the one hand I felt I should 'try to make him talk', while at the same time asking myself how much I should expose him to answer such intimate questions when perhaps he normally avoided speaking about his inner experiences. Was it right to use the interview questions to solicit a thought process that he would not normally have engaged in?

Should I interrupt or postpone the interview, as being possibly too burdensome? On the other hand, he *had* consented to the interview. Might an interruption offend him?

Nevertheless, as short as his sentences were, he clearly told us that, relatively frequently, he wished his sickness would progress more rapidly. He said he had also thought about taking his life. At the same time, he told us he did not want to die, and we understood that this wish to live was predominant. His answers to our questions about the kind of situations in which he did not want to continue living, however, expressed all the ambivalence of his thinking:

Walter: Just that, if I may say so, you die. And perhaps you'd be glad, once it's over, to be able to shut the door, close the chapter. [. . .] But properly closed. [. . .]

Interviewer: But have I understood you correctly now: you would be glad if the door were already shut?

Walter: No, no. It can be open . . . You [have] the feeling time and again, perhaps you'll still find something with which to open the lock. And that it'll be OK again then.

Interviewer: So there's hope.

Walter There's hope. But where do you find . . . hope? [*Pause*] . . . Yes.

The coexistence of opposing and fluctuating wishes in his pondering on his life's end was evident. But the reasons for this were not really clear even to himself:

Walter: That's . . . you just have to find the reason where, I believe, why you want to die at all. [. . .] Because if you know the reasons, then perhaps it's also less, like much less, what you were looking for with that.

On the one occasion on which he told his wife about his wish to die—as he related— she 'actually didn't react much. She actually said: "Don't be so stupid! Yes" '. Reading through the interview transcripts at this point, it seems that telling us about his wife's reaction touched him, as he fell into a long silence after that and only returned to answering our questions after some time.

At the end of the interview, I left Walter with mixed emotions. Even though he claimed to feel fine, I questioned whether I had kept the fine ethical line between investigating a participant's thoughts and respecting his actual need for (non-)communication. Was it right to have talked with him about these intimate ideas, which he apparently found difficult to discuss? What was he actually wishing for and why? What effect had his wife's reaction had on his wish to die? What support would he need to find the answer to the question he raised about the reasons for his wish to die?

Wishes to die

While the ethical challenges in communication between the researcher and the interviewee are different from those between the healthcare professional and the patient, there are similar difficulties and complexities when it comes to talking about sensitive wishes at the end of life: the question of how much to insist when inviting the other to talk, deciphering indirect expressions, offering recognition, opening oneself up to the moral understandings of the other, and the complex mix of one's own ideas and fears at stake in the communication. What we understand from each other in these talks we do so through complex engagements in sense making and social interaction.

For healthcare professionals, exploring the often conflicting feelings and ideas of these patients and responding competently and compassionately requires fine-tuned listening, good communication skills, and knowledge about what patients might experience (Hudson et al. 2006b). Over the last decade, prospective qualitative interview studies involving patients have provided important insights into the experiences, attitudes, and moral beliefs of patients expressing a wish to die (Wilson et al. 2000; Lavery et al. 2001; Kelly et al 2002; Coyle and Sculco 2004; Pearlman et al. 2005; Johansen et al. 2005; Mak and Elwyn 2005; Schroepfer 2006; Nissim et al. 2009). Complementing the body of existing quantitative research on the topic (Breitbart et al. 1996; Chochinov et al. 1998; Kissane et al. 1998; Filiberti et al. 2001; Emmanuel 2002; Suarez-Almazor et al. 2002; Ferrand et al. 2012, among many others), qualitative studies have outlined a much richer moral and psychosocial landscape associated with wish to die statements. These describe the wishes of patients in palliative care as complex and relational phenomena with a multifactorial aetiology, associated with depression and hopelessness. Today we know that under good palliative care, psychosocial and spiritual conditions seem to be more important than physical ones (Monforte-Royo et al. 2012).

Recent interesting reviews have documented a lack of conceptualization, and much work is still needed to understand in detail the needs of dying patients with a wish to die (Hudson et al. 2006a,b; Stiel et al. 2010; Monforte-Royo et al. 2010, 2012). Monforte-Royo and colleagues indicate the difficulty of comparing existing research, because often 'studies have not distinguished clearly between a general wish to die, the wish to hasten death, and requests for euthanasia or physician-assisted suicide' (Monforte-Royo et al. 2012, p. 1). The diversity of terms used (*desire to die, wish to hasten death, request to die*, etc.) and the lack of clear definitions add to this problem (Monforte-Royo et al. 2010). Furthermore, a wish to die might mean different things when expressed at early palliative stages than later on, but current studies often do not disclose the nearness to death at which patients were interviewed.

In clinical practice it is well known that not all wish to die statements imply a wish to hasten death as well (Hudson et al. 2006a,b; Schroepfer 2006); however, much research and ethical discussion concentrates only on the latter. Little is known about the subjective experience of a wish to die and its development over time. Several studies (Johansen et al. 2005; Nissim et al. 2009) have documented the fluctuating character of such statements, which makes investigating and describing them a more complex task. Additionally, social interactions around the wish to die as well as cultural aspects, such as the legal status of assisted dying, might strongly influence what patients allow themselves to wish for.

The goal of our study, which was led by Christoph Rehmann-Sutter and Heike Gudat, was to obtain more insight into the subjective structure, meaning contents, and functions of wish to die statements, including their possible development over time and their constitutive relations to other people, particularly relatives and healthcare professionals. Based on our empirical findings (the main results have been published in Ohnsorge et al. 2012, 2014a,b), this chapter presents a model that describes the various dimensions of wishes to die as they appeared in the statements of the participants we interviewed. This model might help us to understand and conceptualize the wish to die in palliative patients in more detail.

Here, when I refer to a 'wish to die', I mean a wish for death to come. A 'wish to live' is a wish for life to continue. A 'wish to hasten death' is the desire to act in such a way that life will end sooner (Ohnsorge et al. 2014a; for more detail see chapter 15).

Methods

Our study was based on a qualitative research methodology which combined narrative-hermeneutic approaches, interpretive phenomenological analysis (Smith et al. 2009), and grounded theory (Charmaz 2006; Corbin and Strauss 2008). Overall, we interviewed 30 patients in a palliative care situation (hospice, hospital palliative care ward, palliative home care). With patients' consent, we also interviewed their healthcare professionals and relatives (a total of 116 interviews). We included only (1) patients with incurable cancer in (2) a palliative situation (characterized by limited antitumour treatment, predominant use of palliative measures, and limited life expectancy), who (3) had been informed about the incurability of their disease, (4) were cognitively in a condition to be interviewed, (5) whose primary physician had agreed to their enrolment in the study, and who (6) consented to participate. We decided not to limit the sample to patients who had expressed a desire to die because we assumed that not all had previously disclosed their wishes to others.

We had planned to interview all patients at least twice, but as we interviewed in relative proximity to death (the median time between the last interview and a patient's death was 22.5 days) we were in fact only able to interview eight patients more than once.

All patients were tested for depression (Beck and Kovacs 1979; Robinson and Crawford 2005) and three patients were on antidepressant medication at the time of the interview. However, none of the patients seemed to be compromised in their decision-making capacity.

We informed the participants (chosen by theoretical sampling) in writing and verbally that we were investigating the experiences of severely ill patients and their ideas and wishes regarding living and dying. Central questions in the semi-structured interviews were: 'In the course of your illness, did you ever wish your disease to proceed more rapidly?', 'Can you imagine situations in which you would prefer not to continue living?', or 'Have you ever thought of putting an end to your life?' (for the entire interview guide see Ohnsorge et al. 2014a Appendix). For ethical reasons, we used the term 'wish to die' only when it was introduced by the participant, and only participants who said things that could be related to a wish to die were confronted with more concrete questions from the interview guide. Periodically, the interview guide was refined on the basis of the experience gained from the interviews. All interviews were audio-recorded and fully transcribed.

In the interviews with relatives, nurses, and doctors, we wanted to know what they thought about the patient's wishes regarding dying, to what extent they knew about them, and which conversations or reactions were important regarding the patient's wishes. In addition to idiographic data, we also collected the medical records for each of the 30 patients.

Because of the issue at stake, conducting these interviews required a particularly responsible approach. We encouraged participants to interrupt or postpone the interview whenever they felt it appropriate or when they seemed to be tired or burdened. More than once we took up the interview again at a later point. Patients and relatives who had been interviewed were personally followed up by the primary physician shortly after the interview. Patients generally reported no adverse effects (except one who had talked about burdensome childhood experiences during the interview). The study was approved by the Basel research ethics committee (Ethikkommission Beider Basel).

Christoph Rehmann, Heike Gudat, and I analysed the transcripts over the course of the interview process. In a first step, each of us independently coded and interpreted the transcripts of one case unit (patient, relative, healthcare professional). In a second step we compared our coding and interpretations, and discussed them until we found a shared interpretation for each case unit, a list of 'emerging themes', and a list of 'set themes' (stemming from the initial research questions). Triangulating patients' interviews with those of relatives and healthcare professionals served to obtain a richer and more valid interpretation of patients' statements. After 14 patient case studies we created a provisional list of emerging and set themes, which we used as an instrument for further case analysis. This list was continuously refined as additional themes appeared. Theoretical saturation was achieved with regard to the overarching model and to some findings (i.e. intentions) but not to others (i.e. meanings, social interactions, etc.).

Narratives of wishes to die

In investigating the meaning and structure of wishes to die, we assumed, in line with narrative and hermeneutic theory, that wishes to die are—as any type of moral thinking— 'narrative in pattern' (Walker 2007, p. 75), as they select and sum up a process of meaning-making of past and present experiences into evaluative strands that explain why that wish is currently present. Wishes to die are situated within a particular setting between particular people at particular points in time, and are usually embedded into broader moral understandings of people that show how values and commitments are operative in that person's life, and how they are enacted and lived by (see Chapter 13). Similarly, what Hille Haker notices for moral experiencing in general (Haker 2005), wish to die statements have three different narrative characteristics: they are usually *reflective*, as they are deeply woven into how the person who experiences the wish makes sense of what is important to him or her (Ohnsorge et al. 2012; see also Chapter 2); but they are also *evaluative*, as wishes to die express how people evaluate and interpret past and current experiences, options for action, relationships, values, and their deepest commitments (Lindemann 2001, p. 71). And they are *performative*, as the new interpretations that happen when a wish to die is expressed and talked about in turn influence the ways in which this wish is perceived by the people it affects. In the attempt to care for and assist patients expressing such a wish at the end of life it seems most important to develop a closer understanding of the narrative structure and content of wish to die statements. And this was the aim of our study.

Results

The story of Walter is one of many strikingly different narratives in which patients told us about their wishes to live or to die. In this chapter we cannot pay tribute to the richness of these personal stories, experiences, and reflections that patients, families, and healthcare professionals shared with us. In their narratives, however, we identified three dimensions that we found relevant in all accounts. We saw that patients' wishes contained an *intention* that revealed how they wanted to die. In addition, patients' accounts also contained multiple indications of the *motivations* for why this wish was present. And finally, we saw that the wish was constituted in complex and manifold ways through *social interactions*, which often had a significant influence on what the patient was wishing. These three dimensions form a model that we called a 'contextual anatomy of a wish to die' (Ohnsorge et al. 2014b). This model was not used by us as an analytical tool for data analysis but was developed in going back and forth between the empirical data, our interpretation, and our knowledge of the current literature.

Intentions of the wish to die

What we call 'intentions' describes *how* patients wish to die or what they wish for when expressing such a wish. For example, not all patients who wish to die also wish to hasten death. Others have only a hypothetical wish to die in the future, while still others undertake concrete actions to shorten life. These differentiations are important for a more accurate understanding of what the patient is wishing for.

From the patients' narratives, we identified nine different types of intentions inherent in patients' wishes (see Table 8.1; Ohnsorge et al. 2014a). These wishes were of course much more richly nuanced than our synthetic description could capture. We observed two main differences in what patients wished for. First, expressing a wish to die was not automatically associated with a wish to hasten death: a significant group of patients wished to die without also expressing a wish to hasten death. Second, we observed a difference between participants who spoke about their wish to die as a *fantasy* they had about dying without (at the moment) proceeding to take further action, and those patients who actually undertook *actions* that led to, or would lead to, dying. We distinguish therefore between three groups: (1) wishes to die without the wish to hasten death, (2) wishes to die where patients consider hastening death without undertaking actions that lead to it, and (3) wishes to die where patients act to bring about their death (Ohnsorge et al. 2014a). It might be helpful in the clinical context (for overcoming reluctance to deal with such statements) to bear in mind that wish to die statements do not necessarily mean a person also intends to hasten death, and that a patient with a wish to hasten death does not always intend to carry out this wish.

For each of these three groups we found three different intentions (see Table 8.1). For example, among *participants who express a wish to die while not considering hastening death* there were patients who longed to 'go to the other side', because life thereafter (with God) seemed to be more promising than to continue living under the current burdensome circumstances. Others simply wished that the period of their dying would proceed more rapidly. Still others had a strong wish to die, but found hastening death to be a morally unacceptable option. Among *participants who were considering hastening death without undertaking actions that would lead to it* were a larger number of participants who said that they would consider hastening death if, at some point in the future, they felt their life was not valuable (a hypothetical wish to die). Others said they currently had a wish to hasten death but their moral commitments caused them to feel, it

Table 8.1 Intentions towards dying

Patients' statements expressing their wishes about the end of their life can fall into one or more of the following categories:

Wish to live
Acceptance of dying
Wish to die

Not considering hastening death

1. Looking forward to dying

2. Hoping that dying happens more quickly

3. Desiring to die (but hastening death is not considered)

Considering hastening death

4. Hypothetically considering hastening death (in future, if certain things happen)

5. Actually considering hastening death, but at the moment (for moral or other reasons) it is not an option

6. Actually considering hastening death, hastening death is a (moral) option

Will to die

7. Explicit request

8. Refusing life-sustaining support (such as food or treatments) with the intention of hastening death

9. Acting towards dying (such as suicide or assisted dying)

Reproduced from: Intentions in wishes to die: analysis and a typology — A report of 30 qualitative case studies of terminally ill cancer patients in palliative care, K. Ohnsorge, H. Gudat, C. Rehmann-Sutter, *Psycho-Oncology*, 23(9), pp. 1021–26, doi: 10.1002/pon.3524. Copyright © 2014, The Authors. *Psycho-Oncology* published by John Wiley & Sons, Ltd.

was not the right thing to do. Still others considered hastening death at the present moment, but had not (yet) taken action or expressed a request to anyone. Finally, among *participants with a wish to die who acted towards dying* some did so by expressing an explicit request to others for assistance in dying. Several patients refused life-sustaining treatments with the explicit intention of hastening death. Only three patients had taken active steps towards causing death, either by attempting suicide or by entering into the procedures of one of the Swiss organizations offering assisted suicide.

The patients we interviewed often articulated more than one intention when they described their last wishes. Often their wishes to die were composed of various intentions that could exist contemporaneously, sometimes in tension with each other, sometimes not. For example, during the hour of the interview patients could talk of their wish to die as a concrete will to hasten death that they were already taking steps to realize, while the next moment they could frame this wish as only a hypothetical idea should the situation worsen. In many patients, wishes to die also existed alongside wishes to live. While eight out of our 30 study patients held on to their wish consistently throughout the entire research period, for many patients the preferred intention would change over time, sometimes very radically from one day to the other. We interpreted this continuous shifting between different intentions, which in some care contexts might be negatively labelled as an 'ambivalent attitude', as belonging to an inner thought process, inherent to the situation at the end of life, in which patients naturally negotiate different narratives of the self containing various moral commitments and identifications (Ohnsorge et al. 2012).

Motivations of wish to die statements

When we asked patients about *why* they had a wish to die, they referred to three different motivational dimensions. First, patients gave concrete *reasons* for the causes of such a wish. Secondly, however, they also explained, through wider narrative strands implying their personal values, commitments, and moral understandings, why this wish mattered to them. We called these wider narrative strands the '*meanings*' of the wish to die. Thirdly, in some narratives the wish to die statement had a specific intended or unintended *function* or effect, either regarding the patient's own psychological stability or to achieve an effect within their social relationships.

Subjective reasons

The reasons perceived by our study patients as being behind their wish to die in many ways reflected the main aetiological factors found in various other studies (Hudson et al. 2006a; Monforte-Royo et al. 2012). In addition to physical reasons such as acute or chronic pain, nausea, drowsiness, or respiratory distress, patients spoke about psychological burdens such as anxiety, hopelessness, sadness, and the fear of becoming dependent. However, the most important were social reasons, such as the fear of being a burden to others, the experience of loneliness or abandonment by loved ones, social isolation, and a lack of financial support. Spiritual issues, such as experience of the loss of dignity or activity, the incurability and terminal nature of their condition, the uncertainty of the dying process, and loss of a sense of life, played further important roles.

Meanings

Patients' narrative accounts contained much richer explanations about what this wish meant to them. For patients, the wish to die almost always had a much wider significance than just the subjectively perceived reasons, and could therefore not be explained fully through these reasons alone. When we asked them for the broader ideas, values, hopes, and fears underlying their wish, patients mostly referred to personal values, commitments, and moral understandings, which were tightly connected to their sense of identity, existential–spiritual convictions, and how they understood themselves within personal relationships. For example, one patient, who undertook steps to hasten death with EXIT, stated as *reasons* for her wish to hasten death frequent nausea, incontinence, and her poor eyesight, which made it impossible for her to read. But the *meanings* that this wish to die had within her narratives were: her wish to *let death put an end to severe suffering, to end a situation that she saw as an unreasonable demand,* and that in hastening death she saw the possibility of *preserving self-determination in the last moments of life* (detailed case description in Ohnsorge et. al. 2014b).

In the patients' narratives we identified nine different meanings, which can be found in Table 8.2 (details in Ohnsorge et al 2014b). As meanings are very subjectively bound to personal values, this list is probably not exhaustive.

Table 8.2 Meanings and functions of wish to die statements (open list)

Meanings
A wish to die can be a wish:
1. To allow a life-ending process to take its course
2. To let death put an end to severe suffering
3. To end a situation that is seen as an unreasonable demand
4. To spare others from the burden of oneself
5. To preserve self-determination in the last moments of life
6. To end a life that is now without value
7. To move on to another reality
8. To be an example to others
9. To not have to wait until death arrives

Functions
A wish to die can function as:
1. An appeal
2. A vehicle to speak about dying
3. A means for re-establishing of agency
4. A manipulation

Reproduced from: What a wish to die can mean: reasons, meanings and functions of wishes to die, reported from 30 qualitative case studies of terminally ill cancer patients in palliative care, K. Ohnsorge, H. Gudat, and C. Rehmann-Sutter, *BMC Palliative Care*, 13 (38), doi:10.1186/1472–684X-13–38. Copyright © 2014, The Authors. BioMed Central Ltd published by Springer under the Creative Commons Attribution License.

Functions

In some patients' narratives the wish to die also had a function in the sense that patients hoped, consciously or not, for this wish to have a particular effect, either on themselves or on their relationships. Some expressed a wish to die as an *appeal* intended to provoke help or interaction; others used wish to die statements as a *vehicle to speak about dying*, if talking about their imminent death was otherwise too difficult. For still others their wish to die functioned in proximity to death as a means to *win back some space of agency*. And finally, some wishes to die seemed to have a *manipulative function*, i.e. they were expressed to provoke the reactions of others, to attract attention, or simply to shock or induce fear. With the exception of one case, in which a patient used such statements to put psychological pressure on his wife (but had no real wish to die), all wishes to die that had a function also had a meaning.

Constitutive social interactions

From the analysis it emerged that the particular setting and social relationships of patients often had a decisive influence on what the patient was wishing. How patients perceived themselves and others in relationships, and the things that were at stake in these relationships, co-constituted their wishes in subtle ways. This could happen through direct communication with, and the reactions of others, but equally through non-verbal or indirect reactions, or even through a patient's assumptions about possible reactions from important others, including families and friends and their healthcare professionals.

Wishing with respect to others

Interdependence, voluntary or non-voluntary responsibilities, and obligations towards others played an important role in how patients allowed themselves to express their wish to die, or how they evaluated it over time. Many patients balanced in their decisions divers values important to them respecting also the assumed or real feelings and moral understandings of others. Several patients told us, for example, that they distanced themselves over time from their explicit wish to hasten death because they did not want to burden their loved ones who opposed their wish or who would find assisted suicide too difficult. One patient, whose numerous children were initially opposed to it, but then declared they all wanted to be present at the moment their father hastened his death with EXIT, said:

> . . . whether that wouldn't be a total shock for these children, I don't know. I mean, whether I would then really want to expect that [sitting beside me] of them, that's what I don't know. It isn't the right thing.

But hastening death on his own without telling the children also went against his ideas of their mutually caring relationship and of being a responsible father.

While most of these patients respected the moral feelings and values of important others out of an attitude of loving care and their own moral self-understanding, other patients reported being constrained by the negative reactions and contrasting moral values of their families or healthcare professionals. One patient reported significant pressure from her relatives, who had told her that assisted suicide would bring shame on their well-known family.

Constitutive preconceptions of others

Often, the way in which those around understood a patient's wishes contributed morally to how this wish was interpreted. One patient gave up on her attempt to express her wish to die: her best friend and only social contact, whom she told about her idea, as well as one nurse towards whom she made an active request for euthanasia, both refused to listen when she explained she had a wish to hasten death. The friend told her that she believed it was too early for her to have this wish, and let her understand that she was also against assisted dying out of her own Catholic conviction. The nurse answered an active request for euthanasia by stating that it was legally impossible for her to do. By clinging to their preconceptions, both missed the opportunity to acknowledge and explore the patient's ideas. This made the patient withdraw from her few social contacts and apparently added to her suffering. However, the friend and the nurse subsequently interpreted this silence as a change in the patient's thinking, while in the interview the patient told us she still had this wish. In this case, the preconceptions of the friend and the nurse shaped what they believed about the patient's wish to die, failing to recognize how it actually was; and their reaction again had an effect on the patient's wish (the persistence of her wish to die despite their reactions added to her suffering). On the other hand, one can imagine the preconceptions of others influencing a patient's wish to die in a very different way. In our study, we did not observe a case in which others, out of their own moral convictions or fears of dying, prompted patients to think about hastening death. However, the fact that we did not observe it does not mean that this never happens.

Performative aspects

The explicit expression of a wish to die often changed something in the relationships between people. Patients were aware that voicing their ideas would have a strong impact on those around them. Some patients told us that they preferred not to confront their loved ones with their wish to die so as not to burden them. One man who frequently thought about attempting suicide explained that he was not sharing his ideas with his family because he felt that, even if he just spoke about his wishes, his family would feel a responsibility towards him that he did not want them to have. In other cases, we assume that the fear of other people's anticipated negative reactions kept people back from sharing their most intimate ideas. However, others deliberatively used the performative effect of declaring a wish to die to provoke a certain reaction, such as calling for attention from the healthcare professionals or, as already mentioned, to manipulate family members.

Communicating wishes to die often had particular implications for the patients themselves, as new interpretations, which came with explaining their story, again influenced what they wished. Until the interview Walter, for example, had never talked with the hospice team about his reflections on dying. The hospice physician, however, reported retrospectively that, following the interview, Walter opened up to the male nurse and let him know during hygiene care much of what he thought. In the days before he died, Walter became more relaxed. During ward rounds he then gave the physician to understand that he had made up his mind, as the physician told us:

[Physician] And then I had, in the subsequent conversations during ward rounds I had the impression that he was dealing with it internally, because his answers changed. And that culminated in his [. . .] saying: I know what awaits me. I'm ready. I'd actually never heard that from him, that it was actually the endpoint of many considerations. I mean it came, it came out very considered.

Master narratives

Some patients' choices around the wish to die we interpreted as motivated by what Hilde Lindemann (2001) has called 'master narratives'—dominant cultural schemes that make individuals order and frame their experiences in a certain light (see also Chapter 13). For example, as reported in other studies, several of our patients wanted to die because they perceived themselves to be a burden to others. While such a statement might have actual causes in personal interactions, it might also be influenced by dominant societal schemes. Statements like 'old people are an enormous expense to society', repeated frequently by Cyril (whose case is described in detail in Chapter 20), indicate a reflection of wider societal narratives. Being independent, having a task, and being a productive member of the community are dominant virtues and positive identity elements in our societies. For the older generation in particular, these dominant narratives might lead to a desire not to generate care needs or costs. Not wanting to be a burden might be interpreted as an internalized part of this larger social narrative (Agich 2003).

Discussion

What participants told us about their wishes to die showed these wishes to be characterized by complex and dynamic processes of coming to terms with the situation at the end of life. Simple wish to die statements frequently gave insight—when investigated more deeply—into a diversity of wishes with various intentions that existed contemporaneously and were motivated by different reasons, meanings, and functions. Even though there was usually one predominant intention, other, even contradictory, intentions were also important, and patients often changed their focus of preference unexpectedly and over a short time. These oscillating intentions in many narratives capture the ambivalence of a patient's situation near death. Recognizing how they are further influenced by social interactions and communication is what makes up the complexity around last wishes.

Nevertheless, eight out of 30 study patients reported having had a stable wish over the entire research period. Therefore, we cannot conclude that patients' wishes were generally unstable, or that a wish to hasten death can never be called 'persistent'. However, as a high proportion of participants showed oscillations in what they wished, we believe that the concept of the 'stability' of a wish to die is not unproblematic and definitely needs further research, especially before referring to it in ethical debate or legal or normative policies.

We also saw that not all wish to die statements were wishes to hasten death, and of those that were, many remained on the level of fantasy and involved no active steps towards death. This finding is confirmed in more detail by many quantitative studies (Monforte-Royo et al. 2010). We agree with Bregje Onwuteaka-Philipsen (Chapter 10) that it is important to acknowledge that patients with *all sorts of* wishes to die are in need of support and care. Clinical practice, as well as research, is too often focused only on patients who have a wish to hasten death. We therefore suggest that the wish to die is conceptualized as a broad phenomenon that includes a whole spectrum of intentions, and to speak of 'wishes to die' rather than just investigating 'desires to hasten death'.

Many patients were able to explain why they held this wish. They did so not only with reference to subjective reasons, which they saw as causing their wish, but also, most importantly, by explaining what this wish meant to them within their wider framework of moral ideas and identities (meanings). For a full understanding of a wish to die it therefore seems crucial not to take just subjective reasons or objective triggering factors into consideration, but first of all to ascertain the meaning a patient attributes to his or her wish.

Even though these wishes were complex, if explored thoroughly they became intelligible to others—although some of the experiences around these wishes might always escape being expressed in words. The model of intentions, motivations, and social interactions that we propose might help us get closer to what matters to patients and why. These wishes are narratively structured in the sense that they relate to broader contexts of self-interpretations in which patients recount their moral understandings to themselves and others (Taylor 1989; Walker 2007). Patients talked about their wishes to die as consisting of more than one storyline, for example when explaining why they held different intentions at the same time, or by referring to different meanings. All these storylines, however, were deeply connected to what patients saw as being important in that situation (see examples in Ohnsorge et al. 2012). In a wish to die, these narratives can run in parallel and are not always integrated into a single coherent story.

Cheryl Mattingly (2010) proposed that we should view willing in general as a 'process of reorientation' rather than defined points of a decision or choice. Something similar could be true for wishing: rather than taking wishes to die as fixed statements, it might be more fruitful to consider them as 'dynamic, sometimes unstable equilibria' in which patients reorient and recount to themselves and others what matters to them about dying (Ohnsorge et al. 2014a). This is not to say that one might not arrive at a final decision, and of course one can: eight study patients did indeed have a stable wish. But seeing wishes to die as a reflexive process with a narrative structure allows to acknowledge the internal work inherent in these wishes.

Wishes to die are not simple messages sent in a linear way from a sender to a recipient. Rather than being 'declarations' through which a patient informs those around him about his preferences, they need to be understood as communicative acts, which are situated within a particular setting between particular people at particular points in time. Part of the complexity of interactions around wish to die statements comes from the fact that surrounding people hear what the patient says through their own moral understandings, including their personal ideas about a 'good death', their spiritual convictions, and professional codes of conduct. Moral obligations towards others, relational values, and the anticipated or real reactions of how others (might) respond to wish to die statements all go towards influencing the wish, how it is stated, and the social interactions around it in a decisive way. How a wish to die is expressed and talked about, but also what it contains and what functions it has, are partly co-constituted through social relations.

Reacting in a responsive and caring way to wish to die statements implies engaging with the underlying narrative structure of these statements. Caring responsibly for someone with a wish to die cannot be done without thoroughly investigating what people think about when they express such a wish and what meanings, fears, thoughts, and moral understandings in relation to themselves and others have brought them there. It is an ethical imperative that patients should not be 'talked into' or 'talked out of' something that does not belong to their own understanding of themselves or does not reflect their own narrative account. It requires rigorous self-observation to detect the subtle influences that one's own values and convictions (i.e. in favour of or against assisted dying) can have within the dialogue that persuades patients directly or indirectly towards the 'better'. Between imposing one's own moral understandings on the patient and offering creative counterstories that support him or her to arrive at a fresh and yet authentic interpretation of his or her experience, there is—as Marian Verkerk suggests in Chapter 13—a thin ethical line.

The threefold phenomenological structure of the wish to die (intentions, motivations, social interactions) that we suggest here hopefully helps to clarify the basic understanding of a wish to die. Knowledge of how these three dimensions can constitute particular wishes to die is key in asking what patients specifically intend and mean when they express such a wish. It enables us to come to a more comprehensive understanding of a wish to die, and is a basis for responding ethically to that wish. Other elements, especially clinical ones, are obviously important as well.

References

Agich, G. (2003). *Dependence and Autonomy in Old Age: An Ethical Framework for Long-Term Care*. Cambridge: Cambridge University Press.

Back, A. L., Wallace, J. I., Starks, H. E., and Pearlman, R. A. (1996). Physician-assisted suicide and euthanasia in Washington State. Patient requests and physician responses. *Journal of the American Medical Association*, **275**, 919–925.

Beck, A. T. and Kovacs, M. (1979). Assessment of Suicidal Intention. The scale for suicidal ideation. *Journal of Consulting and Clinical Psychology*, **47**, 343–352.

Breitbart, W., Rosenfeld, B., and Passik, S. (1996). Interest in physician assisted suicide among ambulatory HIV-infected patients. *American Journal of Psychiatry*, **153**, 238–242.

Charmaz, K. (2006). *Constructing Grounded Theory. A Practical Guide Through Qualitative Analysis*. London: Sage.

Chochinov, H. M., Wilson, K. G., Enns, M., et al. (1995). Desire for death in the terminally ill. *American Journal of Psychiatry*, **152**, 1185–1191.

Chochinov, H. M., Wilson, K. G., Enns, M., and Lander, S. (1998). Depression, hopelessness, and suicidal ideation in the terminally ill. *Psychosomatics*, **39**, 366–370.

Corbin, J. and Strauss, A. L. (2008). *Basics of Qualitative Research. Techniques and Procedures for Developing Grounded Theory*. Los Angeles, CA: Sage.

Coyle, N. and Sculco, L. (2004). Expressed desire for hastened death in seven patients living with advanced cancer: a phenomenologic inquiry. *Oncology Nursing Forum*, **31**, 699–706.

Emmanuel, E. J. (2002). Euthanasia and physician-assisted suicide: a review of the empirical data from the United States. *Archives of Internal Medicine*, **162**, 142–152.

Ferrand, E., Dreyfus, J. F., Chastrusse, M., Ellien, F., Lemaire, F., and Fischler, M. (2012). Evolution of requests to hasten death among patients managed by palliative care teams in France: a multicentre cross-sectional survey (DemandE). *European Journal of Cancer*, **48**, 368–376.

Filiberti, A., Ripamonti, C., Totis, A., et al. (2001). Characteristics of terminal cancer patients who committed suicide during a home palliative care program. *Journal of Pain and Symptom Management*, **22**, 544–553.

Haker, H. (2005). Narrative Bioethik. In: S. Graumann and K. Grüber (eds), *Anerkennung, Ethik und Behinderung. Beiträge aus dem Institut Mensch Ethik und Wissenschaft*, **Vol. 2**, pp. 113–132. LIT Verlag: Münster.

Hudson, P. L., Kristjanson, L. J., Ashby, M., et al. (2006a). Desire for hastened death in patients with advanced disease and the evidence base of clinical guidelines: a systematic review. *Journal of Palliative Medicine*, **20**, 693–701.

Hudson, P. L., Schofield, P., Kelly, B., et al. (2006b). Responding to desire to die statements from patients with advanced disease: recommendations for health professionals. *Journal of Palliative Medicine*, **20**, 703–710.

Johansen, S., Holen, J. C., and Kaasa, S. (2005). Attitudes towards, and wishes for euthanasia in advanced cancer patients at a palliative medicine unit. *Journal of Palliative Medicine*, **19**, 454–460.

Kelly, B., Burnett, P., Pelusi, D., Badger, S., Varghese, F., and Robertson, M. (2002). Terminally ill cancer patients' wish to hasten death. *Palliative Medicine*, **16**, 339–345.

Kelly, B., Burnett, P., Pelusi, D., Badger, S., Varghese, F., and Robertson, M. (2003). Factors associated with the wish to hasten death: a study of patients with terminal illness. *Psychological Medicine*, **33**, 75–81.

Kissane, D. W., Street, A., and Nitschke, P. (1998). Seven deaths in Darwin: case studies under the Rights of the Terminally Ill Act, Northern Territory, Australia. *Lancet*, **352**, 1097–1102.

Lavery, J. V., Boyle, J., Dickens, B. M., Maclean, H., and Singer, P. A. (2001). Origins of the desire for euthanasia and assisted suicide in people with HIV-1 or AIDS: a qualitative study. *Lancet*, **358**, 362–367.

Lindemann, H. (2001). *Damaged Identities, Narrative Repair*. Ithaca, NY: Cornell University Press.

Mak, Y. Y. and Elwyn, G. (2005). Voices of the terminally ill: uncovering the meaning of desire for euthanasia. *Journal of Palliative Medicine*, **19**, 343–350.

Mattingly, C. (2010). Moral willing as narrative re-envisioning. In: K. M. Murphy and C. J. Throop (eds), *Toward and Anthropology of the Will*, pp. 50–68. Stanford, CA: Stanford University Press.

Monforte-Royo, C., Villavicencio-Chávez, C., Tomás-Sábado, J., and Balaguer, A. (2010). The wish to hasten death: a review of clinical studies. *Journal of Psycho-Oncology*, **20**, 795–804.

Monforte-Royo, C., Villavicencio-Chávez, C., Tomás-Sábado, J., Mahtani-Chugani, V., and Balaguer, A. (2012). What lies behind the wish to hasten death? A systematic review and meta-ethnography from the perspective of patients. *PLoS ONE*, **7**(5), e37117.

Nissim, R., Gagliese, L., and Rodin, G. (2009). The desire for hastened death in individuals with advanced cancer: a longitudinal qualitative study. *Social Science and Medicine*, **69**, 165–171.

Ohnsorge, K., Gudat, H., Widdershoven, G., and Rehmann-Sutter, C. (2012). 'Ambivalence' at the end of life: How to understand patients' wishes ethically. *Nursing Ethics*, **19**, 629–641.

Ohnsorge, K., Gudat, H., and Rehmann-Sutter, C. (2014a). Intentions in wishes to die: analysis and a typology. A report of 30 qualitative case studies of terminally ill cancer patients in palliative care. *Psycho-Oncology*, **23**, 1012–1026.

Ohnsorge, K., Gudat, H., and Rehmann-Sutter, C. (2014b). What a wish to die can mean. Reasons, meanings and functions of wishes to die, reported from 30 qualitative case studies of terminally ill cancer patients. *BMC Palliative Care*, **13**(38), doi: 10.1186/1472-684X-13-38

Pearlman, R. A., Hsu, C., Starks, H., et al. (2005). Motivations for physician-assisted suicide. *Journal of General Internal Medicine*, **20**, 234–239.

Robinson, J. A. and Crawford, G. B. (2005). Identifying palliative care patients with symptoms of depression: an algorithm. *Journal of Palliative Medicine*, **19**, 278–287.

Rosenfeld, B., Breitbart, W., Galietta, M., et al. (2000). The schedule of attitudes towards hastened death. Measuring desire for death in terminally ill cancer patients. *Cancer*, **88**, 2868–2875.

Schroepfer, T. A. (2006). Mind frames towards dying and factors motivating their adoption by terminally ill elders. *Journals of Gerontology Series B: Psychological Sciences and Social Sciences*, **61**, 129–139.

Seale, C. and Addington-Hall, J. (1994). Euthanasia: why people want to die earlier. *Social Science and Medicine*, **39**, 647–654.

Smith, J., Flowers, P., and Larkin, M. (2009). *Interpretive Phenomenological Analysis*. Los Angeles: Sage.

Stiel, S., Elsner, F., Pestinger, M., and Radbruch, L. (2010). Wunsch nach vorzeitigem Lebensende. Was steht dahinter [A wish to hasten death: what is behind it]. *Schmerz*, **24**, 177–189.

Suarez-Almazor, M., Newman, C., Hanson, J., and Bruera, E. (2002). Attitudes of terminally ill cancer patients about euthanasia and assisted suicide: predominance of psychosocial determinants and beliefs over symptom distress and subsequent survival. *Journal of Clinical Oncology*, **20**, 2134–2141.

Taylor, C. (1989). *Sources of the Self: Making of Modern Identity*. Cambridge: Cambridge University Press.

Walker, M. U. (2007). *Moral Understandings. A Feminist Study in Ethics*, 2nd edn. Oxford: Oxford University Press.

Wilson, K. G., Scott, J. F., Graham, I. D., et al. (2000). Attitudes of terminally ill patients toward euthanasia and physician-assisted suicide. *Archives of Internal Medicine*, **160**, 2452–2460.

Chapter 9

Acting on a wish to die at the end of life: the Swiss situation

Alexandre Mauron

Introduction: the Swiss situation

Wishing to die at the end of life in the Swiss context is crucially determined by the legality of acting on that wish with the help of others, in the form of assisted suicide. Moreover, compared with other countries in which euthanasia and/or assisted suicide are legal, the Swiss situation is unique in several respects. The most visible and most discussed is that assisted suicide is not merely legal in specific circumstances but is often provided by organizations that are themselves legal and operate openly. Highly publicised cases of people travelling to Switzerland to obtain assistance with suicide, which they would not be able to obtain legally in their home countries, have raised much media attention. International news reporting and ethical controversy often focus on this 'death tourism' (Avery 2003; Sokol 2008). Nevertheless, in order to understand the conceptual and legal background, historical development, and current societal debates, it is necessary to analyse practices in Switzerland itself. That is the focus of this chapter, which will include a brief description of the current Swiss situation as regards assisted suicide and concentrate on present discussions, especially regarding open ethical, legal, and policy questions. These are exemplified by ongoing debates in jurisprudence, as well as the *de facto* coexistence between palliative care models and organized assisted suicide. Various aspects of the Swiss model of assisted suicide have been described (Bosshard et al. 2002; Hurst and Mauron 2003; Guillod and Schmidt 2005), sometimes with a view to promoting it as a well-founded framework for enabling autonomous decision-making at the end of life (Ziegler 2009) or denouncing it as a case of 'inadvertent' liberalism based on a loophole exploited by right-to-die movements (Andorno 2013). In fact, producing an in-depth and reasonably unbiased account of the Swiss situation is quite difficult, if only because it results from the interplay of complex historical and political contingencies. These include legal discussions spanning more than a century, a strong liberal tradition as regards individual freedom, and a tradition of 'lean' legislation that tends to rely heavily on low-level regulatory arrangements rather than specific statutes (Swiss National Advisory Commission on Biomedical Ethics 2005). This is traditionally praised in Swiss political discourse as allowing fluid adjustments to novel situations. On the other hand, it can also make controversial social practices less transparent and less predictable for the individual citizen, an issue that has recently regained urgency concerning assisted suicide in view of the 2013 judgement of the European Court of

Human Rights in the case of *Gross v. Switzerland* discussed in the section 'The current Swiss situation and its legal environment' (European Court of Human Rights 2013). In addition, this informality implies that there is little open or mutual engagement of palliative care practitioners with organizations for assisted suicide.

The current Swiss situation and its legal environment

In Switzerland, volunteer-based right-to-die organizations provide suicide assistance to individuals wishing to end their life for health-related reasons. Volunteers play a major role in the process as they are typically involved in extensive discussions with the applicant, bring the fast-acting barbiturate to the applicant's home, witness the death, and take an active role in the legal proceedings that follow. As is the case for every suicide, assisted or not, the police or judicial authorities must be immediately notified. The ensuing inquest is concluded rapidly as soon as it is clear that no breach of the law has taken place.

The regulatory framework of assisted suicide is rather slim as regards federal law, since it is basically limited to article 115 of the Federal Penal Code (there is an important local exception in the new law on assisted suicide recently adopted in Canton de Vaud; see 'Organized assisted suicide: from legalization to control?'). Article 115 defines the offence of aiding and abetting suicide as an action inspired by a 'selfish motive'. The logical consequence, consistently supported by case law, is that a person providing suicide assistance for altruistic reasons does not commit the offence referred to in article 115 and cannot be prosecuted on these grounds. In order to avoid prosecution, assisted suicide organizations must not be profit-making ventures and must make sure that the applicant is legally competent and fully understands the implication of her or his request (Guillod and Schmidt 2005). Typically they also screen applicants in order to assess the severity of suffering resulting from their illness as well as the constancy of their will to die.

These criteria vary between assisted suicide organizations, which is significant in view of the persisting controversy about whether access to assisted suicide should be contingent on illness-related criteria and what these should be. For instance, EXIT A.D.M.D., which is active in French-speaking Switzerland, requires medical evidence of 'an incurable disease and either a lethal prognosis or severe disability', to which 'disabling polypathologies of old age' were recently added (EXIT A.D.M.D. 2014). Swiss German Exit emphasizes 'a prognosis without hope of improvement, or unbearable suffering, or disability' (EXIT Deutsche Schweiz 2013). As long as they operate within the law, such organizations are free to choose self-limiting criteria and to apply them as they see fit. On the other hand, formal ethical guidelines have been issued by the Swiss Academy of Medical Sciences, setting more stringent limits to physicians' involvement in assisted suicide, which should only be considered for patients with a terminal disease (Swiss Academy of Medical Sciences 2013, p. 9). These guidelines exert a degree of moral pressure on the medical profession but are not legally enforceable. They are important insofar as they apply not only to physicians who collaborate with assisted suicide organizations but also to physicians who enter a private arrangement to help a patient end his or her life. This is legal for the same reasons already presented and was the usual form of physician involvement in assisted suicide before organizations appeared on the scene in the 1980s.

These complex criteria tend to limit access to assisted suicide to an extent that is not easily predictable. They also illustrate the fact that there is no entitlement to receive suicide assistance in the Swiss system in its present configuration. On the other hand, it can be argued that the Swiss practice implies a form of what in Hohfeldian terminology would be considered a *claim right* (Wenar 2013) as regards suicide assistance, i.e. at minimum, a right not to be prevented outright from obtaining it. An across-the-board prohibition of assisted suicide would abrogate that right, and would be widely perceived as antithetical to the Swiss liberal tradition. A prohibitionist policy has never been put to a nationwide vote, but in one local vote it was resoundingly defeated (Zürcher Oberländer 2011). Nevertheless, the nature and extent of this right is far from clear and has not been analysed in depth in legal scholarship. In addition, the failure of several legislative proposals to change the status quo in either a more liberal or a more restrictive direction gave the impression that public debate was hopelessly bogged down and leading nowhere (Andorno 2013). Yet recent events have shown that the issue will not go away. In fact, the debate *de lege ferenda* has now been reactivated in a ruling of the European Court of Human Rights that reprimanded Switzerland for the lack of clear conditions of access to assisted suicide (*Gross v. Switzerland*; European Court of Human Rights 2013). The court heard the case of an applicant for assisted suicide who had been repeatedly refused suicide assistance for various reasons. The court found that this person had been wronged, not necessarily for not obtaining suicide assistance but for being unable to receive a clear and principled answer to what the court's jurisprudence had repeatedly considered a legitimate request under article 8 of the European Convention of Human Rights protecting the right to private life (on appeal this ruling was overturned on a technicality but the basic legal question of due process remains). This case vividly illustrates that the Swiss situation cannot be understood on the sole basis of federal law since a variety of guidelines and informal regulatory arrangements are important parts of the regulatory environment. These informal rules make a decisive contribution to shaping the actual practice of assisted suicide in Switzerland and to making it rather more complex, and less liberal, than it is often made out to be in the scholarly literature as well as in the media.

A comparative and historical perspective

Two major differences that set Switzerland apart from all other jurisdictions that allow euthanasia and/or assisted suicide need additional commentary. First, there are no provisions in federal law on the role of healthcare professionals in suicide assistance, neither to prohibit it nor to prescribe and regulate it. The concept of 'physician-assisted suicide' has no legal existence, even if in current practice physicians are usually involved with writing the prescription for the lethal substance. Second, the present situation results from a century-old historical development, initiated well before the 'modern' social conversation on patient autonomy in terminal illness that motivated the legal changes in other countries. Article 115 has been the law of the land since the Federal Penal Code came into force in 1942, and the discussions that influenced the legislative process actually date back to the beginning of the twentieth century (a detailed historical account is given by the Swiss National Advisory Commission on Biomedical Ethics, 2005). In fact, much of the basic legislation of modern Switzerland emerged at that time and was strongly shaped by the liberal and secular values of the then dominant Radical Party. One important aspect of these discussions was related to the consequences of the fact that suicide had been decriminalized. It became clear at the time that complicity in suicide as such, i.e. without further specification, was a conceptual impossibility since one cannot be complicit in an action that is not defined as criminal. Therefore, aiding and abetting suicide could not be made punishable without further action, i.e. unless some specific malfeasance was involved. This led to making a selfish motive a defining element of illegal suicide assistance in article 115. Interestingly, other European countries had the same problem, especially those outside the Anglo-Saxon common law tradition, in which suicide remained an offence until much later. For instance, to this day, France and Germany do not have a statute expressly prohibiting assisted suicide, and one may well ask why there is no open practice of assisted suicide in these countries. The reason is that in France and Germany, providers of suicide assistance would in many cases fall foul of 'good Samaritan laws'—applicable to all citizens or specifically to healthcare personnel, on the reasoning that a person asking for assistance with suicide ought to be seen as in need of being saved from suicide—or to legislation on the prescription of controlled substances. In other words, one may say that in France and Germany there exists a Hohfeldian *liberty-right* or *privilege* (Wenar 2005) as regards assisted suicide, since there is no universally valid duty to abstain from this action. Yet this liberty-right amounts to very little in reality since most cases of assisted suicide would be indictable for other, secondary, reasons. In Switzerland, legal thinking developed in a quite different direction, and several examples discussed by early legal authorities involved assisted suicides, which in their view ought to be legal. These examples involve a variety of suicide motives, some of which appear exotic to the modern mind, such as suicides of honour, but they also include suffering due to incurable disease. In recent times, the public debate on assisted suicide has converged with similar societal debates in other countries, and the ethical and political arguments exchanged about active aid in dying are largely similar. However, this must be qualified on account of three important Swiss specificities, which can be summarized as follows:

- The distinction between assisted suicide and voluntary euthanasia is essential. This is understandable since the Swiss liberalism about assisted suicide originated from a discussion concerning suicide itself. Attempts to legalize voluntary euthanasia have been unsuccessful so far. This sets Switzerland apart from other liberal European countries (the Netherlands, Belgium, Luxembourg).

- There is no need to 'demedicalize' assisted suicide, since it is not thought of as a medical matter in the first place. This is a point argued forcefully by the Swiss Academy of Medical Sciences and reflected in the practice of assisted suicide organizations, which rely heavily on non-medical volunteers. The current problem is rather how to specify the proper role of health professionals in assisted suicide since they have a privileged access to the pharmacological means of non-violent suicide. In this respect the Swiss situation is different from jurisdictions that make the participation of a physician a legal requirement for assisted suicide, as in Oregon, Washington, Montana, and Vermont in the United States.

◆ Finally, there is no explicit, positive, and legal framework for the practice of assisted suicide, and this sets Switzerland apart from all other liberal jurisdictions. This does not imply that assisted suicide operates in a normative vacuum, as we have seen, but it does imply that the Swiss liberalism is inherently fragile, as shown for instance by the recent case of *Gross v. Switzerland* mentioned earlier. Furthermore, the very informality of the Swiss model makes it difficult to compare with other systems and also makes it more difficult for professionals involved in end-of-life care, especially palliative care specialists, to come to terms with the practice of assisted suicide in an explicit and clearly defined way.

Assisted suicide and palliative care

Euthanasia and assisted suicide are an obvious challenge for palliative care, at least as regards the official philosophy as stated in the bylaws of the European Association of Palliative Care (art. 4.1; European Association of Palliative Care 2011), which are opposed to active aid in dying. This does not preclude a certain commonality of values, especially the emphasis on preserving and fostering the autonomy of patients in the face of death (Hurst and Mauron 2006). Nor does it obviate the need to continuously reflect on the demarcation between euthanasia and other actions that may be life-shortening, such as palliative sedation—a difficult question being actively investigated by palliative care organizations (Cherny and Radbruch 2009). Nevertheless, the philosophy of palliative care is traditionally antagonistic to active aid in dying, and the fact that the latter is lawful in liberal countries does not in itself invalidate this basic philosophical commitment. Yet once a country has moved decisively towards legalizing euthanasia and/or assisted suicide, it would seem that palliative care specialists need to deal with this new predicament. They have to decide, explicitly or informally, how they will deal with the open, legal practice of active aid in dying, both in terms of handling patients' requests for it and in deciding the kind of relationship with providers of euthanasia and/or assisted suicide that they are willing to countenance. The palliative care literature provides some guidance in this respect. There is a considerable body of research on 'desire to die statements' among patients with advanced illness using a range of methodologies and patient populations (Breitbart et al. 2000; Emanuel et al. 2000; Lavery et al. 2001; Rodin et al. 2007; Monforte-Royo et al. 2011, 2012) as well as normative reflection and guidance about how to handle requests for euthanasia and/or assisted suicide (Hudson et al. 2006). That such a request should be discussed with the patient in an empathic and non-judgemental way, with a view to clarifying the request and exploring alternatives, is not controversial. However, there is a sense in which the request itself is necessarily moot in places where assisted aid in dying is illegal: it is in effect akin to ordering steak in a vegetarian restaurant. As a result, and since much of this literature originates from prohibitionist countries, its insights are not necessarily applicable to the situation in liberal jurisdictions, at least not without some critical examination. One can therefore ask if similar investigations that would explicitly take on board the possibility of assisted suicide have been conducted within the Swiss context. Few studies along those lines have been published so far (but see Gamondi et al. 2013; Ohnsorge et al. 2014).

In liberal European countries other than Switzerland, the legality of euthanasia and assisted suicide is based on an explicit and detailed legal framework that gives both substantive and procedural guidance to healthcare professionals. This may not make choices easier for palliative care personnel but at least it provides a clear-cut normative context to contend with. Furthermore, the notion that palliative care and active aid in dying are mutually exclusive policy choices is not substantiated in practice. There is evidence that in Belgium, after the legalization of euthanasia, use of palliative care increased—what did decrease is the incidence of life-ending action without explicit request, an outcome that ought to be welcomed by all parties to the debate (Pardon et al. 2013). Studies about end-of-life care in Belgium point to the reality of an integrated approach, of which palliative care and euthanasia are both legitimate components (Van den Block et al. 2009; Pardon et al. 2012). This suggests that a constructive collaboration between palliative care and active aid in dying is a workable proposition. For instance, in Flanders a multidisciplinary working group devised a guideline on end-of-life care for general practitioners. This document was developed in a focus group-based process with considerable involvement of the public and of palliative care specialists, as well as a frank consideration and practical guidance for euthanasia as a concrete end-of-life option (Deschepper et al. 2006). There is little published evidence about such collaborations in Switzerland (but see Preisig 2013), which suggests that the mere fact that assisted suicide is legal is not decisive in shaping the relationship—or lack thereof— between palliative care and assisted suicide. As we have seen, the distinguishing feature of the Swiss situation is the major role of assisted suicide *organizations*, rather than the legality of assisted suicide itself. Therefore, the specific question to be asked is how the legality of assisted suicide organizations shapes the views of palliative care practitioners and of patients confronted with choices at the end of life.

There is published and ongoing research into the desire to die of patients who went through assisted suicide in Switzerland (Fischer et al. 2009; Imhof et al. 2011). Attitudes of Swiss physicians towards assisted suicide have been documented as part of the EURELD study comparing physicians' attitudes to a range of end-of-life issues in six European countries (Fischer et al. 2006). That study suggests a rather complex link between the legal status quo and doctors' attitudes towards active aid in dying. While half of the physicians in Switzerland accept the administration of drugs at lethal doses upon the explicit request of a patient in extreme pain, it is not clear that the legally crucial distinction between self-administration by the patient, i.e. assisting suicide, and direct administration of the drug by the physician plays a major role in shaping these attitudes. The same study included a few items related to palliative care. For instance, 69% of the Swiss physicians in the study agreed or strongly agreed with the following statement: 'Sufficient availability of high-quality palliative care averts almost all requests for euthanasia or assisted suicide.' However, in order to understand the specific attitudes of palliative care specialists one has to fall back either on official statements or on published accounts and opinions of palliative care practitioners or teams. The bylaws of the Swiss Association for Palliative Care (recently renamed 'palliative ch') clearly state that palliative care implies 'respect for life and its natural end' (art. 3; Swiss Association for

Palliative Care 2007). On the other hand, palliative ch commissioned a survey among its members on active aid in dying, with rather mixed results. A rather slim majority (56%) opposed assisted suicide, whereas refusal of active euthanasia was clearer (69%) (Bittel et al. 2002). These results suggest that the controversy is alive in palliative care circles, even though there have been no policy changes by palliative.ch so far. Other data suggest a will on the part of some palliative care practitioners to demarcate themselves sharply from the practice of assisted suicide (Pereira et al. 2008).

Organized assisted suicide: from legalization to control?

To the extent that this can be inferred from public information, the worlds of palliative care and organized assisted suicide appear to be largely foreign to each other in Switzerland. Obviously, this does not preclude the possibility of informal contacts and arrangements as described by Preisig (2013), but it is safe to say that, overall, there is little approval of, or trust in, assisted suicide organizations on the part of the palliative care community. Contrasting this situation with the more positive picture in Belgium suggests that the peculiarly informal and libertarian spirit in which assisted suicide organizations deploy their activities in Switzerland is a powerful obstacle to their recognition by many healthcare professionals as genuine partners. This brings us back to the limits of liberalism alluded to earlier in the section 'The current Swiss situation and its legal environment'. The failure to regulate assisted suicide organizations by explicit legislation means that they operate in a kind of libertarian limbo, which may seem a good thing to them but it effectively prevents their recognition as fulfilling a socially valid role. Self-regulation is a poor substitute for legal intervention, because self-regulatory efforts are necessarily heterogeneous and often lack recognized professional authority. Furthermore, these organizations have not been able to sufficiently distinguish their activist role on the political scene from their informal and yet real responsibility as providers of a public service. Their freedom of action is considerable, guaranteed as it is by a negative right to non-interference by the state, but the price they pay for it is huge. Rather than as legitimate players in end-of-life care, the authorities tend to see assisted suicide organizations as a merely societal phenomenon, at best neutral, at worst shocking or freakish, but one which must be tolerated in view of the considerable public support they enjoy and the political difficulty of building a consensus around specific legislation. Assuming that assisted suicide has a legitimate place in end-of-life care, this is an unsatisfactory predicament.

This brings us back to the issue of explicit regulation. The year 2013 was a turning point in this respect, not only because of the conclusions of the European Court of Human Rights in the Gross case, but also because one Swiss canton, Vaud, did pass a law on assisted suicide (Canton de Vaud 2013). The practical consequences will probably be quite limited since the law applies only to requests for suicide assistance from patients in public hospitals and public retirement homes. Nevertheless, the law could serve as model for additional local or federal legislation because it answers several of the issues raised here. A detailed discussion of this law is beyond the scope of this chapter, but in short it provides patients and physicians with both substantive and procedural guidance. In order to be considered, a request for suicide assistance must meet three criteria: the patient must be legally competent; his or her wish to die must be persistent after a careful exploration of alternatives such as appropriate palliative care; and the suffering must be caused by a severe and incurable illness and/or its consequences. The physician receiving the request has a number of procedural obligations including the duty to verify these criteria and to provide a detailed written answer to the patient within 4 weeks. In addition, the law stipulates an appeals procedure. This legislation represents a major change from the status quo at the federal level in a number of ways, of which only one will be mentioned: The patient now has a recognized *claim right* to have the request considered and to receive a principled positive or negative answer. On the other hand, the patient does not have a claim *to* suicide assistance against the individual physician receiving the claim, on account of the physician's right to conscientious objection. Whether the patient has a less stringent claim to suicide assistance against the healthcare system, as opposed to a claim against a particular person, is not really clear at this time. Such clarification is obviously of major importance.

This law—and others that may follow—represents a challenge not only to the medical profession but to assisted suicide organizations as well. The latter are not mentioned in the new law, unlike the initial proposal from which the legislative debate originated. If, in the future, assisted suicide in Switzerland is legislated along the lines discussed here, the question of corresponding institutional arrangements would need to be discussed anew. The function of organizations as providers of assisted suicide would have to be re-examined critically (their role as right-to-die societies bringing specific concerns to the political debate is obviously not in question; indeed the president of EXIT A.D.M.D has stated that '[he] would like to see EXIT disappear because assisted suicide would be regulated and accepted socially and politically'; Sobel 2009). Finally, this would also be a challenge and an opportunity for the palliative care community to rethink their place in end-of-life care in a way that would be more responsive to societal evolution as regards autonomous choice at the end of life.

References

Andorno, R. (2013). Nonphysician-assisted suicide in Switzerland. *Cambridge Quarterly of Healthcare Ethics*, **22**, 246–253.

Avery, D. (2003). Assisted suicide seekers turn to Switzerland. *Bulletin of the World Health Organization*, **81**, 310.

Bittel, N., Neuenschwander, H., and Stiefel, F. (2002). 'Euthanasia': a survey by the Swiss Association for Palliative Care. *Supportive Care in Cancer*, **10**, 265–271.

Bosshard, G., Fischer, S., and Bar, W. (2002). Open regulation and practice in assisted dying—how Switzerland compares with the Netherlands and Oregon. *Swiss Medical Weekly*, **132**, 527–534.

Breitbart, W., Rosenfeld, B., Pessin, H., et al. (2000). Depression, hopelessness, and desire for hastened death in terminally ill patients with cancer. *Journal of the American Medical Association*, **284**, 2907–2911.

Canton de Vaud (2013). *Etat de Vaud: Directive et loi sur l'Assistance au Suicide*. Available at: <http://www.vd.ch/themes/sante/professionnels/assistance-au-suicide/> (accessed 10 January 2014).

Cherny, N. I. and Radbruch, L. (2009). European Association for Palliative Care (EAPC) recommended framework for the use of sedation in palliative care. *Palliative Medicine*, 23, 581–593.

Deschepper, R., Vander Stichele, R., Bernheim, J. L., et al. (2006). Communication on end-of-life decisions with patients wishing to die at home: the making of a guideline for GPs in Flanders, Belgium. *British Journal of General Practice*, 56, 14–19.

Emanuel, E. J., Fairclough, D. L., and Emanuel, L. L. (2000). Attitudes and desires related to euthanasia and physician-assisted suicide among terminally ill patients and their caregivers. *Journal of the American Medical Association*, 284, 2460–2468.

European Association of Palliative Care (2011). *Bylaws*. Available at: <http://www.eapcnet.eu/Corporate/AbouttheEAPC/EAPCofficaldocuments/EAPCBylaws.aspx> (accessed 10 January 2014).

European Court of Human Rights (2013). *Case of Gross v. Switzerland*. Available at: <http://hudoc.echr.coe.int/sites/fra/pages/search.aspx?i=001-119703#{%22itemid%22:[%22001-119703%22]}> (accessed 10 January 2014).

EXIT A.D.M.D. (2014). Conditions pour obtenir une assistance au suicide. Available at: <http://www.exit-geneve.ch/conditions.htm> (accessed 10 February 2015).

EXIT Deutsche Schweiz (2013). Für wen kommt eine Begleitung in Frage? Available at: <http://www.exit.ch/freitodbegleitung/bedingungen/> (accessed 18 December 2013).

Fischer, S., Bosshard, G., Faisst, K., et al. (2006). Swiss doctors' attitudes towards end-of-life decisions and their determinants—a comparison of three language regions. *Swiss Medical Weekly*, 136, 370–376.

Fischer, S., Huber, C. A., Furter, M., et al. (2009). Reasons why people in Switzerland seek assisted suicide: the view of patients and physicians. *Swiss Medical Weekly*, 139, 333–338.

Gamondi, C., Pott, M., and Payne, S. (2013). Families' experiences with patients who died after assisted suicide: a retrospective interview study in southern Switzerland. *Annals of Oncology*, 24, 1639–1644.

Guillod, O. and Schmidt, A. (2005). Assisted suicide under Swiss Law. *European Journal of Health Law*, 12, 25–38.

Hudson, P. L., Schofield, P., Kelly, B., et al. (2006). Responding to desire to die statements from patients with advanced disease: recommendations for health professionals. *Palliative Medicine*, 20, 703–710.

Hurst, S. A. and Mauron, A. (2003). Assisted suicide and euthanasia in Switzerland: allowing a role for non-physicians. *British Medical Journal*, 326, 271–273.

Hurst, S. A. and Mauron, A. (2006). The ethics of palliative care and euthanasia: exploring common values. *Palliative Medicine*, 20, 107–112.

Imhof, L., Bosshard, G., Fischer, S., and Mahrer Imhof, R. (2011). Content of health status reports of people seeking assisted suicide: a qualitative analysis. *Medicine Health Care and Philosophy*, 14, 265–272.

Lavery, J. V., Boyle, J., Dickens, B. M., Maclean, H., and Singer, P. A. (2001). Origins of the desire for euthanasia and assisted suicide in people with HIV-1 or AIDS: a qualitative study. *Lancet*, 358, 362–367.

Monforte-Royo, C., Villavicencio-Chavez, C., Tomas-Sabado, J., and Balaguer, A. (2011). The wish to hasten death: a review of clinical studies. *Psycho-Oncology*, 20, 795–804.

Monforte-Royo, C., Villavicencio-Chavez, C., Tomas-Sabado, J., Mahtani-Chugani, V., and Balaguer, A. (2012). What lies behind the wish to hasten death? A systematic review and meta-ethnography from the perspective of patients. *PLoS ONE*, 7, e37117.

Ohnsorge, K., Gudat, H., and Rehmann-Sutter, C. (2014). Intentions in wishes to die: analysis and a typology—a report of 30 qualitative case studies of terminally ill cancer patients in palliative care. *Psycho-Oncology*, **23**, 1021–1026.

Pardon, K., Deschepper, R., Vander Stichele, R., et al. (2012). Expressed wishes and incidence of euthanasia in advanced lung cancer patients. *European Respiratory Journal*, **40**, 949–956.

Pardon, K., Chambaere, K., Pasman, H. R. W., Deschepper, R., Rietjens, J., and Deliens, L. (2013). Trends in end-of-life decision making in patients with and without cancer. *Journal of Clinical Oncology*, **31**, 1450–1457.

Pereira, J., Laurent, P., Cantin, B., Petremand, D., and Currat, T. (2008). The response of a Swiss university hospital's palliative care consult team to assisted suicide within the institution. *Palliative Medicine*, **22**, 659–667.

Preisig, E. (2013). Médecine palliative et assistance au décès. *Primary Care*, **13**, 397–398.

Rodin, G., Zimmermann, C., Rydall, A., et al. (2007). The desire for hastened death in patients with metastatic cancer. *Journal of Pain and Symptom Management*, **33**, 661–675.

Sobel, J. (2009). *Mythes et Réalités du Suicide Assisté en Suisse: Interview*. Swissinfo, 3 January 2009. Available at: <http://www.swissinfo.ch/fre/actualite/Mythes_et_realites_du_suicide_assiste_en_Suisse.html?cid=542196> (accessed 10 January 2014).

Sokol, D. K. (2008). Paving the way for assisted suicide. *British Medical Journal*, **337**, a3010.

Swiss Academy of Medical Sciences (2013). *End-of-life Care Guidelines*. Available at: <http://www.samw.ch/en/Ethics/Guidelines/Currently-valid-guidelines.html> (accessed 18 December 2013).

Swiss Association for Palliative Care (2007). *Bylaws*. Available at: <http://www.palliative.ch/professionnels/lassociation/statuts/> (accessed 10 February 2015).

Swiss National Advisory Commission on Biomedical Ethics (2005). *L'Assistance au Suicide. Prise de Position no. 9/2005*. Available at: <http://www.nek-cne.ch/fileadmin/nek-cne-dateien/Themen/Stellungnahmen/fr/suizidbeihilfe_fr.pdf> (accessed 10 February 2015).

Van den Block, L., Deschepper R., Bilsen, J., Bossuyt, N., Van Casteren, V., and Deliens, L. (2009). Euthanasia and other end of life decisions and care provided in final three months of life: nationwide retrospective study in Belgium. *British Medical Journal*, **339**, b2772.

Wenar, L. (2005). The nature of rights. *Philosophy and Public Affairs*, **33**, 223–252.

Wenar, L. (2013). The nature of claim-rights. *Ethics*, **123**, 202–229.

Ziegler, S. J. (2009). Collaborated death: an exploration of the Swiss model of assisted suicide for its potential to enhance oversight and demedicalize the dying process. *Journal of Law, Medicine and Ethics*, **37**, 318–330.

Zürcher Oberländer (2011). *Deutliche Abfuhr für Sterbehilfe Initiativen*, 15 May 2011. Available at: <http://www.zol.ch/ueberregional/kanton-zuerich/Deutliche-Abfuhr-fuer-SterbehilfeInitiativen/story/21581442> (accessed 10 January 2014).

Chapter 10

Understanding older people's wish to die

Bregje Onwuteaka-Philipsen

Introduction to understanding older people's wish to die

In all countries where this topic has been investigated in population-based studies, it has consistently been found that there is a group of older people who have thoughts and wishes about wanting to die (Forsell et al. 1997; Rao et al. 1997; Barnow and Linden 2000; Scocco and De Leo 2002; Yip et al. 2003; Skoog et al. 1996; Ayalon 2011; Rurup et al. 2011a; Almeida et al. 2012). Incidences of such thoughts and wishes vary, but are never higher than in one in five older adults. The variations found are possibly due to characteristics of individual countries, but certainly also partly due to differences in study designs, such as the questions used in assessing death thoughts and wishes and the study population. In several studies, death thoughts and wishes were measured using (variations of) questions developed by Paykel et al. (1974) and Beck et al. (1979). In these questions death thoughts and wishes are both considered to be components of suicidal ideation. Beck et al. (1979) define a suicidal ideator as a person who has seriously thought, planned, or wished to commit suicide. These questions make it possible to distinguish different situations within a group of people who had or have suicidal ideation. The Dutch population-based study by Rurup et al. (2011a), for instance, found that the 18.7% of older people with death thoughts and wishes consisted of the following groups:

- older people who had ever had death thoughts and/or wishes, but had not wished to die within the past week and had a moderate to strong wish to live in the past week (15.3%),

- older people who had only a weak wish to live in the past week, but no wish to die in the past week (1.2%),

- older people who had no wish to live in the past week and/or a weak wish to die in the past week (1.4%),

- older people who had a moderate to strong wish to die in the past week (0.8%).

This suggests that death thoughts and wishes occur in a small but substantial group of older people who need attention from society and the healthcare system, for example by developing interventions to prevent or diminish wishes to die in older people. For this to happen it is essential that more is known about the development of death wishes, the consequences of wishes to die for older people who have them, and the possible ways that people themselves see for diminishing their wish to die. This chapter addresses these questions, drawing mostly on a study in the Netherlands of wishes to die in older people. More information on that study is given in Box 10.1.

Box 10.1 Methods of study of older people's wish to die

This chapter draws on results of a study of older people's wish to die that was conducted in the Netherlands. The study consisted of two parts. First, a quantitative study investigated the incidence of wishes to die in older Dutch people and the factors associated with having a wish to die. Second, a qualitative study was carried out to obtain a better understanding of how wishes to die developed and what it meant for a person's life to have a wish to die. These studies have been reported previously in Rurup et al. (2011a,b,c).

Methods for the quantitative study

The quantitative study was based on the Longitudinal Aging Study Amsterdam (LASA), and involved a representative cohort of older people in the Netherlands (Huisman et al. 2011). Measurement waves took place every 3 years using face-to-face interviews and a self-administered questionnaire. The respondents were asked about a broad spectrum of physical, psychological, and social aspects of their life. In the fifth wave (2005/2006), questions about wishes to die derived from Paykel et al. (1974) were included. A total of 1794 older people aged 58–98 years were asked about these questions and about other factors such as basic demographics, social functioning, physical and mental health, functional limitations, life events, and mastery, all of which might be related to wishes to die.

Methods for the qualitative study

Respondents were included from two cohort studies, the LASA study and the Advance Directive Cohort (ADC) (van Wijmen et al. 2010). The latter cohort consisted of a representative sample of people who had made one or more of the most common advance directives in the Netherlands. They had received a questionnaire every 18 months since 2005, and in the 2007 wave, 3754 respondents answered the questions about wishes to die (similar to those in LASA). Using purposive sampling, 16 older people were identified from each cohort who, in the questionnaire or interview, had indicated that they had had only a weak wish, or none at all, to continue living in the past week and/or a weak wish to die in the past week (47 for LASA, 320 for ADC), or that they had had a moderate or strong wish to die in the past week (14 for LASA, 86 for ADC). Of these 32 people, 29 agreed to be interviewed. Two pilot interviews were also used, taking the number of respondents to 31 (13 men and 18 women ranging in age from 49 to 99 years). Of these, according to the responses they gave in the cohort study, 16 respondents had a moderate or strong wish to die and no wish

---

Box 10.1 Methods of study of older people's wish to die (continued)

to live, while the others had other variations of responses to questions on wishes to die. The in-depth interviews took place in the person's home (except one, which took place in a conference room) and lasted between 30 minutes and 2 hours 45 minutes. After an opening question about their thoughts on life and death, compared with what they had filled in earlier, questions were based on the participants' responses, using a topic list as a reminder of the issues that needed to be addressed. The interviews were recorded and fully transcribed. Through sequential analysis, using open and inductive coding, recurring themes were identified. The code list was extended by analysing more interviews, but most codes were created in the analysis of the first 15 interviews. The study procedure was approved by the Ethics Committee of the VU University Medical Center (Amsterdam, the Netherlands).

That this study is qualitative implies that it provides better understanding of reasons and processes, but does not give frequencies of these. When looking at the results, readers should bear this in mind. In light of this it would be right, when presenting the findings, to talk of respondents instead of older people. However, in order to enhance readability in this chapter, respondents are referred to as older people.

Which factors are associated with having a wish to die?

One way of obtaining more information on the development of death wishes is to look for factors that are associated with death thoughts and wishes. This has been done in several studies in different countries. The most frequently studied factor in relation to death wishes is depression. Behind this might be the idea that one must be depressed to have a death wish. All studies have indeed found a relationship between depression and death wishes (Forsell et al. 1997; Rao et al. 1997; Barnow and Linden 2000; Scocco and De Leo 2002; Yip et al. 2003; Skoog et al. 1996; Ayalon 2011; Rurup et al. 2011a; Almeida et al. 2012; Han et al. 2014). However, the strength of the association varies. This can partly be attributed to whether major depression or depressive symptoms were measured. In the Dutch study described in Box 10.1 we found, for instance, that 20% of the older people with a current wish to die had major depression and 67% had depressive symptoms (versus 0.3% and 9% in the group that had never had death thoughts or wishes). Although it is clearly incorrect to assume the presence of depression in older people with a wish to die, the association found shows that the presence of a death wish should trigger an inquiry into the presence of major depression or depressive symptoms. If depression is present, treating it might help diminish the death wish.

In addition to depression, other factors have been examined for their relationship to death wishes in older people, although less thoroughly; factors found to be associated with death wishes in several studies include:

- increased disability in daily living (Jorm et al. 1995; Forsell et al. 1997; Dennis et al. 2007),

- living in an institution, such as in residential care (Jorm et al. 1995; Forsell et al. 1997),

- having a visual or hearing impairment (Jorm et al. 1995; Forsell et al. 1997; Yip et al. 2003),

- having poor self-rated health (Jorm et al. 1995; Dennis et al. 2007; Almeida et al. 2012),

- being widowed, not married, or divorced (Dennis et al. 2007; Jorm et al. 1995; Rurup et al. 2011a),

- having lower (perceived) social support (Dennis et al. 2007; Rurup et al. 2011a; Almeida et al. 2012; Ra and Cho 2013),

- being in pain (Jorm et al. 1995; Almeida et al. 2012),

- being under financial strain (Rurup et al. 2011a; Almeida et al. 2012; Gilman et al. 2013).

Our knowledge about these factors indicates that their presence in older people should possibly encourage a healthcare professional to inquire into a person's feelings about living and dying. However, knowledge of these associated factors does not really provide insight into the interventions that might diminish wishes to die. For that, more in-depth knowledge is necessary. The rest of this chapter will draw on the results of a qualitative study of older people with death wishes (Rurup et al. 2011a,b).

What triggers the development of a wish to die?

From the qualitative study (Box 10.1), five triggers of the development of a wish to die emerged. These triggers are situations that can lead to the development of a death wish.

A first group consisted of older people who had already developed serious thoughts about death at a very young age after a serious traumatic life event, such as abuse or war experiences. While their death wish had been present to some extent throughout their lives, it became more pronounced later due to negative life events (such as loss of a partner or disease) or when important roles in life such as raising children or employment had ended.

For people in the second group, a traumatic life event late in life triggered the development of a wish to die. This was typically the loss of a partner due to death or divorce, but could also be loss of their job due to retirement or illness.

A third group described a life of general adversity and distress that had gradually caused a wish to die to develop. This could be the combination of unrelated problems, such as the loss of several partners, a road accident, or financial problems. As with the other triggers, this was recognized as such by the research team. For this trigger, the evaluation of adversity and distress by the respondents themselves influenced the development of the wish to die. One respondent explained that in other people's lives everything seemed to fit beautifully, with something going wrong only every now and then, while in his life there were too many things that were not as they should have been, and that were not under his control: 'my life is a story imagined by a madman'.

In a fourth group, death wishes had developed as a consequence of ageing or illness that resulted in a diminished quality of life. People in this group typically described how they used to be able to do everything themselves but were now increasingly unable to do so. This could include limitations in personal care, daily activities, or mobility.

Finally, there was a fifth group who suffered from recurring episodes of depression or burnout. They had developed a death wish during one of these episodes. They typically described ups and downs in their feelings towards living and dying.

How does a wish to die develop in older people?

The five types of trigger do not in themselves provide an explanation of how the wish to die developed. Figure 10.1 shows a framework that illustrates how death wishes generally seem to arise. It shows that, after certain life-events or increased impairment due to ageing or illness, people realized that they were in a situation that they did not consider acceptable. Their real situation was too different from their desired situation. People often perceived that they had a lack of control over their lives, which is in line with the finding of the quantitative study that mastery was negatively associated with having a wish to die (Rurup et al. 2011a). They experienced their situation in such a way that it was impossible for them to be content with how life was going. Some situations and

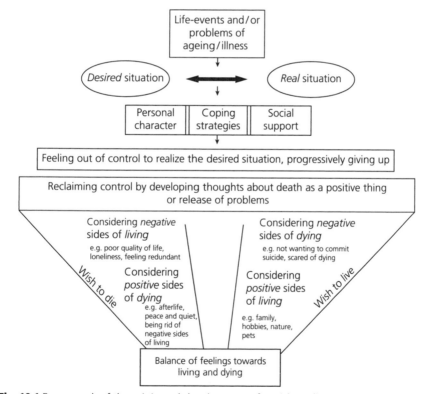

Fig. 10.1 Framework of the origin and development of a wish to die.

Used with permission from M. L. Rurup, H. R. W. Pasman, J. Goedhart, D. J. H. Deeg, A. J. F. M. Kerkhof, and B. D. Onwuteaka-Philipsen, Understanding why older people develop a wish to die, *Crisis: The Journal of Crisis Intervention and Suicide Prevention*, 32(4), pp. 204–216, doi: 10.1027/0227–5910/a000078 Copyright ©2011, Hogrefe Publishing <http://www.hogrefe.com/>

traumatic events described were so exceptional that it seemed likely that many people in such a situation would think of death as a solution. In other situations this seemed less likely, and for those people in particular the development of a wish to die could only be understood in the context of someone's personality, their coping strategies, and the characteristics of their social support system.

For many older people the development of a wish to die seemed to be a conscious or subconscious way of reclaiming control over their lives. They seemed to be unable to influence their lives in such a way that they could change their real situation into something more acceptable and more closely resembling their desired situation, but they felt that at least with death the real situation would end. Once these thoughts of death as a positive way out had developed, the respondents considered the positive and negative sides of both life and death. These considerations were mostly much more elaborate than the original trigger of the wish to die. For instance, growing dependency and impairments were frequently a negative side of living, for people for whom those had not been the actual trigger. Other negative aspects of living could be having financial problems, experiencing their care as poor, or having lost faith in other people. In addition to the positive side of dying—that it would solve their problems—people might believe in an afterlife, where for instance they would be reunited with loved ones, or they would associate death with peace and tranquillity. Negative sides of dying could be practical, for example the inability to consider suicide as an option, or relational in terms of not wanting to end their lives for the sake of their children or other loved ones. Some described a fear of death or dying. Generally, people could also see positive sides of living, especially through a partner, children, or grandchildren if they had good contact. Other positive sides could be related to pleasant activities, and for some people the hope of living to see a certain event such as the birth of a grandchild.

Together, these negative and positive sides formed a balance of feelings towards living and dying. For some this could be very stable, for instance when people said they wished to be dead but would not commit suicide, but more people experienced this balance as less stable.

Recurring themes in older people with a wish to die

Several themes emerged from the analysis of personal characteristics and situations that might influence whether or not older people felt that they had lost control and could not turn their real situation towards their desired one. First, intolerance of dependency seemed important. People who were grieving over losing their partner or their health could feel that their impairments prevented them from overcoming their loss. They could, for instance, feel they were too sick or impaired to find a new purpose in life. Secondly, not being able to be useful to relatives or friends or even to society was an important issue for several older people with a wish to die. Thirdly, having high expectations of other people could play a part in having a death wish. For example, people could have taken care of their own parents in old age, or had generally often been very helpful, and were now disappointed that others did less than they thought they themselves would have done. Finally, experiencing a lack of social contacts seemed important to the development of a wish to die. This could be through a shrinking network due to death of their partner, friends, and acquaintances, or due to having contacts but experiencing these contacts as not very close (as they might have had with a partner). Some people had always had difficulty making friends.

Experienced burden of having a wish to die

There were some older people who described their wish as obsessive. However, older people did not generally consider their wish to die to be very burdensome in itself. It was present more or less in the background. Some people thought about it every day, others less frequently. Some described waves of thinking more or less about it. That being said, everybody thought a lot about the situation that had led to the development of thoughts about death, such as their impairments, the loss of a loved one, financial problems, or a traumatic event they had experienced in childhood. They were sad and/ or disappointed about their situation.

Many older people felt they could not be totally open to loved ones about their wish, and found this burdensome. Many did not tell their children or other loved ones about their wish to die, or told them a watered down version of their thoughts on life and death. Reasons for this could be that they did not want to burden loved ones with their feelings, that they thought it was not a topic for discussion, that they did not want to spoil the atmosphere when they had visitors, or that they thought their loved ones would become angry or sad. This could go together with the feeling that there was no need to discuss their wish with their loved ones because they could not do anything to improve their situation in any case. Some people, even when they thought seeing their children more often would help them, felt that discussing this would be pointless.

Thinking of suicide

As it was a study among living people with a wish to die, the qualitative study could provide no information on older people with a wish to die who had committed suicide. Virtually all older people with a strong wish to die included in the study had seriously considered suicide and possible methods of ending life, and some had also made one or more suicide attempts. There was also a group of people who had collected medication with which to end their life when they thought the right moment had come. Yet most people with a strong wish to die did not have plans to end their life in the near future. They could have several reasons for not considering suicide to be good option for themselves. A very important one was that it would be too painful for their children or other loved ones or for others who would become involved, such as the physician who would prescribe the medication without knowing its real purpose, the train driver if they were planning to jump in front of a train, or the person who would find them after hanging or taking an overdose. These were reasons why a group of people with a strong wish to die would still find suicide unacceptable. There was also a group who generally took the above reasons into consideration but who still wanted to end their life. They did not commit suicide because they were afraid to perform it or afraid of surviving with serious impairments as a consequence. Finally, these reasons could be combined with having reasons to live. These reasons could be indeterminate, in the sense that people were not sure what still bound them to life. This could be described as 'not being allowed to give up'. However, other older people could name specific positive reasons for wanting to stay alive, such as contact with their partner or other loved ones or having pets. Other positive aspects of life, such as having hobbies or cultural activities, were generally looked upon as pleasant ways to pass the time and not as a reason to stay alive. For some people, finding ways to pass time was a strategy to make life as bearable as possible while hoping that death would come quickly. This was especially necessary when they knew that they would not have help in committing suicide or when they wanted to postpone suicide because, for example, they did not want to burden loved ones with it.

In the Netherlands there has been discussion about a 'suicide pill': while such a pill does not exist, should it be possible that older people who are tired of life should have access to medication outside the scope of the euthanasia law (in which unbearable suffering must stem from a medically classifiable illness)? Since such a pill might take away some of the objections that older people with a wish to die have against suicide, participants were asked what their opinion on a 'suicide pill' was (Rurup et al. 2011c). Generally they thought it would be good if such a pill became available under conditions that would prevent people taking it on impulse. There was also a group who thought such a pill would be a good solution for them, either because they would have used it or because they would like to have it just in case. While there were older people who rejected suicide in general but thought the suicide pill to be a good option, there were also people who had similar concerns about a suicide pill to those about suicide by other means. This especially concerned being a burden to others, and also the aspects that made life still worth living, such as contacts with loved ones.

Thoughts about the future

Older people with a wish to die typically avoided thinking about the future. They talked about the future without animation, indicating that they lived from day to day and just waited to see what the future would bring. Generally, they did not seem to have fears about the future that contributed to their current wish to die. However, there was a group who thought that the balance of all the positive and negative aspects of living and dying would make them change their preference towards dying if something particular were to change. This change could be the death of a loved one or further physical deterioration. There was a group who hoped for a serious illness, such as cancer. They saw it as an easy solution to their situation in which ending their life would become legitimate (in light of the euthanasia law). Yet there was also reserve about this scenario in people who did want to die, but not at any cost—not with physical suffering.

What could diminish the wish to die?

When questioned about what might diminish their wish to die, older people could not generally name a situation in which this would happen. There were things or actions that would theoretically improve their situation (Rurup et al. 2011c), but in general they did not consider these feasible in practice. These things or actions could be:

- social, such as getting a new partner, new friendships, restoring/improving contact with children or grandchildren,
- physical, such as hearing better, being more independent and mobile, and having more energy,
- other, such as having more money, travelling, doing (voluntary) work, or living somewhere else.

Looking at this list, some things seem more feasible than others. Some of these options might be considered unfeasible as the result of previous unsuccessful attempts to make new friends or to do voluntary work, for example. Some people considered themselves to be too old to make substantial changes, and others did not feel the need for any further change.

Older people with a wish to die differed in their ideas about obtaining treatment (medical or otherwise) from a general practitioner, psychologist, or psychiatrist. Some people had had such treatment and felt it had helped diminish their wish to die. Others did not feel treatment would be useful because earlier treatments had not helped. When older people had previously discussed their wish to die with the general practitioner this had often led to a psychiatric referral. When this was not wanted, for instance because it felt like they were being considered as 'crazy', or when it did not lead to anything, people would be reluctant to look for help a second time. General practitioners did not always take the initiative to discuss the wish to die again, and while some older people did not expect or want this anymore, others would have liked their general practitioner to initiate discussion. Finally, there was a group who did not want treatment because they felt that it would be unnatural, and that the wish to die was part of who they were. Some people, for instance, felt that their depressive feelings were part of their character or normal within their circumstances; taking antidepressants would not solve their real problems.

In conclusion

There are several practical implications of understanding the wishes to die described in this chapter. Having a wish to die was not necessarily related to a risk of suicide. Nevertheless, this does not mean that the problems of this group do not need attention. While there are many triggers that can cause a wish to die to develop, the feeling of having no control seemed to be an important contributor to the development of a wish to die. This might be a starting point for intervention. Although it is clear that depression plays a role in only some of the older people with a wish to die, and that people with a wish to die are not always eager to receive treatment for depression, it might be helpful for some. Thus, caregivers need to keep an open mind. They should assess psychopathology and comorbidity and the extent to which they are treatable. At the same time they should be open to the independent nature of death wishes that reflect legitimate evaluations of the quality of life. Caregivers should realize that the experiences of older people who had experienced previous unsuccessful attempts by caregivers to treat their problems were important in the development of the wish to die, and this can make them reluctant to try new alternatives. Caregivers' active attention to the wish to die might diminish such negative experiences. Finally, it is important to realize that death wishes can be self-protective by nature. When everything else is out of their control, the wish to stop living is someone's final autonomous protection against the threat of continued life.

References

Almeida, O. P., Draper, B., Snowdon, J., et al. (2012). Factors associated with suicidal thoughts in a large community study of older adults. *British Journal of Psychiatry*, 6, 466–472.

Ayalon, L. (2011). The prevalence and predictors of passive death wishes in Europe: a 2-year follow-up of the Survey of Health, Ageing, and Retirement in Europe. *International Journal of Geriatric Psychiatry*, 26, 923–929.

Barnow, S. and Linden, M. (2000). Epidemiology and psychiatric morbidity of suicidal ideation among the elderly. *Crisis*, 21, 171–180.

Beck, A. T., Kovacs, M., and Weissman, A. (1979). Assessment of suicidal intention: the scale for suicidal ideation. *Journal of Consulting and Clinical Psychology*, 47, 343–352.

Dennis, M., Baillon, S., Brugha, T., Lindesay, J., Stewart, R., and Meltzer, H. (2007). The spectrum of suicidal ideation in Great Britain: comparisons across a 16–74 year age range. *Psychological Medicine*, 37, 795–805.

Forsell, Y., Jorm, A. F., and Winblad, B. (1997). Suicidal thoughts and associated factors in an elderly population. *Acta Psychiatrica Scandinavica*, 95, 108–111.

Gilman, S. E., Bruce, M. L., Ten Have, T., et al. (2013). Social inequalities in depression and suicidal ideation among older primary care patients. *Social Psychiatry and Psychiatric Epidemiology*, 48, 59–69.

Han, B., McKeon, R., and Gfroerer, J. (2014). Suicidal ideation among community-dwelling adults in the United States. *American Journal of Public Health*. 104, 488–497.

Huisman, M., Poppelaars, J., van der Horst, M., et al. (2011). Cohort profile: the Longitudinal Aging Study Amsterdam. *International Journal of Epidemiology*, 40, 868–876.

Jorm, A. F., Henderson, A. S., Scott, R., Korten, A. E., Christensen, H., and Mackinnon, A. J. (1995). Factors associated with the wish to die in elderly people. *Age and Ageing*, 24, 389–392.

Paykel, E. S., Myers, J. K., Lindenthal, J. J., and Tanner, J. (1974). Suicidal feelings in the general population: a prevalence study. *British Journal of Psychiatry*, 124, 460–469.

Ra, C. K. and Cho, Y. (2013). Differentiated effects of social participation components on suicidal ideation across age groups in South Korea. *BMC Public Health*, 13, 890.

Rao, R., Dening, T., Brayne, C., and Huppert, F. A. (1997). Suicidal thinking in community residents over 80. *International Journal of Geriatric Psychiatry*, 12, 337–343.

Rurup, M. L., Deeg, D. J. H., Poppleaars, J. L., Kerkhof, A. J. F. M., and Onwuteaka-Philipsen, B. D. (2011a). Wishes to die in older people: a quantitative study of prevalence and associated factors. *Crisis*, 32, 194–203.

Rurup, M. L., Pasman, H. R. W., Goedhart, J., Deeg, D. J. H., Kerkhof, A. J. F. M., and Onwuteaka-Philipsen, B. D. (2011b). Understanding why older people develop a wish to die. *Crisis*, 32, 204–216.

Rurup, M. L., Pasman, H. R. W., Kerkhof, A. J. F. M., Deeg, D. J. H., and Onwuteaka-Philipsen, B. D. (2011c). Older people who are 'weary of life': their expectations for the future and perceived hopelessness. *Tijdschrift voor Gerontologie en Geriatrie*, 42, 159–169 [in Dutch].

Scocco, P. and De Leo, D. (2002). One-year prevalence of death thoughts, suicide ideation and behaviours in an elderly population. *International Journal of Geriatric Psychiatry*, **17**, 842–846.

Skoog, I., Aevarsson, O., Beskow, J., et al. (1996). Suicidal feelings in a population of non-demented 85-year-olds. *American Journal of Psychiatry*, **153**, 1015–1020.

van Wijmen, M. P., Rurup, M. L., Pasman, H. R., Kaspers, P. J., and Onwuteaka-Philipsen, B. D. (2010). Design of the Advance Directives Cohort: a study of end-of-life decision-making focusing on advance directives. *BMC Public Health*, **10**, 166.

Yip, P. S., Chi, I., Chiu, H., Chi Wai, K., Conwell, Y., and Caine, E. (2003). A prevalence study of suicide ideation among older adults in Hong Kong SAR. *International Journal of Geriatric Psychiatry*, **18**, 1056–1062.

Chapter 11

Dialogue intermezzo: I

CHRISTOPH REHMANN-SUTTER: A wish to die rather than live is a remarkable phenomenon of human agency that still disturbs many clinicians, relatives, and philosophers—and may also, in some circumstances, be difficult for the patients who are experiencing and expressing such wishes to understand. But is the language of 'experience and expression' the right language to use here? Is a wish to die an 'experience' at all, like hunger or pain? Or should such wishes be better understood as elements of purposive action, like a plan?

YASMIN GUNARATNAM: You are right about end-of-life wishes being a remarkable phenomenon. I am not sure that they are a single thing, and it is because of this indeterminacy that care and ethics can become so fraught and challenging: 'Is she saying that she wants to die because she is trying to convey something about how unbearable her physical and existential pain is at this moment, or is this wish a considered choice and request?' More prosaically, there are also the contradictions and changes that can occur in the narration of the self at times of dying: 'She has always believed that her life is in God's hands but she is now asking for help to die.' Do we act on the continuities of her former self—what Ricoeur would call 'narrative identity'—or do we act on what she is saying right now?

I have come to think of an end-of-life wish as what Roger Luckhurst (2002) has called a 'hybrid object', that is, a phenomenon that is a subjective experience and expression but one that is also known and produced in its journeying across different conceptual, disciplinary, and diagnostic borders. For me, as a social scientist, at the level of ontology or how things are, I think there are two main challenges in trying to understand a person's wishes. First, I do worry about literal interpretations of what people say and ask for because this can privilege an overly rational and decontextualized model of subjectivity. The social science mantra is that subjectivity is always relational, produced with regard to others and social contexts; but (!) this touches on the second point, which is that I think the biochemistry of the body can disrupt subjective experience in ways that we don't fully understand. Crucially, what this means is that care practitioners and researchers have to take risks in how they interpret an end-of-life wish, orienting to both the biographical history of someone's life, which can include advance care plans, and to newer, perhaps surprising, expressions. So in the realm of care and research I think we need to keep in mind an ontology of the end-of-life wish that is open to the disjunctures and transitions of experience, especially when disease, pain, and suffering can make such great incursions into personhood and experience.

ALEX MAURON: 'Experience' or 'plan'? Probably both, and there's the rub. Healthcare professionals are better equipped to deal with the former than the latter. Indeed, to listen with empathy to an expressed wish to die and to hear the various subtexts that may underpin the patient's request is an important skill in end-of-life care. The patient may be conveying existential anguish and despair, or signalling exhaustion due to poorly controlled pain and discomfort. These must be heard and acted upon accordingly. Yet to acknowledge seriously the purposive request for aid in dying, when that is in fact the patient's message: that is more difficult and necessarily coloured by the professional's personal values as well as the normative context in which she or he operates. The temptation may well be to practice *acharnement herméneutique*, hermeneutical obstinacy (Mauron 2006), by over-interpreting the patient's expressed wish in such a way that its literal meaning is never allowed to surface. If one is serious about the right to control one's death, one cannot smother the patient's voice under a layer of interpretive creativity, however well-meaning and sincere.

TRACY SCHROEPFER: I think that a wish to die can be many things. In talking with terminally ill patients who express a wish to die, I have found that at times their emotional, spiritual, and social pain is so overwhelming that they simply want to find a way to end that pain. At other times, I have found that a wish to die is a cry for someone to listen—to truly listen and be willing to hear the emotional pain with which the individual is struggling and not try to 'fix' his/her feelings. I have also found that the love of family and friends can lie at the heart of the wish. The fear of what lies ahead in their dying process and what that will mean for their families is often too much for the individual to bear. Finally, I have also found that a wish to die can be simply the need to die with dignity. To be allowed the control over one's own body and have the right to simply say, 'I am done and I am ready to go now.'

HEIKE GUDAT: We might raise the question of why we always understand a wish to die as an expression of 'failure'. Aren't there ill people who see the right moment has come to let a good life end, or who think that letting the natural history of illness happen allows a last phase of life with more dignity (instead of a phase of symptoms, deficits, and frailty)? Many physicians have difficulties in accepting this attitude. Some answer with 'a layer of interpretive creativity', as Alex Mauron mentions, some with antidepressants. What must be done so that physicians or medicine in general can let ill people develop their own form of *ars moriendi*?

GARY RODIN: I agree with Alex, both that the wish to die cannot be collapsed into a single experience and that we should allow literal meanings to emerge. However, in my experience, it is the literal meanings that are most often privileged in medical settings. I agree with Heike about the multiple and contextual meanings of human communication, and about the complex and contradictory nature of human experience and desire—the 'hybrid' Luckhurst mentions. We studied this in longitudinal qualitative research with Rinat Nissim, exploring the desire for hastened death (DHD) in patients with metastatic cancer. We found that for some of these patients, the DHD reflected despair and the wish for life to be shortened, for others it represented a hypothetical plan B, the contemplation of which provided a sense of cognitive mastery, and for others, or for some at other times, it was linked to death acceptance. The

DHD in such patients rarely reflected a clear and purposeful plan. We also know that the majority of some populations endorse assisted dying—perhaps its endorsement bolsters the sense of agency—while only a small minority pursue this as a purposeful plan. Reflective space and an engaged other are needed for such multiple meanings to emerge; these features are not necessarily available in busy medical settings.

References

Luckhurst, R. (2002). *The Invention of Telepathy: 1870–1901*. Oxford: Oxford University Press.

Mauron A. (2006). La médecine moderne et l'assistance au suicide en Suisse. Synthèse du point de vue de la CNE. Symposium de Zürich 17 & 18 Septembre 2004, pp. 309–319. In: C. Rehmann-Sutter, A. Bondolfi, J. Fischer, and M. Leuthold (eds), *Beihilfe zum Suizid in der Schweiz, Beiträge aus Ethik, Recht und Medizin*. Bern: Peter Lang Publishers.

Part III

Ethics

Chapter 12

Caring and killing in the clinic: the argument of self-determination

Lars Johan Materstvedt

Palliative care versus assisted dying

Following what has become the international convention, I take 'assisted dying' to comprise the voluntary forms of euthanasia, physician-assisted suicide (PAS) and (non-physician) assisted suicide (Materstvedt 2012). According to the World Health Organization (WHO), 'Palliative care is an approach that . . . affirms life' and that does not intend 'to hasten . . . death' (World Health Organization 2015), whereas euthanasia is medicalized 'killing on request' (Griffiths et al. 1998, p. 17). By intentionally hastening death by means of lethal injection, rather than affirming life, the latter approach *rejects* life (Materstvedt 2012). So, in these conceptions, palliative care and euthanasia are like fire and water.

Yet both palliative care and assisted dying are found side by side in some palliative care institutions in Belgium (Bernheim et al. 2008). Furthermore, a number of nursing homes all over Switzerland, and a few hospitals in the French-speaking part of the country, have allowed assisted suicide to be performed on their premises in recent years (Pereira et al. 2008). From a purely practical point of view, then, these opposite practices can obviously coexist.

However, several serious issues are associated with this combination of caring and killing. For instance, patients in such wards may lose the will to live, and they may come to think that it is their duty to request assisted dying. It also increases the danger that palliative care becomes a neglected concern in times of economic crisis, with the emphasis shifting to the less costly alternative of assisted dying—I deal with these and related issues in Materstvedt (2013) and in Materstvedt and Bosshard (2015).

Autonomy as self-determination

From an ethical point of view, justifying the combination of palliative care and assisted dying would require a different outlook on palliative care from that of the WHO. It is noteworthy that the WHO definition makes no reference to patient autonomy, whereas what I shall call 'the argument of autonomy' is a key issue for those who defend assisted dying. A persuasive one, the argument has been found to enjoy support even among terminally ill patients at a palliative medicine unit (Johansen et al. 2005).

'Autonomy' stems from the Greek *auto* [self], and *nomos* [law]. Thus it means self-legislation: one gives oneself the 'laws' by which one chooses to live. In other words: I myself determine how to lead my life. We may therefore speak of the triangularity of the concepts of autonomy/self-legislation/self-determination; they can be taken to cover the same phenomenon.

Kant on suicide—and on physician-assisted suicide and euthanasia

First and foremost, the German philosopher Immanuel Kant (1724–1804) is the 'father' of autonomy in the sense of being the originator of the way that autonomy is thought of and spoken about in modern Western society. Furthermore, within Kant's ethical system, 'autonomy [*Autonomie*] is the ground of the dignity [*Würde*] of human nature and of every rational nature' (Kant 1981, p. 436/41)[1]. The impact of Kant's thinking on Western societies, both with respect to individual freedom—including laws regulating such freedom—and conceptions of what constitutes right and wrong conduct in very many areas, can hardly be overrated (Materstvedt 2011).

In one of the most influential works of ethics, *Grounding for the Metaphysics of Morals* [*Grundlegung*], Kant discusses the issue of suicide [*Selbstmord*] twice. He begins by expressing great understanding towards people who contemplate killing themselves, referring to a man who experiences hopelessness [*Hoffnungslosigkeit*] and 'feels sick of life' (Kant 1981, p. 421/30). Despite these sentiments, Kant goes on, this person 'is still so far in possession of his reason [*Vernunft*]' (Kant 1981, p. 422/30) that he 'will ask himself whether his action can be consistent with the idea of humanity as an end in itself [*als Zweks an sich selbst*]. If he destroys himself in order to escape from a difficult situation, then he is making use of his person merely as a means so as to maintain a tolerable condition till the end of his life. Man, however, is not a thing and hence is not something to be used merely as a means: he must in all his actions always be regarded as an end in himself. Therefore, I cannot dispose of man in my own person by mutilating [*verstümmeln*], damaging [*verderben*], or killing him' (Kant 1981, p. 429/36).

Suicide thus runs against the second formula of the categorical imperative, or the moral law—in Kant a distinctive feature of a human being's transcendental, practical reason, regardless of time in history, culture, ethnicity, sex, or race—which states: 'Act in such a way that you treat humanity, whether in your own person or in the person of another, always at the same time as an end and never simply as a means [*Mittel*]' (Kant 1981, p. 429/36).

By the same token, I believe, Kant would have taken *physician-assisted* suicide and *assisted* suicide to be immoral. Additionally, both categories emerge as self-contradictory and irrational because one makes use of one's autonomy to put an end to that very autonomy. This is Kant's core logical argument against suicide. The argument may be extended to include euthanasia by the following reasoning: 'Unlike physician-assisted suicide, euthanasia requires that the physician intends the patient's death' which, it is further observed, 'is, in both cases, triggered *by the patient's own voluntary and competent request*. Morally, the event is then suicide assisted by another. The extent to which the patient can physically co-operate makes no moral difference' (Pogge 2003; italics in original).

A duty to stay alive?

Would this argument also apply to patients who refuse life-sustaining treatment or want it discontinued (i.e. who demand that such treatment is withheld or withdrawn)? I pose this question because sometimes a non-treatment decision (NTD) can result in a shorter lifespan than might follow from continued treatment. So, for example, when a competent dying patient decides to stop taking antibiotics his or her life might well be shortened as a consequence. If this happens, the 'destruction' of his or her autonomy for the additional period of time they might have enjoyed with continued treatment follows from this autonomous decision. Based on the Kantian conception, is there then a moral duty to stay alive for as long as possible for the sake of exercising one's autonomy until the (natural) end (Materstvedt and Bosshard 2010)?

Regardless of the answer, there is this additional issue: would a duty to never decline, or always demand, life-prolonging treatment be imperfect or perfect? Practical (as opposed to theoretical) reason informs us that a perfect duty must always be observed because it cannot be refused without contradiction. By contrast, an imperfect duty is 'wide', meaning that 'it determines nothing about the kind and extent of actions themselves but allows a latitude for free choice [*freien Willkür*]' (Kant 1991a, p. 446/240). Not so with refraining from committing suicide, which in the *Doctrine of Virtue* [*Tugendlehre*] is an example of a perfect duty to oneself (Kant 1991a, p. 421/218). Here it is claimed that 'Killing oneself is a crime [*Verbrechen*] (murder [*Mord*]). It can also be regarded as a violation of one's duty to other human beings (the duty of spouses to each other, of parents to their children, . . .)' (Kant 1991a, p. 422/218).

Saying no to life-sustaining treatment would *not* be on a par with killing oneself; rather, in this case it is the illness that kills—one lets nature take its course. Accordingly, death is not hastened even though life is sometimes thereby *shortened*—it is pivotal that these two phenomena be kept separate, as they are not the same (Materstvedt 2013). In conclusion, then, even supposing that there is, from a Kantian point of view, a duty to always stay alive, this would never amount to a perfect duty.

On morality and legality

Furthermore, Kant draws a fundamental distinction between morality [*Moralität*] and legality [*Legalität*], and this distinction is also of relevance to the question 'What would Kant have said?' All things that according to reason are immoral cannot at the same time be illegal, Kant argues, or else one would witness 'the moralization of the law' (Materstvedt 1997). In modern terms, this would be akin to a Taliban regime, under which people are, for example, thrown into jail for being unfaithful to their spouse; without a distinction between morality and legality, lying to your partner about having an affair would carry a sentence. Such an arrangement would violate the (human) right to freedom and would thus fail to treat people as 'ends in themselves'. Hence, there can be no free society without room for the legal performance of immoral acts.

But where do you draw the line? Although murder will be both immoral and illegal, interestingly in our context suicide appears to qualify only as the former within the Kantian system. The Norwegian philosopher Nils Gilje writes: 'Force can be used . . . in order to make one meet one's legal obligations. In contrast, moral obligations cannot be enforced. Kant allocates the moral prohibition on suicide, for instance, to this category' (Gilje 1989, p. 304; my translation).

Kant does not state this explicitly, hence it is an interpretation of his political philosophy; a correct interpretation, I believe. What brings me to this conclusion is the basic scheme of duties delineated by Kant in *The Metaphysics of Morals*, the doctrine of right [*Rechtslehre*], which distinguishes between moral duties [*Tugendpflichten*] and legal duties [*Rechtspflichten*] (Kant 1991a, pp. 239–40/25–6). In the same vein, the prominent Kant scholar Paul Guyer observes: 'Kant . . . argue[s] that the only proper aim of coercive juridical legislation is the prevention of injury to the person and property of *others*' (Guyer 1998; italics added). Hence, what you do to *yourself* is not a matter for legislation. In this respect, Kant is a very modern thinker for his time—or, more precisely, he is way ahead of his time.

Still, what Kant writes elsewhere seems to contradict this highly individualistic liberalism. For instance, he unambiguously states that 'everyone has his inalienable rights [*unverlierbaren Rechte*], which he cannot give up even if he wishes to' (Kant 1991b, p. 304/84), and that 'no-one can voluntarily renounce his rights by a contract or legal transaction [*rechtliche Handlung*] to the effect that he has no rights [*keine Rechte*] . . . .' (Kant 1991b, p. 292/75). The implementation of assisted dying entails that a patient gives up his or her right to life. Having signed away this ultimate right, the patient is left with no rights whatsoever. By implication, it appears to follow that a patient may not enter into a contract with his or her doctor about assisted dying.

At the very least, such a prohibition does not sit well with Kant's insistence that a state that tries to make its citizens happy according to *its* idea of happiness would be 'the greatest conceivable *despotism*', treating the subjects 'as immature children [*als unmündige Kinder*] who cannot distinguish what is truly useful or harmful to themselves' (Kant 1991b, pp. 290–1/74; italics in original).

Kant on assisted dying: is it legally acceptable?

I have argued that since killing oneself is morally repugnant to Kant, the same holds for a doctor injecting a patient with lethal substances at his or her voluntary and competent request, or a doctor or layperson helping a patient commit suicide (as practised in Switzerland). But whereas what according to the Dutch penal code qualifies as medical murder, i.e. non-voluntary and involuntary drug-induced ending of life (Griffiths et al. 2008; Materstvedt 2012), will no doubt be outlawed by Kantian standards, this might not be the case for assisted dying, by the same token that 'normal' suicide is not deemed illegal due to the distinction between moral duties and legal duties. Indeed, I believe this distinction to be so important in Kant's system that it outweighs his view on inalienable rights; the distinction commits him to discard these rights—they must give way.

However, should assisted dying entail a *threat* to the life of other patients, Kant would have rejected it as illegal. For then the practice would breach 'the universal principle of right' [*Allgemeines Prinzip des Rechts*] found in the doctrine of right, which spells out that 'Any action is *right* [*recht*] if it can coexist with everyone's freedom in accordance with a universal law, or if on its maxim the freedom of choice [*Willkür*] of each can coexist with everyone's freedom in accordance with a universal law' (Kant 1991a, p. 230/56). And elsewhere: '*Right* [*Recht*] is the restriction of each individual's freedom so that it harmonises with the freedom of everyone else (in so far as this is possible within the terms of a general law [*allgemeinen Gesetze*])' (Kant 1991b, pp. 289–90/73).

This is reminiscent of the position of another great liberal, namely the English philosopher John Stuart Mill (1806–1873), who was born 2 years after Kant's death. Mill's 'harm principle' reads as follows: 'The only purpose for which power can be rightfully exercised over any member of a civilised community against his will, is to prevent harm to others. . . . Over himself, over his own body and mind, the individual is sovereign' (Mill 1991, p. 78).

The formal meaning of both Kant's and Mill's principle is that the area of my freedom borders on yours: my freedom of action stops where yours begins, and vice versa. What, then, are the *real* boundaries of individual freedom? This will be determined by law; and should our interests happen to 'collide', the dispute is accordingly a matter for the courts to decide.

Leading researchers from the Netherlands and the United States have insisted that legalized assisted dying does not put vulnerable patients at risk (Battin et al. 2007). I have argued elsewhere that, by its very nature, the available quantitative evidence cannot support this claim; nor do we currently have access to the sort of *qualitative* evidence that might have underpinned it (Materstvedt 2009, 2013). The fact of the matter, then, is that all we have are anecdotes. We are accordingly not in a position to assess this claim against the principles put forward by Kant and Mill.

J. S. Mill on assisted dying: is it morally acceptable?

While Kant, as we have seen, would have rejected assisted dying on moral grounds, it is not clear whether or not Mill would have done the same. The Utilitarian maxim of 'the greatest happiness of the greatest number' (Mill 1991) speaks in favour of pursuing the minimization of pain and other suffering, the 'volume' of which would indeed be smaller if *eradicated* by way of assisted dying. Morally speaking, the principle of utility therefore appears to open the door to assisted dying.

It has been claimed that Mill's psychological hedonism entails that 'pleasure is not only all we do desire, but all we can desire, as a matter of necessity' (Benn 1998, p. 68). Now, if that were completely true it would seem to entail that all who experience severe and persisting suffering as they approach the end of life would request assisted dying. But the large-scale studies of the Dutch practice carried out in 1990, 1995, 2001, 2005, and 2010 have consistently shown that even when assisted dying is available this kind of request is made by relatively few (Onwuteaka-Philipsen et al. 2003, 2012; van der Heide et al. 2007).

Self-ownership and assisted dying: Locke and Nozick

The argument of self-determination is a strong one in the debate on assisted dying. This argument is stronger still if it is based on the idea that people *own* themselves; for if they do, it would seem that what they do with their bodies is entirely a matter for their own discretion. Self-ownership is an idea that originates with one of the most prominent philosophers within the liberal tradition, namely the Englishman John Locke (1632–1704). Also a physician, Locke wrote that 'every Man has a *Property* in his own *Person*. This no Body has any Right to but himself' (Locke 1988, §27/287; italics in original).

Born nearly a hundred years before Kant, Locke's influence on Western thought, politics, society, and legislation is paramount. For example, the US Declaration of Independence of 1776 adopts the political philosophy of Locke's *Second Treatise of Government* (1698) in one of its most famous passages, namely: 'We hold these truths to be self-evident, that all men are created equal, that they are endowed by their Creator with certain unalienable Rights, that among these are Life, Liberty and the pursuit of Happiness' (Declaration of Independence 1776).

One key formulation here is 'certain unalienable Rights', which can only mean that there is a limit to what you can do to yourself; according to Locke, you may not rescind the right to life, for instance. Hence, 'every one . . . is *bound to preserve himself*, and not to quit his Station wilfully . . .' (Locke 1988, §6/271; italics in original). And elsewhere, Locke confirms this stance: 'For a Man, not having the Power of his own Life, *cannot*, by . . . his own Consent . . . put himself under the . . . Power of another, to take away his Life . . . No body can give more Power than he has himself; and he that cannot take away his own Life, cannot give another power over it . . .' (Locke 1988, §23/284; italics in original). And so assisted dying is ruled out.

In Locke, self-destruction is not an available option because self-ownership is limited by the 'big' owner of us all, God, who created humanity and who decides for each and every one of us when it is time to leave this world. But the semi-Lockean US philosopher Robert Nozick (1938–2002), whose *Anarchy, State, and Utopia* (1974) remains one of the classics of the twentieth century, is unhampered by such religious metaphysics (for a detailed exposition and discussion of Nozick's political philosophy see Materstvedt 1997). Nozick's conception of self-ownership justifies total control over oneself (Nozick 1974, p. 58; italics in original):

> A person may choose to do himself, I shall suppose, the things that would impinge across his boundaries [i.e. violate his rights] when done without his consent by another. (Some of these things may be impossible for him to do to himself.) Also, he may give another permission to do these things to him (including things impossible for him to do to himself). Voluntary consent opens the border for crossings. . . . My nonpaternalistic position holds that someone may choose (or permit another) to do to himself *anything*, unless he has acquired an obligation to some third party not to do or allow it.
>
> Reproduced from Robert Nozick, *Anarchy, State, and Utopia.* Wiley-Blackwell, Oxford Copyright © 2001, Wiley-Blackwell

It is clear that this position makes assisted dying morally permissible: your being in total possession of yourself means that you may also treat and even dispose of yourself like any other commodity. Interestingly, in 1997 Nozick became involved in the campaign for legalization of physician-assisted suicide in the United States—which with the Oregon Death with Dignity Act was indeed legalized later in the same year. Listing a number of famous American philosophers as co-authors—Ronald Dworkin, Thomas Nagel, John Rawls, Thomas Scanlon, and Judith Jarvis Thomson—Nozick published a piece called 'Assisted suicide: the philosophers' brief' in *The New York Review of Books* (Rawls et al. 1997). The basic argument of the article is the individual's right to autonomy or self-determination.

Still, reserving physician-assisted suicide for the terminally ill, which is what both the brief and the Oregon law prescribe, runs afoul of the non-paternalistic[2] position declared by Nozick several years earlier in *Anarchy, State, and Utopia*. Why is that? Because it represents disrespect of the self-ownership of those who are *not* terminally ill but who might nevertheless want access to assisted dying. According to Nozick's conception in his book, a state imposing such a limitation on people's individual rights practices 'partial slavery' since it acts as if it owns shares in you and is thus entitled to decide for you or partake in your decisions. Hence the following position of the philosophers' brief would also fail the slavery 'test': 'States may be allowed to prevent assisted suicide by people who—it is plausible to think—would later be grateful if they were prevented from dying' (Rawls et al. 1997). Quite the contrary, states may *not* be allowed to do so.

The Oregon law states that 'The attending physician shall: . . . (h) Inform the patient that he or she has an opportunity to rescind the request at any time and in any manner, and offer the patient an opportunity to rescind at the end of the 15 day waiting period pursuant to ORS 127.840' (Oregon law on physician-assisted suicide 1997). But this kind of requirement is explicitly rejected by Nozick: '. . . nor may lesser paternalistic restrictions geared to nullify supposed defects in people's decision processes be imposed—for example, compulsory information programs, waiting periods' (Nozick 1974, p. 324). It follows that if judged according to Nozick's conception of individual freedom this law would constitute 'paternalistic aggression', which he defines as 'using or threatening force for the benefit of the person against whom it is wielded' (Nozick 1974, p. 34).

Indeed, not even the laws in the Netherlands and Belgium would escape this characterization. For although in both countries assisted dying as a legal option in principle also includes the chronically and psychiatrically ill, the patient must suffer 'unbearably and hopelessly' in a medical sense in order to qualify (Materstvedt and Bosshard 2015). According to the Nozickean conception, you would not need to be ill at all, for 'whose body is it anyway?'.

Nozick's conception would doubtlessly underpin the view that so-called 'tiredness of life' in the old, without any accompanying serious somatic or psychiatric disease, ought to be sufficient ground for assisted dying. This view has recently been found to have considerable support among the Dutch public (Raijmakers et al. 2015), although the Dutch Supreme Court has ruled that such suffering is not covered by the euthanasia law (Rurup 2012). That said, to Nozick even this is too narrow, for *any* requirement that entails non-consented restrictions would be paternalistic: why only in the old; why would one need to be 'finished with life' or to be suffering from 'life fatigue', as it has also been called?

Are people really 'the best judges of their own interests'?

The philosopher Derek Parfit remarks that 'we are paternalists when we make someone act in his own interests' (Parfit 1984, p. 321). It has been observed that 'paternalism runs against the main currents of liberal thinking, for typically liberals insist that each person is the best judge of his or her own welfare' (Miller 1991, p. 368)—an idea which is central to the assisted dying debate. In the same vein, it has been claimed that people 'are independent and rational beings, who are the sole generators of their own wants and preferences, and the best judges of their own interests' (Lukes 1973, p. 79).

However, the question is whether one's own best interest is always what one judges it to be. Besides, how can we possibly *know* that people are the best judges of their own interests; how would one go about assessing the truth or falsity of this claim? But let us, for the sake of argument, assume that it is true. From this it then appears to follow that *nobody else*, only the person in question, can have the correct knowledge about that person's own interests: other people are in principle incapable of gaining direct access to this sort of information since it can only be possessed 'from within' by the person themselves. That is why any person is said to be the *best* judge of his or her own interests; in comparison, other people's judgements concerning these interests are not as good.

Now this person might well proceed to *tell* others what constitutes his or her real interests, thus providing 'outsiders' with an indirect route to the information—but this does not mean that others are in a position to *know*. For one thing, the person could be lying. But more fundamentally, people's (allegedly) exclusive, direct access to the truth about their own interests means that others cannot 'check' whether a person's interpretation, insight, introspection, or whatever we want to call it, is correct. Accordingly, others are never in a position to know *for sure*. And 'who would call that *knowing*?', a rejoinder might go. But even granting that this sort of knowledge is personal, can anyone be sure that *they* have got it right, even if they have the most direct access to their own minds? How do they know that they know, and so on—indefinitely (ad infinitum).

Whether or not the best-judges doctrine is true or false, seen from the perspective of ordinary, everyday, non-philosophical life I believe that our self-image encapsulates the view that we are *generally* the best judges of our own interests. By implication, we admit that in some instances this is not the case. For example, one sometimes hears people complaining that they did not know their own interests at specific past points in time. This is probably why our best thoughts are said to be *after*thoughts—especially those thoughts which emerge after we have done (what we now take to be) stupid things.

But even so, a person might be wrong in thinking now that they acted contrary to their own interests at that other time. Looking back, they might be exercising misguided self-criticism. Also, they might misunderstand what constitutes their own interests *at the present time*. So while for the moment they might feel confident that '*now* I see', they might be wrong this time around, too—and, in theory, they might remain equally misguided for the rest of their life.

A person may have several reasons, then, for doubting that they are the best judge of their own interests *at specific points in time*, although not doubting their own judgement at a general level. For we will be reluctant to let go of the idea that we know best—'after all, *I* am the best judge of my own interests'—even if we might acknowledge that a close friend, say, at a particular point saw more clearly than we did what was best for us.

But notice that even in holding a friend's judgement to be 'better' than mine, the standard of measurement is defined by *me*: my best interests as *I myself* see them. It is against the background of these interests, i.e. against the background of what I *conceive* them to be, that I now think a friend made a better assessment back then.

Self-determination in practice: how wishes to die tend to fluctuate

This leaves us with a perhaps surprising conclusion: the idea that 'I know what is best for me' is actually hard to defend both in principle and in practice. In the context of palliative care, this idea becomes all the more dubious. The autonomous faculties can be impaired in the seriously ill—sometimes severely so—due to factors such as clinical depression, hopelessness (Beck scale), pain, dyspnoea, nausea, delirium, fatigue, cachexia, perceived meaninglessness, and existential crisis/suffering. Additionally, dementia might be an issue.

As far as autonomy is concerned, this means that while patients have a *right* to decide for themselves, they will sometimes lack sufficient *capacity* to do so. It is thus crucial to distinguish between ethical and empirical autonomy, respectively, as I have denoted these different levels elsewhere (Materstvedt 2011).

In the assisted dying debate, the philosopher Neil Campbell has taken the argument of empirical (as opposed to ethical) autonomy to extremes. Regarding a rule that allows euthanasia in cases of unbearable suffering, he questions whether such patients are in a situation conducive to making a free choice: 'If the pain and suffering are by definition unbearable, then it seems clear enough that the decision to die is not freely chosen but is compelled by the pain.' He asks us to 'consider the analogy of the prisoner who is tortured for information', and proposes that 'the natural conclusion to draw from this is that there can be no such thing as voluntary euthanasia' (Campbell 1999).

This argument goes to the heart of the euthanasia laws in the Netherlands and Belgium: in both countries it is required that the patient's suffering must be 'unbearable'. At the same time, a request for assisted dying must be 'voluntary', or if you like, free (Netherlands' law on euthanasia 2002; Belgian law on euthanasia 2002). But how can the requirements of 'unbearable suffering' and 'voluntary' choice ever coincide? If they cannot coincide, it would seem that those laws thereby contain contradictory elements.

We know that there is much fluctuation in the will to live in the terminally ill (Chochinov et al. 1999). The same goes for the wish to hasten death. As a post-doctoral fellow with the Norwegian Cancer Society (<https://kreftforeningen.no/en>), I carried out research on the relationship between palliative medicine and euthanasia, which included conducting interviews with terminally ill cancer patients at a palliative medicine unit about their attitudes towards assisted dying (Johansen et al. 2005). A frequent finding was that patients uttered the *possibility* of wishing for assisted dying—some time in the future, never now, and thus only as a hypothetical possibility.

Furthermore, some wishes were inconsistent—as illustrated by the following conversation taken from the interview with patient 6 in Johansen et al. (2005) (the quoted text has been slightly amended by me for the present context):

'I have big ups and downs', states the patient. 'Some days, I just want to disappear. There have been several occasions where I have felt that I wanted help to do just that. But at other times, everything is different.' The interviewer then asks if the patient has ever thought of taking his own life. 'Never', he responds. The interviewer goes on to inquire whether the patient has never had any concrete wishes to get such help from a doctor, 'Yes, I have', he answers, 'but you know, when the situation arrives and you are faced with the reality of it, I don't think I would have gone through with it anyway. You want to postpone.'

We found clear differences between attitudes, wishes, and requests. We also unravelled what seem to be the characteristics and nature of wishes for assisted dying: ambivalence, fluctuation, and hypotheticalness. Furthermore, such wishes may represent a kind of emergency plan, a possible future 'solution' or way out; they may thus have a positive psychological impact in that they create a feeling of control and consolation. The hypothesis that such wishes may actually represent a coping strategy should be further explored in future research.

Given the many possible meanings of an expressed wish for assisted dying (see Chapters 3 and 8), the obvious and highly dangerous scenario is the doctor who responds to patients' appeals for such hastened death as if they were actual requests. Because of the irrevocable nature of assisted dying, it is of the utmost importance that healthcare workers are aware of the apparently ambivalent nature of patients' stated wishes for assisted dying, and that these statements may mean something completely different from an actual request for hastened death. Another observation is that even if a seriously ill patient is in favour of assisted dying in principle, this does not, according to our results, signify that the person wants to request it, that he or she has personal wishes for it to apply to their own person, or that they want it legalized (Johansen et al. 2005).

Furthermore, many clinicians working within palliative care have occasionally experienced that an apparent request (i.e. not only a wish) for euthanasia turns out to be something else altogether. It could be a cry for help or better pain management, or perhaps an expression of a strong desire for social and psychological support: the patient wants to be 'seen' and recognized as a valuable person in his or her own right, someone whose life is worth living, even if miserable, and who is important to other people.

So what do patients actually want when they request assisted dying? If in the context of a dinner party I ask for a glass of water, it is obvious to others that I am thirsty. If in the context of terminal care I ask for a lethal injection, it can be a lot harder to tell whether this is in fact what I really want. Interestingly, less than half of all requests for assisted dying are granted by Dutch physicians (Onwuteaka-Philipsen et al. 2012).

Concluding remarks

From an ethical point of view, it has been noticed that self-determination is being used as a crucial argument in the current assisted dying debate: 'the principle of autonomy is one of the most important arguments of those who are in favor of the legalization of euthanasia' (Griffiths et al. 1998, p. 168). Kant's theory of autonomy is the key theory on this topic by a wide margin. As we have seen in this chapter, this theory does not lend straightforward support to the legalization of assisted dying, rather, it points in two separate directions. Morally speaking, within Kant's system the argument of autonomy does not hold water as support for assisted dying. Legally speaking, though, Kant's view of autonomy—as this writer understands it—would in fact underpin assisted dying, presuming that its legalization does not in practice run foul of 'the universal principle of right' (Kant 1991a, p. 230/56).

From an empirical point of view, the combination of caring and killing, practised in certain institutions in Belgium, carries with it a number of dangers and is fraught with hugely difficult issues regarding patient autonomy and, at a deeper level, whether or not a person can know what his or her best interests are. All of these issues have become much more relevant with the very recent legalization of euthanasia in Québec, Canada, where the law requires that 'Every institution must adopt a policy with respect to end-of-life care', and that its annual 'report must also state, where applicable, the number of times . . . medical aid in dying were administered . . . *in the premises of a palliative care hospice* by a physician' (Québec law on euthanasia 2014; italics added). In other words, the law explicitly paves the way for a practice akin to the Belgian 'integral' model (Bernheim et al. 2008; Materstvedt 2013).

As a final point, I would like to bring attention to the Orwellian Newspeak permeating the topic of assisted dying. For example, the Québec law uses the euphemism 'care' as a substitute for voluntary killing by lethal injection: '"medical aid in dying" means *care* consisting in the administration by a physician of medications or substances to an end-of-life patient, at the patient's request' (Québec law on euthanasia 2014; italics added). Whereas care will be given up until the point at which euthanasia is performed, euthanasia quite obviously is not care and thus the law's statement is false. Indeed, euthanasia is not medical treatment, even though it is a medical *act* (Materstvedt and Bosshard 2010).

It is further claimed that 'medical aid in dying' is carried out 'in order to *relieve* . . . suffering by hastening death' (Québec law on euthanasia 2014; italics added). This way of putting it is fundamentally flawed and involves what philosophers call a category mistake: euthanasia is not about relieving suffering, it is about ending life as a way to *stop* suffering (Materstvedt and Bosshard 2009; Materstvedt 2012).

The Oregon statute also contains notable examples of Newspeak: a patient who qualifies, it states, 'may make a written request for medication for the purpose of ending his or her life in a humane and dignified manner' (Oregon law on physician-assisted suicide 1997). Nowhere in the statute is there any mention of 'physician-assisted suicide'.[3] To end one's life 'in a humane and dignified manner' surely sounds better than committing suicide aided by a doctor, yet such wording does not change the fact of the matter. Whatever one thinks of killing patients at their voluntary request or helping them kill themselves, these are serious acts and should be described accordingly. Using palatable terms to gloss over the stark reality is both misleading and unhelpful.

And whatever one thinks of euthanasia in the Netherlands, the Dutch deserve credit for being frank about what euthanasia is: '"Euthanasia" in the strict—and in the Dutch context the only proper—sense refers to the situation in which a doctor kills a person who is suffering "unbearably" and "hopelessly" at the latter's explicit request (usually by administering a lethal injection) . . . "euthanasia" is in the Netherlands reserved for killing on request' (Griffiths et al. 1998, p. 17). Finally, there are many who readily acknowledge the problems associated with the practice, such as physician and philosopher Gerrit Kimsma, a well-known Dutch advocate for and practitioner of euthanasia: 'I ended the unacceptable suffering of a terminal patient with brain tumor by injection in 1977; this was my first time . . . I still feel ambivalent about it . . . From early on I have been aware of the "open ends", risks, and dangers of these irreversible interventions by physicians' (Kimsma 2012).

Notes

1 The page numbers in the references to quotations from Kant are from the German Akademie-Ausgabe edition and the particular English translation of the work used, respectively.

2 Notice that while being non-paternalistic, Nozick's position is not *anti*-paternalistic: it is not against paternalism as such, provided it is voluntary. And so anyone is free to enter into any paternalistic arrangement over himself or herself. A legal ban on entering into such arrangements would violate a person's self-ownership. For a comprehensive account and critical discussion of this topic, see Materstvedt (1997).

3 Not even the name of the statute itself uses this expression; it is called 'The Oregon Death with Dignity Act'. However, both in the reference here and in other places in the present chapter, as well as and in the reference list, I have chosen to call it what it undeniably is: a law on physician-assisted suicide.

References

Battin, M.P., van der Heide, A., Ganzini, L., van der Wal, G., and Onwuteaka-Philipsen, B.D. (2007). Legal physician-assisted dying in Oregon and The Netherlands: evidence concerning the impact on patients in 'vulnerable' groups. *Journal of Medical Ethics*, **33**, 591–597.

Belgian law on euthanasia (2002). The Belgian Act on Euthanasia of May, 28th 2002. *Ethical Perspectives*, **9**(2–3), 182–8. URL: <http://www.ethical-perspectives.be/viewpic.php?lan=e&table=ep&id=59>

Benn, P. (1998). *Ethics. Fundamentals of Philosophy Series*. London: University College London Press.

Bernheim, J. L., Deschepper, R., Distelmans, W., Mullie, A., Bilsen, J., and Deliens, L. (2008). Development of palliative care and legalisation of euthanasia: antagonism or synergy? *British Medical Journal*, **336**, 864–867.

Campbell, N. (1999). A problem for the idea of voluntary euthanasia. *Journal of Medical Ethics*, **25**, 242–244.

Chochinov, H. M., Tataryn, D., Clinch, J. J., and Dudgeon, D. (1999). Will to live in the terminally ill. *Lancet*, **354**, 816–819.

Declaration of Independence (1776). *The Declaration of Independence: A Transcription*. URL: <http://www.archives.gov/exhibits/charters/declaration_transcript.html>

Gilje, N. (1989) *Det naturrettslige kontraktparadigmet. En teorihistorisk analyse av naturretts-filosofi og kontrakttenkning i tradisjonen fra Hobbes til Kant*. Skriftserien no. 11. Bergen: Centre for the Study of the Sciences and the Humanities, University of Bergen. URL: <http://www.fou.uib.no/drgrad/1990/533001/> [in Norwegian]

Griffiths, J., Weyers, H., and Bood, A. (ed.) (1998) *Euthanasia and Law in the Netherlands*. Amsterdam: Amsterdam University Press.

Griffiths, J., Weyers, H., and Adams, M. (ed.) (2008) *Euthanasia and Law in Europe*. Oxford: Hart Publishing.

Guyer, P. (1998, 2004). Kant, Immanuel. In: E. Craig (ed.), *Routledge Encyclopedia of Philosophy*. London: Routledge. Available at: <http://www.rep.routledge.com/article/db047sect10>

Johansen, S., Hølen, J. C., Kaasa, S., Loge, J. H., and Materstvedt, L. J. (2005). Attitudes towards, and wishes for, euthanasia in advanced cancer patients at a palliative medicine unit. *Palliative Medicine*, **19**, 454–460. [Appendix 'Themes and questions from the interview guide – entire list of questions' available at: <http://folk.ntnu.no/larsmat/SLB_study_ english_version_questions.pdf>; written information and informed consent form for the study available at: <http://folk.ntnu.no/larsmat/SLB_study_written_information_and_ informed_consent_form.pdf>]

Kant, I. (1981). *Grounding for the Metaphysics of Morals* [Grundlegung zur Metaphysik der Sitten], transl. J. W. Ellington. Indianapolis: Hackett Publishing.

Kant, I. (1991a). *The Metaphysics of Morals: Doctrine of Right & Doctrine of Virtue* [Metaphysische Anfangsgründe der Rechtslehre & Metaphysiche Anfangsgründe der Tugendlehre], transl. M. Gregor. Cambridge: Cambridge University Press.

Kant, I. (1991b). On the common saying: 'This may be true in theory, but it does not apply in practice' [Über den Gemeinspruch: Das mag in der Theorie richtig sein, taugt aber nicht für die Praxis]. In: H. Reiss (ed.), *Kant's Political Writings*, pp. 61–92. Cambridge: Cambridge University Press.

Kimsma, G. K. (2012). Preface. In: S. J. Youngner and G. K. Kimsma (eds), *Physician-Assisted Death in Perspective. Assessing the Dutch Experience*, pp. vx–xvii. Cambridge: Cambridge University Press.

Locke, J. (1988). *Two Treatises of Government: In the Former, The False Principles, and Foundation of Sir Robert Filmer, and His Followers, Are Detected and Overthrown. The Latter Is an Essay Concerning The True Original, Extent, and End of Civil Government*. Cambridge: Cambridge University Press.

Lukes, S. (1973). *Individualism*. Oxford: Basil Blackwell.

Materstvedt, L. J. (1997). *Rights, Paternalism, and the State. A Kantian Exploration of Nozick's Political Thought*. Doctoral (dr.art.) dissertation, Department of Philosophy, Faculty of Arts, Norwegian University of Science and Technology (NTNU), Trondheim (submitted 1996). URL: <http://folk.ntnu.no/larsmat/dravh_ljm.pdf>

Materstvedt, L. J. (2009). Inappropriate conclusions in research on assisted dying. *Journal of Medical Ethics*, **35**, 272.

Materstvedt, L. J. (2011). What is this thing called medical ethics? A Kantian interpretation. In: S. G. Carson, J. Knowles, and B. K. Myskja (eds), *Kant: Here, Now, and How. Essays in Honour of Truls Wyller*, pp. 207–233. Paderborn: mentis Verlag.

Materstvedt, L. J. (2012). Intention, procedure, outcome and personhood in palliative sedation and euthanasia. *BMJ Supportive and Palliative Care*, **2**, 9–11.

Materstvedt, L. J. (2013). Palliative care ethics: the problems of combining palliation and assisted dying. *Progress in Palliative Care*, **21**, 158–164.

Materstvedt, L. J. and Bosshard, G. (2009). Deep and continuous palliative sedation (terminal sedation): clinical-ethical and philosophical aspects. *Lancet Oncology*, **10**, 622–627.

Materstvedt, L. J. and Bosshard, G. (2010). Euthanasia and physician-assisted suicide. In: G. Hanks, N. Cherny, N. Christakis, M. Fallon, S. Kaasa, and R. Portenoy (eds), *Oxford Textbook of Palliative Medicine*, 4th edn, pp. 304–319. Oxford: Oxford University Press.

Materstvedt, L. J. and Bosshard, G. (2015). Euthanasia and palliative care. In: N. Cherny, M. Fallon, S. Kaasa, R. Portenoy, and D. Currow (eds), *Oxford Textbook of Palliative Medicine*, 5th edn, pp. 314–322. Oxford: Oxford University Press.

Mill, J. S. (1991). *Utilitarianism, On Liberty, Considerations on Representative Government*. London: Everyman's Library.

Miller, D. (ed.) (1991). *The Blackwell Encyclopaedia of Political Thought*. Oxford: Basil Blackwell.

Netherlands' law on euthanasia (2002). *Termination of Life on Request and Assisted Suicide (Review Procedures) Act*. Netherlands Ministry of Foreign Affairs International Information and Communication Department in cooperation with the Ministry of Health, Welfare and Sport and the Ministry of Justice. URL: <http://www.bioeticanet.info/eutanasia/LleiEuHol.pdf >

Nozick, R. (1974). *Anarchy, State, and Utopia*. Oxford: Basil Blackwell [reprinted 2001].

Onwuteaka-Philipsen, B. D., van der Heide, A., Koper, D., Keij-Deerenberg, I., Rietjens, J. A., Rurup, M. L., et al. (2003). Euthanasia and other end-of-life decisions in the Netherlands in 1990, 1995, and 2001. *Lancet, 362*, 395–399.

Onwuteaka-Philipsen, B. D., Brinkman-Stoppelenburg, A., Penning, C., de Jong-Krul, G.J., van Delden, J.J., and van der Heide, A. (2012). Trends in end-of-life practices before and after the enactment of the euthanasia law in the Netherlands from 1990 to 2010: a repeated cross-sectional survey. *Lancet, 380*, 908–915.

Oregon law on physician-assisted suicide (1997). Oregon Public Health. *Oregon Death With Dignity Act*. URL: <http://public.health.oregon.gov/providerpartnerresources/evaluationresearch/deathwithdignityact/pages/index.aspx>

Parfit, D. (1984). *Reasons and Persons*. Oxford: Clarendon Press.

Pereira, J., Anwar, D., Pralong, G., Pralong, J., Mazzocato, C., and Bigler, J. M. (2008). Assisted suicide and euthanasia should not be practiced in palliative care units. *Journal of Palliative Medicine, 11*, 1074–1076.

Pogge, T. W. (2003). From New York City. *Palliative Medicine, 17*, 119.

Québec's law on euthanasia (2014). *Quebec's Bill 52—Right to Die*. URL: <http://www.scribd.com/doc/228378011/Quebec-s-Bill-52-Right-to-Die>

Raijmakers, N. J., van der Heide, A., Kouwenhoven, P. S., van Thiel, G. J., van Delden, J. J., and Rietjens, J. A. (2015). Assistance in dying for older people without a serious medical condition who have a wish to die: a national cross-sectional survey. *Journal of Medical Ethics, 41*, 145–150.

Rawls, J., Thomson, J. J., Nozick, R., Dworkin, R., Scanlon, T., and Nagel, T. (1997). Assisted suicide: the philosophers' brief. *The New York Review of Books*, March 27. URL: <http://www.nybooks.com/articles/archives/1997/mar/27/assisted-suicide-the-philosophers-brief/>

Rurup, M. (2012). Being 'weary of life' as cause for seeking euthanasia or physician-assisted suicide. In: S. J. Youngner and G. K. Kimsma (eds), *Physician-Assisted Death in Perspective. Assessing the Dutch Experience*, pp. 247–262. Cambridge: Cambridge University Press.

Van der Heide, A., Onwuteaka-Philipsen, B. D., Rurup, M. L., Buiting H. M., van Delden, J. J., Hanssen-de Wolf, J. E., et al. (2007). End-of-life practices in the Netherlands under the Euthanasia Act. *New England Journal of Medicine, 56*, 1957–1965.

World Health Organization (2015). *WHO definition of palliative care*. URL: <http://www.who.int/cancer/palliative/definition/en/>

Chapter 13

Towards responsive knowing in matters of life and death

Marian A. Verkerk

The beauty that could not last

She was a woman of 45. She had that kind of a delicate beauty that looks very natural but, one suspects, takes quite some time every morning to get the right result. Her clothing was very sophisticated. You could see that physical appearance was very important to her.

It was about 6 months ago when she came to my practice and told me that she had a lump in her breast. After I examined her briefly, I got worried and sent her to the oncologist at the nearby hospital. Two weeks later very bad news arrived: she was suffering from stage 4 breast cancer and she probably had only a few months to live. We talked through the terrible diagnosis at her home. I explained to her that chemotherapy would lengthen her life by a few more months. I also told her that there were ways to combat the pain symptoms with radiation therapy. She listened to me quietly. I could see that she was shocked and that she had difficulty digesting the bad news. We agreed that we would meet in a couple of days and talk again.

And so a week later she called for an appointment. Almost immediately after she sat down in my consulting room she told me that she had made up her mind. She did not want any treatments whatsoever. She wanted euthanasia instead, and what is more, she requested it for the following week. She said: 'I know I'm going to die, doctor, and that's terrible. But more frightening to me is the prospect of watching myself deteriorate in the coming months. At this moment I still look good and I want to be remembered that way. I don't want to look like somebody who is very ill— scrawny, wasted, ugly, and pathetic. My beauty has always been central to my life. I have put so much effort into being beautiful. This is who I am. The idea that I could lose that identity causes me unbearable suffering. And so I want you to help me before I lose myself.'

As a general practitioner I have accepted several requests for euthanasia in the last couple of years. I am not against it and I do not have moral objections to it in principle. On the other hand, I want to convince myself that the person who requests euthanasia is actually suffering unbearably. And that is not only because of the legal requirements that surround the practice of euthanasia in the Netherlands. It is a moral thing: I could not assist anyone in dying who is not actually suffering at that moment. And so there was this difficulty: although my patient was diagnosed with an incurable disease and was going to die within the coming months, she did not seem to me to be ill at that point. Nor, in my opinion, did she seem to be depressed, nor did she have a history of psychiatric disorders. In fact, her reasoning was quite sound. She was married and she had two daughters aged 16 and 18. I asked her if she had discussed this with her family. She told me that she had and that her family was very, very sad about the diagnosis as well as about her request. But they also respected her wish. 'It's my life doctor, and so it's also my death.'

I told her that I wanted to think about it and that I needed an independent consult from another doctor. She understood that there were legal requirements. She also understood that I needed time to think about it. On the other hand, she insisted that she did not have much time left, as she reckoned she would soon become ill.

Since then, I visited her a couple of times. During these visits we spoke intensely with each other about death, about life, about her family. In the meantime a colleague has visited and spoken to her too. This independent consultant understood the difficulty I had with her request. But he too was convinced that this woman was suffering intolerably at the prospect of losing her beauty. And so, finally, I honoured her request. She died 3 weeks after the first diagnosis and she was still very beautiful.

Euthanasia in the Netherlands

'The beauty that could not last' is an actual case that I encountered some years ago when I was a member of one of the euthanasia review committees in the Netherlands. When we read the paperwork on the case it struck us as so unusual that we invited the doctor and the independent consultant to tell us more in a face-to-face conversation. And so they did.

In the Netherlands, euthanasia is understood to mean 'termination of life by a doctor at a patient's specific request'. It can be distinguished from simply desisting from treatment, in consultation with the patient and his or her family, when further intervention is pointless. Withholding or withdrawing treatment is accepted medical practice, as is palliative or terminal sedation, which is understood as 'the intentional lowering of consciousness of a patient in the last phase of his or her life in order to relieve suffering'. By contrast, euthanasia is considered a criminal offence, but the criminal code has been amended to exempt doctors from criminal liability if they report their actions and show that they have satisfied the due care criteria formulated in the Act on the Termination of Life on Request and Assisted Suicide (WTLVHZ 2014).

The actions of doctors in such cases are assessed retrospectively by the review committees (of which there are five regional ones), each of which consists of a doctor, a lawyer, and an ethicist appointed by the Minister of Security and Justice and the Minister of Health, Welfare, and Sport. Where a doctor has reported a case and a review committee has decided on the basis of the case file that he or she has acted with due care, the Public Prosecution Service will not be informed and no further action will be taken.

When dealing with a patient's specific request for euthanasia or assisted suicide, doctors must observe the following due care criteria (WTLVHZ 2014, chap. II, art. 2; translated from the Dutch). They must:

(a) be satisfied that the patient's request is voluntary and well-considered;

(b) be satisfied that the patient's suffering is unbearable, with no prospect of improvement;

(c) inform the patient of his or her situation and further prognosis;

(d) discuss the situation with the patient and come to the joint conclusion that there is no other reasonable solution;

(e) consult at least one other physician with no connection to the case, who must then see the patient and state in writing that the attending physician has satisfied the due care criteria listed in the four points above; and

(f) exercise due medical care and attention in terminating the patient's life or assisting in his or her suicide.

Only after the criteria (a)–(e) have been fulfilled may the physician proceed to perform euthanasia or assist the patient in committing suicide.

And so this case was reported and we as a review committee had to decide whether the due care criteria were satisfied. Our queries focused on the nature of this woman's suffering.

Unbearable suffering

In this particular case we had no doubts about the voluntary nature of the patient's request. Of course we asked both physicians whether they were under the impression that the woman was suffering from depression or any other psychiatric disorder. Both of them were convinced that that was not the case. Nor did we have any doubts about the prognosis. Our difficulties had to do with whether the woman was suffering unbearably at that time with no prospect of improvement, and also whether there was no other reasonable solution to her situation. As in most cases of reported euthanasia and assisted dying, the discussion in the committee concentrated on the nature of suffering. But this particular case was more difficult than others.

The Act on the Termination of Life on Request and Assisted Suicide (WTLVHZ 2014) stipulates that the suffering must be 'without prospect of improvement' in the prevailing medical opinion, as assessed by the attending physician—that is, doctors must agree that the patient's condition will not improve. The doctor and patient must discuss every possible alternative treatment since, as long as a feasible alternative is available, there is, in a medical sense, a prospect of improvement. It is harder to establish objectively whether suffering is 'unbearable', for this is essentially a person-related notion. As stated in the Act, the physician must find the patient's suffering to be unbearable (WTLVHZ 2014, chap. II, art. 2) The question here is not whether people in general or the physician would find suffering such as the patient's unbearable, but whether it is unbearable to that specific patient. The physician must therefore be able—so says the Act—to *empathize* not only with the patient's situation, but also with the patient's point of view' (WTLVHZ 2014, chap. II, art. 2). For the review committee, then, the task is to examine each individual case to establish whether the doctor could reasonably conclude that the patient was suffering unbearably.

But what is suffering anyway? According to Eric Cassell's classic formulation, suffering can be defined as 'the state of severe distress associated with events that threaten the intactness of the person' (Cassell, 1982). It is awareness of the disintegration, or the danger of disintegration, of one's sense of self. So suffering refers to a person and a person's identity: it is the person who suffers, not only the body.

In line with this definition one could say that the woman in this case was suffering beyond any doubt. It is clear that she felt that by losing her beauty, she risked disintegration; she would lose sense of herself, so to say. But is her suffering unbearable, and, if so, how do we know? One answer to that last question could be: it is unbearable when the person who suffers says it is unbearable. Again, it is the *person* who suffers *unbearably*. There is no objective way to determine 'the unbearability of suffering'; we always need to refer to the person who suffers and finds that suffering unbearable.

At the same time the fact that the person says she suffers unbearably is not enough to render her request for euthanasia legitimate. It is the doctor who—as the Act says—has to find the patient's suffering to be unbearable.

Moral imagination

In judging whether a patient is suffering unbearably, the physician must be able—according to the Act—'to *empathize* not only with the patient's situation, but also with the patient's point of view'. Empathizing can be understood as entailing the use of one's moral imagination (for a similar view see Gelhaus 2012). It is important to stress here that when making a judgement on whether euthanasia would be appropriate, a *rational moral understanding* of the patient's situation is insufficient. In other words, it is not enough to have an adequate grasp of the relevant facts and features of the situation and to assess these in the light of some sort of evaluative criteria. One also has to imagine oneself in someone else's situation and perspective. But, as Jackie Leach Scully points out in *Disability Bioethics*, there are different conceptions of moral imagination. One of them is 'putting oneself in someone's else shoes'. In that case I imagine myself being in the situation of that other person. As Scully puts it: 'I enact the narrative that I imagine I would enact if it were me' (Scully 2008, p. 54). Applied to our case here, the physician must imagine him- or herself in the shoes of the woman and try to understand what it means to be in the woman's situation. What the physician asks mainly is: what would I do if I were in that situation? But this form of moral imagination is not what is meant by the Act. Using the moral imagination here means 'imagining myself, not as me, but as *that* person'. And so it is not only about the facts and features of this particular situation, it is also about someone's perspective on life. For that form of moral imagination one needs to know more about the person's identity, about what makes 'her' be her.

It is an open question as to how far this notion of moral imagination as empathetic imagining (Goldie 2000; Scully 2008) can reach. Is it possible to leave our own perspectives behind and genuinely adopt the other's thoughts, feelings, and emotions? In that I agree with Scully when she says that imaginative projection will always involve a mixing of the other person's perspective with one's own. And in the case discussed above, one wonders whether our moral imagination is not stretched too far.

Moral ambivalence

When I was first confronted by this case, I felt shocked. I certainly felt a moral ambivalence towards the nature of this woman's suffering. On the one hand I could imagine that for her the idea of deteriorating within the coming months, and thereby losing her beauty, caused her suffering, and was probably intolerable. On the other, I felt that maybe this woman had become a victim of her own beauty ideals. I had difficulty imagining that beauty could be such an essential theme in the narrative of her life. I asked myself whether this case could not be seen as the perfect example of what Zygmunt Bauman (1997) has called post-modern dying, in which death and dying are often negated.

That was me, judging the case from my own perspective. But as the ethicist of the review committee I had to judge this case in a different way. I had to judge whether the doctor could reasonably come to the conclusion that the patient was suffering unbearably. For that, I needed to know whether and how the doctor came to a moral understanding that did justice to the patient. In other words, had there been a practice of responsive knowing between doctor and patient? And if so, how could I know?

In the rest of this chapter I will elaborate on the conditions in which euthanasia can be seen as a justified moral practice. This question of justification emerges in both judgmental perspectives, the doctor's as well as my own. For that, I will first unpack the idea that the moral conversation between doctor and patient ought to be seen as a practice of responsive knowing. And although in my role as a member of the review committee my judging of this case remains necessarily marginal, as a philosopher and ethicist I can learn lessons from that for future research related to euthanasia.

Responsive knowing

The term 'responsive knowing' is at home in what I call a naturalized bioethics. In 2008 my colleagues Hilde Lindemann, Margaret Walker, and I published an anthology about naturalized bioethics (Lindemann et al. 2008). In line with feminist theory, we—together with other ethicists and philosophers—explored ways of developing a more situated and self-reflexive ethics. The term 'naturalized' can have several distinct meanings. Minimally, naturalism in ethics is committed to understanding moral judgement and moral agency in terms of natural facts about ourselves and our world (Walker 2008). Our naturalism, however, does not privilege institutionally organized natural and social scientific knowledge but embraces the experience of individuals in personal, social, and institutional life as well. This naturalized approach to ethics is based on the idea that morality is a living practice, a continual interpersonal process of holding ourselves and others to account for what we value, negotiating responsibilities, making ourselves morally intelligible, and constructing and reconstructing our moral views of how best to proceed together.

How we think about a good death can be interpreted as a moral practice, and the moral conversations that we have with each other about death and dying must be seen as *situated moral discourses*. Naturalizing ethical thinking about a good death implies that we do not only use scientific knowledge about dying, for example knowledge about pain relief or how to keep the patient physically as comfortable as possible. We also need to know the experiences of individuals about what it means to die and what a good death might mean. This knowledge can only be obtained in a practice of what I would call *responsive knowing*. The practice of responsive knowing contains certain presuppositions concerning the moral discourse between doctor and patient about someone's request for euthanasia. Both doctor and patient are situated and have their own socially and culturally shaped presuppositions about what makes life meaningful. For patients, views and ideas about how they want to die are often deeply held moral convictions about what is essential in life. For doctors, it will always be difficult to empathize fully with the patient. As we stated earlier, imaginative projection will always involve a mixing of the other person's perspective with our own. And what is more, the doctor should also be seen as situated in this moral conversation. He or she also has his or her own deeply held convictions and perspective on life. 'Responsive knowing' therefore implies that as situated persons we need to be attentive and responsive towards each other. We need to be attentive to what is said by the other, so that we grasp the aspects of that irreducible particularity of that individual person in his or her concrete context. Adequate responsiveness—that is, 'giving what is needed by the patient's vulnerable situation'—requires attentiveness. Only when we are attentive to that particular person can we respond to him or her in a way that does justice to the particularity of that person. Narrative appreciation, including empathic imagining, should be part of this. Responsive knowing implies, therefore, that we are epistemically just towards each other.

Epistemic justice

In her book *Epistemic Injustice*, Miranda Fricker (2007) discusses two forms of injustice: testimonial and hermeneutical injustice. Both forms of injustice appear in caring practices. Testimonial injustice refers to the situation in which some voices are not heard or receive a deflated degree of credibility, owing to prejudice on the hearer's part. In the case at hand, it is possible that we are being unjust towards the woman's request if we simply dismiss it as a neurotic attitude towards beauty: it cannot be so important that losing one's beauty would cause unbearable suffering. Hermeneutical injustice, on the other hand, is the result of a more structural prejudice: we cannot make sense of an experience because we lack the moral narratives for it. Fricker herself gives the example of the difficulty of making sense of homosexual desire as a legitimate sexual orientation in a cultural–historical context where homosexuality is interpreted as perverse or shameful. Again, it could be the case that a negative reaction to the woman's request is an example of hermeneutical injustice: in a society in which emphasis on beauty is seen as shallow, the request runs the risk of not being taken seriously by the doctor.

Exercising epistemic virtues of attentiveness and responsiveness can prevent testimonial injustice. Exercising attentiveness and responsiveness implies that we grasp the particularity of that person. By trying to appreciate her story, with any luck we can respond to what she needs. So the doctor needs to attend to what the woman says: is this really what she wants or is she just scared? Is her beauty indeed such a powerful part of what makes life meaningful to her, or is she frightened that her husband and children will not recognize her any more as the person she is once she falls ill? When exercising attentiveness, we can at least 'hear' the story that is told by the woman and recognize her as the woman she is. But what about situations of hermeneutical injustice?

Hermeneutical injustice

There are voices in the debate about euthanasia in the Netherlands who say that we lack structural moral narratives about death and dying. These voices are in line with ethicists such as Emanuel and Emanuel, who stated that dying and death are approximated from a sociocultural attitude that first and foremost negate dying and death (Emanuel and Emanuel 1998). The ideal of youth seems to be much more important than old age. Youthful longevity is often desired, and still seems to be the cornerstone of progress of health care. The focus, as the Emanuels say, has been on avoiding problems and stopping bad interventions rather than on a positive ideal of a good death. And so, according to Emanuel and Emanuel, we face a paradox: increasing concern about death and dying, tremendous technical capacities to relieve symptoms and improve care, and persistent suffering of dying patients, all combined with the continued denial of death. This raises the question of how to fulfil the promise of a good death.

We seem to miss the narratives that give meaning to death and dying. For the sociologist Zygmunt Bauman, the absence of meaningful narratives about life and death leads to two other observations (Bauman 1997). First of all, care for the dying has become a speciality for professionals. For laypeople, death has become something shameful; something that we would rather not talk about. Our primary confrontation with death and dying is in films and on television, where death is dangerous but also entertaining.

And if it is true that we lack narratives for giving meaning to death, then there is the danger that we are unjust towards others as well as towards ourselves, hermeneutically speaking. We somehow seem to lack the narratives to give meaning to experiences of dying and death. In at least two ways, this phenomenon of lacking moral narratives can lead to hermeneutical injustice in the case under examination. On the one hand, it is possible to read the case as one in which the woman herself cannot give any meaning to her approaching death. Because she lacks the moral resources that would allow her to give meaning to her new situation, she sticks to what she knows. The injustice is therefore done in the first place by herself. And if a doctor goes along with her, he or she also commits injustice towards her by not being able to give her structurally meaningful stories about dying that might allow her to see the situation in a different light. This interpretation would be in line with Bauman's view. On the other hand, it also possible that this individually meaningful story of the women herself is too easily dismissed as shallow because there is cultural prejudice against her story. And in not recognizing her story as a meaningful one, we commit a hermeneutical injustice towards the woman.

Responsive knowing is about counterstories

For now it is sufficient to point out the need for narratives that give meaning towards such important events in one's life. Although one's identity is constituted by one's self-narrative, we are never more than co-authors of our life narratives (Nelson 2001, p. 81). So, although the woman is sincere in her idea that beauty is the most important thing in life, one should not dismiss the thought that this narrative might be the result of an oppressive master narrative in which women are depicted as 'creatures of beauty'. By developing counterstories (Nelson 2001) of what makes life and death meaningful, we can combat this form of hermeneutical injustice.

In developing counterstories about meaningful death, we need to be alert to the danger of sentimentalizing it. There seems to be something terribly wrong when death appears. Death seems often to be misplaced. There is an ambivalence towards death—some lurking, ineradicable sense of its wrongfulness, juxtaposed against all rational arguments for its inevitability and even preferability (Burt 2005). And so, whatever story we develop, privately or publicly, it may be impossible to find a sufficient and satisfying story about death and dying. As Paul Ramsey once said, 'Death is the biggest insult to life' (Ramsey 1970). Death elicits feelings of awe, grief, and pain (Sachs 2000). A good counterstory would capture this ambivalence, facing it squarely rather than concealing or denying it as the master narratives currently in circulation do.

A research agenda

Responsive knowing in matters of life and death implies that we are epistemically just towards each other. When applied to the moral conversations between doctors and patients, this means that doctors need to be as attentive as they can towards the needs of their patients and their own prejudices. But both parties should also be aware of the fact that their private discourse is always a socially and culturally situated one. And so they need to be aware of oppressive master narratives about what makes life meaningful. It is not only doctors who have an epistemic responsibility here. Patients have a responsibility as well. One could say that assigning a responsibility towards the patient him- or herself might be too harsh: the patient, after all, is dying. On the other hand, if we want to consider euthanasia as a moral practice in which patients practise their autonomy with regard to death, then we also need to acknowledge the responsibility they bear.

Responsive knowing aims to help us prevent hermeneutical and testimonial injustice. I have tried to argue for the need to see the moral conversation between doctor and patient as a responsive practice that is socially and culturally situated. As a member of the review committee, I need to convince myself that the particular conversation between doctor and patient has been one that is epistemically just. Of course that will not be easy. I am always evaluating the conversation in retrospect: I was not there at the specific moment. My evaluation will therefore be marginal in one way. On the other hand, from my experience as a review committee member I can insist on the need for more knowledge, personal and experiential, about dying. We need a research agenda in which more counterstories are developed and studied in order to attain a practice of responsive knowing.

References

Bauman, Z. (1997). Immortality, postmodern version. In: Z. Bauman (ed.), *Postmodernity and its Discontents*. Cambridge: Polity Press.

Burt, R. A (2005). The end of autonomy. *Hastings Center Report*, **35**, 9–13.

Cassell, E. (1982). The nature of suffering and the goals of medicine. *New England Journal of Medicine*, **306**, 639–645.

Emanuel, E. J. and Emanuel, L.L. (1998). The promise of a good death. *Lancet*, **351**, SII21–SII29.

Fricker, M. (2007). *Epistemic Injustice*. Oxford: Oxford University Press.

Gelhaus, P. (2012). The desired moral attitude of the physician: (I) empathy. *Medicine, Health Care and Philosophy*, **15**, 103–113.

Goldie, P. (2000). *The Emotions: a Philosophical Exploration*. Oxford: Oxford University Press.

Lindemann, H., Verkerk, M., and Walker, M. U. (2008). *Naturalized Bioethics. Toward Responsible Knowing and Practice*. Cambridge: Cambridge University Press.

Nelson, H. L. (2001). *Damaged Identities, Narrative Repair*. Ithaca, NY: Cornell University Press.

Ramsey, P. (1970). *The Patient as Person*. New Haven, Conn.: Yale University Press.

Sachs, G. A. (2000). Sometimes dying still stings. *Journal of the American Medical Association*, **284**, 2423.

Scully, J. L. (2008). *Disability Bioethics*. Lanham, MD: Rowman & Littlefield Publishers.

Walker, M. U. (2008). Introduction: Groningen naturalism in bioethics. In: H. Lindemann, M. Verkerk, and M. U. Walker (eds), *2008 Naturalized Bioethics. Toward Responsible Knowing and Practice*. Cambridge: Cambridge University Press.

WTLVHZ [Wet Toetsing Levensbeëindiging op Verzoek en Hulp bij Zelfdoding] (2014). Wet Toetsing Levensbeëindiging op Verzoek en Hulp bij Zelfdoding. URL: <http://wetten. overheid.nl/BWBR0012410/geldigheidsdatum_24-06-2014>

Chapter 14

Dealing with dilemmas around patients' wishes to die: moral case deliberation in a Dutch hospice

Guy Widdershoven, Margreet Stolper, and Bert Molewijk

Introduction

In the Netherlands, end-of-life decisions have been an issue of debate for several decades. Euthanasia has been an important topic in the debate. Physicians have played a central role in putting euthanasia on the agenda and in developing criteria for good care, the so-called due care criteria (Kennedy 2002). These criteria have received a legal status, first in jurisprudence and since 2002 in the euthanasia law. The euthanasia law is based on the legal notion of a conflict of duties. When a patient expresses a wish to die in a situation of unbearable suffering, the physician experiences a conflict between the duty to refrain from administering lethal medication on the one hand and the duty to help the patient by stopping the suffering on the other. This conflict takes the form of a moral dilemma. In a moral dilemma, a person has to choose between two options, knowing that each of them involves doing harm. If the physician decides to perform euthanasia, the moral duty not to end a patient's life is harmed. If the physician decides not to follow the patient's wish, the moral harm is that suffering will continue. The euthanasia law does not solve this dilemma, but provides a legal context in which the physician can, and is expected to, make a decision based on moral concerns.

Physicians play a central role in Dutch euthanasia practice. They are the only professionals who can be legally exempt from punishment in a case of assisted dying. Thus, the decision to respond to a patient's wish to die can only be made and put into practice by a physician. Yet other professionals will also often be involved. Euthanasia can only come at the end of a longer process of care of a patient in a serious condition. In this process, complex care arrangements will often be required, involving physicians, nurses, and other care professionals. This is especially the case in palliative care at the end of life, for example in hospices.

Over the last two decades, palliative care has become more prominent in the Netherlands. This is in part a consequence of the legalization of euthanasia. One of the due care criteria entails that the physician and the patient should have come to the conclusion that no other reasonable solution remains. This conclusion can only be drawn if palliative care options have been explored. Complementary to the legal regulation of euthanasia, the Dutch government has set up a programme to stimulate palliative care. Palliative care is well developed in the Netherlands, both in consultation teams and hospices. Consultation teams for palliative care are multidisciplinary, and include nursing expertise. In hospices, nurses are crucial for the day-to-day care of patients.

Whereas euthanasia and palliative care used to be clearly distinct, both in theory and in practice, the two are now becoming more related in the Dutch debate and in Dutch health care. Palliative sedation is more often regarded as an alternative which should be explicitly considered before the decision for euthanasia can be taken. Palliative care settings, which for ideological motives used to exclude euthanasia as an option, are now more open to euthanasia, but refrain from making this widely known. In hospices, patients expressing a wish to die and requesting euthanasia may give rise to dilemmas for both the medical and the nursing staff.

In this chapter we first elaborate on the legal situation around end-of-life decisions in the Netherlands, focusing on euthanasia and physician-assisted suicide (PAS), and their relationship to palliative care. Next, we discuss the basic principles of moral case deliberation as a way of offering clinical ethics support to healthcare professionals. Then we present an example of an actual moral case deliberation meeting about euthanasia in the context of a palliative care setting. We show that moral case deliberation helps to make the normative orientations of various professionals explicit, and enables the participants to exchange views and learn from one another in a process of dialogue. We conclude that moral case deliberation helps to clarify the views of all professionals and to give them a role in deliberations about end-of-life care, even if the final decision about whether or not to go along with the patient's wish to die remains at the discretion of the physician. This final decision, crucial as it may be from a legal perspective, can only be taken in the context of a process of good care, taking into account the perspectives and responsibilities of all those involved.

Medical decisions in response to a wish to die in the Netherlands

Various kinds of medical decisions at the end of life

When a patient expresses a wish to die, various medical decisions can be relevant. In this chapter we will describe these types of decisions, and provide information on their occurrence in end-of-life situations in the Netherlands in 2010 (Onwuteaka-Philipsen et al. 2012).

First, a physician may decide to end or not to start treatment, which may result in a hastening of death. In 2010, 18% of all deaths involved a medical decision to end or not to start treatment. Secondly, a physician may start palliative care, which aims to make the process of dying comfortable for the patient. In general it will not lead to a shortening of the patient's life, although this may be an (unintended) side effect. In 2010, palliative care interventions were present in 36% of deaths. One example of palliative care is palliative sedation or continuous deep sedation, in which heavy sedatives are administered to make the patient unconscious so that he or she no longer feels any pain. In the Netherlands, palliative sedation is only indicated for patients with a life expectancy of less than 2 weeks, so that death is not the result of stopping artificial fluids and nutrition after sedation (Janssens et al. 2012). In 2010, palliative sedation was administered in 12% of all deaths.

These medical decisions should be regarded as part of normal medical practice. If the patient's wish to die is formulated as an explicit request for active ending of life the physician may perform euthanasia or PAS. In the Netherlands these two medical interventions are not regarded as normal medical practice, and are regulated by a special law which exempts physicians from prosecution under the criminal law prohibiting assisted suicide, provided that specific criteria are met. In 2010, euthanasia was performed in 2.8% and PAS in 0.2% of deaths.

The Netherlands was the first country in which euthanasia (i.e. the active termination of life by a physician at the request of the patient) and PAS were legally permitted under specific circumstances (Griffith et al. 1998). However, controversies remain over the moral legitimacy of assistance in dying if this involves actively and deliberately shortening the life of the patient at the patient's request (Battin 1994; Keown 1995; van Delden 1999; Hendin 2002; Cohen-Almagor 2004; Gill 2009). This is particularly the case if patients do not (or do not only) suffer from somatic illnesses but (also) from mental disturbances, as in case of chronic mental illness or Alzheimer's disease (Berghmans 2010).

The legal context of euthanasia and PAS

In Dutch law, euthanasia and PAS are defined as ending of the patient's life by a physician at the explicit request of the patient. This means that the physician's action originates in the patient's wish. According to Dutch law, euthanasia and PAS can be acceptable if a number of conditions—the so-called due care criteria—are met. For euthanasia or PAS to be acceptable, physicians must (WTLVHZ 2014, chap. II, art. 2; translated from the Dutch):

(a) be satisfied that the patient's request is voluntary and well-considered;

(b) be satisfied that the patient's suffering is unbearable, with no prospect of improvement;

(c) inform the patient of his or her situation and further prognosis;

(d) discuss the situation with the patient and come to the joint conclusion that there is no other reasonable solution;

(e) consult at least one other physician with no connection to the case, who must then see the patient and state in writing that the attending physician has satisfied the due care criteria listed in the four points above; and

(f) exercise due medical care and attention in terminating the patient's life or assisting in his or her suicide.

A case of euthanasia or PAS should be reported to one of the five existing regional euthanasia review committees in the Netherlands. After a retrospective assessment of the case—on the basis of the due care criteria—the committee judges whether the case was acceptable or not. If the case is judged acceptable, no further legal action is taken. If not, the case is sent to the health inspectorate and the public prosecutor who may decide that it will be brought before the criminal court. Between 1998, the year the committees were appointed, and 2009, 23,268 reported cases were reviewed, of which a mere 50 were judged to have been 'not careful' (van Dijk and van Wijlick 2010).

Importance of palliative care

As already pointed out, the practice of palliative sedation (or continuous deep sedation) is much more frequent than euthanasia and PAS together. This illustrates the important role of palliative care at the end of life, as palliative sedation is one of the practices carried out in the context of palliative care. Palliative care and euthanasia are related, as palliative care may be an alternative option before euthanasia can become acceptable. In this sense, good palliative care may prevent the need for euthanasia because it can decrease or take away the suffering. This does not mean that all requests for and cases of euthanasia or PAS can be prevented; neither can it be claimed that such requests and cases are indications of a lack (or of a low quality) of palliative care.

Hospice care and euthanasia

Basically, and traditionally, there is a tension between palliative care and hospice practices on the one hand and euthanasia on the other. The philosophy behind palliative care and its goals are: (1) the recognition that dying is an intrinsic part of life; (2) that neither the acceleration nor the postponement of death is an aim of palliative care; (3) that palliative care aims to lessen pain and other burdensome symptoms; (4) that palliative care is designed to help patients become as active and autonomous as possible; and (5) that palliative care supports the family in coping with the disease and death of their loved one (Olde-Rikkert and Rigaud 2010). Some of these elements are in conflict with the goal and practice of euthanasia (particularly 2), while others are clearly reconcilable with euthanasia (in particular 1 and 4). In the Netherlands, the majority of physicians providing palliative care accept euthanasia as a means of last resort. In other countries there is no consensus that euthanasia should be excluded from palliative care (ten Have 2010). Data from the Dutch right to die society NVVE (Nederlandse Vereniging voor een Vrijwillig Levenseinde) show that 80% of Dutch hospices allow euthanasia and PAS if performed within the framework of the law. Palliative sedation is practised in all hospices, and in 98% of hospices the patient may consciously stop eating and drinking during the terminal stage without an intervention other than keeping the patient comfortable.

What is moral case deliberation?

A moral case deliberation is a meeting of a group of healthcare professionals who systematically reflect on a moral issue emerging in a clinical case from their practice (Steinkamp and Gordijn 2003, 2004; Molewijk et al. 2008). The group usually consists of healthcare professionals from different fields, such as, doctors, nurses, and social workers, either in an existing team or from various wards or settings (van der Dam et al. 2011). The focus of the deliberation is a moral question. This question could be: 'What should we consider as the morally right thing to do in this specific situation and how should we do it in a morally right way?' In addition to focusing on arguments (for example for behaving in a certain way), a moral case deliberation may also focus on emotions and on what it means to be a morally good person.

A moral case deliberation meeting, which usually takes between 1 and 2 hours, is facilitated by an ethicist or someone who is trained in conversation methods for moral case deliberation. The facilitator structures the meeting by means of a conversation method (Steinkamp and Gordijn 2003; Verkerk et al. 2004). The expertise of the facilitator consists in keeping an eye on the moral dimension of the case, supporting the joint deliberation process, and helping the group in planning actions to improve the quality of care.

The primary goal of a moral case deliberation is to foster a constructive dialogue among the participating healthcare professionals in order to create a critical and respectful moral inquiry into both the moral issues in a clinical ethics case and the way participants feel and reason. The aim of the dialogue is to reflect on the professional quality of the participants' work, their ideas about professional behaviour, and their presuppositions about good care at the case level and the organizational or institutional level (Abma et al. 2009). The facilitator does not give advice and does not morally justify or legitimize a specific decision (Widdershoven and Molewijk 2010).

Moral case deliberation is based on the assumption that good care is not given beforehand but becomes defined and redefined in concrete situations. Confronted with difficult situations, caregivers cannot just sit back and think about their practice. There is an urgency to act and to find answers to the particular needs of the situation (Abma et al. 2009). In moral case deliberation, views on what constitutes good care are explored and scrutinized in a deliberative process. By highlighting the different perspectives of the relevant persons involved, and exploring their values and norms, healthcare professionals become aware of conflicting values and ideas in the case. Healthcare professionals explore their own ideas about good care in the specific context, compare their ideas with those of others, and jointly develop a new and more encompassing view. The outcome of a moral case deliberation depends on what the group defines as being the goal of the meeting. Healthcare professionals may aim to understand each other's ideas and emotions better. In an urgent situation they may need to come to a decision about the morally right action. In a moral case deliberation there is ideally equality among the healthcare professionals. This means that views and ideas are explored irrespective of professional hierarchy, expertise, or status. Each voice is important and counts. Still, there are different responsibilities in a team that have to be acknowledged, and consensus is not always possible in the decision-making process.

A moral case deliberation concerning a patient with a wish to die in a hospice

In this section we will present an example of a moral case deliberation in a hospice in the west of the Netherlands. Up to now, the hospice has had a non-euthanasia policy. A physician, who herself had been involved in a case of euthanasia before she came to work in the hospice, has put the non-euthanasia policy on the agenda by arranging a moral case deliberation. She expects that in the near future some patients in the hospice might want to explore the option of or even ask for euthanasia. She has organized a moral case deliberation with an external facilitator. The meeting takes place after working hours and all the staff are invited. They all attend, and the group consists of fifteen participants: two physicians, eleven nurses, and two former volunteers who are employed as cleaners. The physician who organized the meeting brings up a case that happened in another hospice where she worked a year before:

A terminal patient, a woman aged 56, is suffering unbearably and asks for euthanasia. The hospice where she is staying is on an island, where the patient has lived all her life and has played an active role in the community. The hospice has a non-euthanasia policy. On admission, patients are informed about this policy; the woman has also been informed. A couple of days ago, she was in great pain and she screamed loudly for a long time. With medication we were able to reduce the pain for a while. Afterwards, the patient said that she did not want to experience such pain anymore. The question arose: shall we change our policy, or do we tell the patient that for euthanasia she will have to be transferred by helicopter to a hospital on the mainland?

As a first step in the moral case deliberation, the person who brings up the case is asked to describe the situation in the form of a dilemma, with the help of the other participants. The physician formulates the following dilemma:

Are we willing to perform euthanasia or are we going to transfer the patient?

To clarify what is at stake in the dilemma, the facilitator asks the group to elaborate the negative consequences of each of the options. What will happen if the first option is chosen (and consequently the second option cannot be realized), and vice versa?

If we perform euthanasia it may lead to individual conscientious objections, loss of volunteers, and emotional problems for healthcare professionals.

If we transfer the patient this may cause mental instability and physical burdening because of the transfer; we disappoint a patient who has already stayed here for a couple of weeks; and we will be taking her out of her personal environment.

The next step is to analyse the norms and values in the situation. First, a list is made of perspectives that are relevant in the case. These include the people who are involved in the case (stakeholders) but also wider perspectives (for instance the institution or society at large). For each perspective, the group investigates the values behind the views and actions and the norms that make these values concrete. For example, one value may be 'sanctity of life', and the corresponding norm 'the physician should not end life actively'. Sometimes the same value is chosen by two different participants, but translated into two different norms. Values and norms are not derived from ethical theory, rules, or guidelines, but are explicit expressions of the implicit orientations and rules of each of the stakeholders involved. This requires an interpretation of the views and concerns of the stakeholders, both those who are present at the meeting and those who are absent. The parties present, for example the physician or the nurses, can directly confirm interpretations by the group. The values and norms relevant for the stakeholders who are not present, for example the patient and the family, can also be explored by the group: those who know them well can inform the others by giving information and telling stories about them, highlighting orientations and actions.

For the physician, two fundamental values are identified: care for the patient and concern for other people involved. These are made concrete in two norms: 'I have to end the patient's suffering' and 'I have to be aware of the emotions and values of nurses and other patients'. For the nurses, one important value is respect for autonomy, with the corresponding norm: 'We have to respond to the wishes of the patient'. A second value mentioned by the nurses is 'solidarity with the physician', which leads to the norm: 'We should support the physician in a difficult situation and back her up'. A third value is 'concern for the image of the hospice', which is translated into the norm: 'We should be careful not to acquire the image of an institution that does not hold on to the ideas of palliative care'. The nurses express specific worries related to the last value: 'If people notice that we perform euthanasia, more terminal patients will probably come with the same wish, knowing that it is possible here'. The cleaners, who used to be volunteers, say the hospice is a place where euthanasia does not belong. This is expressed in the value 'peace' and the corresponding norm: 'A radical intervention such as euthanasia should not be performed in our hospice'. For the patient, two values relevant to the situation are identified: 'dying peacefully' and 'being part of the community'; the corresponding norms are: 'I should be helped not to die in agony' and 'I should be allowed to die where I have always lived and feel at home'. The patient's family is motivated by concern for the patient's well-being. This implies that their values and norms are in line with those of the patient.

After exploring all the perspectives and corresponding values and norms, each participant in the moral case deliberation meeting is asked to make an individual choice about what he or she considers to be the morally right action in this case. They can choose one of the two sides of the dilemma (performing euthanasia or transferring the patient) or an alternative. They are asked to answer the question: 'What would you do and based on which value and norm would you act?' A further question is: 'What value that you deem important would not be realized, and how would you repair this moral damage?'

Both of the physicians say that they decide in favour of euthanasia, because they want to end the patient's suffering, and are most concerned about invoking emotions in the nursing staff and among the volunteers. They want to try and repair this by talking extensively with these groups. The nurses are divided. Some decide in favour of euthanasia, referring to the values of care and alleviating suffering, although they are worried about the turmoil that might result and the stress on other nurses and volunteers. They would try to respond to these negative consequences by clearly stipulating the policy of giving everyone the option not to be involved in any way. Others decide against euthanasia because of their concern for other patients and volunteers in the hospice. They would try to explain this to the patient and reassure her that she would receive optimal pain medication. Both cleaners decide against euthanasia, because they regard it as being incompatible with palliative care values. They would explain to the patient that euthanasia is not a good death.

The last step is to compare individual choices and investigate the differences, in order to understand each other better and to see whether new ways of dealing with the situation can be found that do justice to crucial values and take all perspectives into account as far as possible.

While comparing individual choices and underlying values and norms, the group recognizes that not allowing euthanasia at all will lead to moral problems, because the physician will not be able to make his or her own judgement, and some patients will have to go elsewhere at a moment of great distress. However, allowing euthanasia in the hospice will inevitably have a great impact.

Euthanasia in the hospice setting is not only a matter for the physician. Nurses will be involved in the process much more than in cases of euthanasia at home; they will have to take care of the patient constantly, while knowing that the patient's life will be ended by the physician within a few days or even hours. They will have to be informed beforehand and allowed to opt out of caring for the patient any longer. Nurses and other staff will always know about the upcoming euthanasia, and have to be sure that the physician will act responsibly, even if they are not involved in the process in any way. Thus, the physician will have to explain and share his or her views with the nurses and other staff, not about the individual case, but more generally. This need for explanation takes a concrete form during the deliberation, when one of the cleaners expresses her sincere worries about the impact performing euthanasia will have on the physician herself. She directly addresses the physician who presented the case, saying: 'How can you ever sleep again after doing such a thing?' The group is impressed by her concern for the physician, and the physician shows gratitude for her sympathy. The physician explains that euthanasia for her is always difficult, but that she feels relieved afterwards, if all has gone well and the patient has died peacefully. The value of peace, which the cleaner deems so important, is crucial for her as well, albeit in another way. The cleaner still has difficulty understanding the physician's view, but she is happy that the physician has sincerely explained how euthanasia works out for her, and no longer feels distressed by the idea that the physician would not be able to sleep again after performing euthanasia.

At the end of the moral case deliberation, which lasted for over two and a half hours, the group formulated the following conclusions: performing euthanasia should not be totally prohibited in the hospice; it should always be an exception, to be considered only after seriously examining the patient's wish to die and possible alternative ways of relieving the patient's suffering; the procedure should be explained carefully to the staff; nurses or other staff should not be obliged to participate in the care of the patient; other patients and volunteers should not be informed or involved in any way; a debriefing should be organized for the healthcare professionals involved.

Discussion

This case example shows that a moral case deliberation enables the participants to investigate normative aspects of a situation in which a patient expresses a wish to die, and find ways of dealing with them. By making explicit the values and norms related to various perspectives and courses of action, and exchanging views and concerns, the participants gain an understanding of the moral dimensions of the case and the moral orientations and convictions of all those concerned. In the process of investigating and exchanging values and norms, participants have an opportunity to ask questions, to examine presuppositions, and to give explanations—for example the physician who explained her experiences around performing euthanasia to the cleaner who showed concern for her well-being. During the deliberation the participants show a growing understanding of and concern for each other and for the people not present, such as the patient and the volunteers. This process of understanding each other's perspectives and showing concern for each other's values and emotions is especially important in settings like a hospice, in which people have to cooperate closely in the care of patients in difficult circumstances.

During the moral case deliberation, the patient's wish to die was examined by the participants and found to be related to the realistic expectation that the pain might recur, even with optimal medication. The participants agreed that the patient's wish should be critically investigated. This is in line with the Dutch euthanasia law, which states that the physician has to discuss the wish to die with the patient, and, together with the patient, come to the conclusion that there are no other reasonable options for relieving the patient's suffering. In a hospice setting, other professionals, such as nurses, will also be included in this process. They will often be the first to hear the wish to die in the daily process of care, and to discuss this with the patient. They will also discuss this with the physician, and give their view on the background and meaning of the patient's wish. Thus, the interpretation of the patient's wish to die requires in-depth communication between various professionals and an exchange of views on the nature of the patient's wish.

A moral case deliberation gives a voice to all parties involved and enables them to be open about what they care about and what they experience as difficult. In moral case deliberations in a hospice not only physicians but also nurses, other professionals, and volunteers play a role. Their experiences in the care process and their values have a prominent place. In this case, the views of the nurses and the cleaners contained important issues and concerns. The nurses were divided. This was regarded by the other participants as an expression of the problematic nature of the situation. The nurses were not forced to take a side, but were enabled to express their different views. The group concluded that differences should be acknowledged and respected. The cleaners were very concerned about the idea of euthanasia being performed in the hospice. Their concerns were taken seriously. Their arguments were not scrutinized from an abstract, theoretical point of view, but they were invited to explain their worries and concerns. This enabled the physician to understand them, and to elaborate on the emotions that euthanasia invoked in herself. In the process of exchanging experiences and responding to emotions, the participants in the group all had an equal position and were empowered as moral subjects.

Facilitating a moral case deliberation presupposes an awareness of power differences, and requires specific interventions to deal with them, such as inviting participants to ask each other questions for explanation instead of making judgements about what the other says, and ensuring that all participants have the same opportunity to express their views and experiences. This does not mean that all stakeholders have the same legal position or the same role in end-of-life decisions. The legal decision about whether the patient's request for euthanasia is granted is left to the physician. However, within a moral case deliberation every participant will have to take into account the consequences of any decision for all stakeholders, and take everybody's values and emotions into consideration.

The outcome of this moral case deliberation was not only a growth in understanding of each other's views and concerns, but also a move towards a new institutional policy. Euthanasia was no longer regarded as totally wrong in the context of hospice care. In exceptional cases it might be the only alternative left for the patient. This conclusion is actually in line with Dutch euthanasia law. Euthanasia can be considered only if all reasonable alternatives have been explored. In a hospice setting, more medical and spiritual alternatives are available than in a patient's home. Thus, euthanasia will be very exceptional. Euthanasia in a hospice requires specific safeguards, for instance in relation to other patients and volunteers. The need for careful practice, which is fundamental in all euthanasia cases, is especially prominent in a hospice setting. By becoming more open towards the possibility of euthanasia, the professionals working in the hospice are not forced to relinquish the values of palliative care. Rather, fundamental values such as 'mutual trust', 'acceptance of dying', and 'providing support in difficult situations' become even more important if euthanasia is considered. The new institutional policy concerning euthanasia implied a change for the hospice, in that some views became less self-evident, especially the idea that the active ending of life is against the very notion of palliative care and therefore always wrong. Yet this also implied a new view of euthanasia, emphasizing not the patient's right to die but the need for help if all other options have failed, and of the requirements of careful practice, which in an interdisciplinary setting requires attention to the needs and emotions of all stakeholders.

Conclusion

Euthanasia and palliative care have a different history, and embody different values and norms. They come from different traditions, are organized differently in healthcare practice, and have a different legal position. However, traditions, practices, and legal systems are not isolated. They touch upon each other and coexist in modern society in general, and health care in particular. This may cause frictions, for instance when euthanasia is put on the agenda in a hospice. Such frictions clearly have a normative dimension.

Decisions around the end of life require attention to the experiences, values, and emotions of physicians, nurses, and other professional and non-professional caregivers. Moral case deliberation gives all participants a voice and invites them to take part in a joint process of moral investigation. By including nurses and other professionals in the deliberation, they are empowered and their values and concerns are put on the agenda, resulting in a widening of the dialogue. Moral case deliberation may help participants to explore moral views and concerns and to help find responsible ways of dealing with dilemmas in healthcare practice.

In a moral case deliberation, the perspectives of all parties involved in a dilemma are investigated. What values are at stake for the patient who expresses a wish to die? What values are important for the physician and other professionals involved? How can these values be taken into account in the final decision about whether or not to assist the patient in dying? The aim is to better understand the views and experiences of all stakeholders, and to examine possible ways of dealing with them. This implies that a patient's wish to die is neither discarded nor accepted as given. It is regarded as a moral appeal, requiring interpretation and deliberation. What exactly does the patient ask of the physician and the other professionals involved? How can they respond in a meaningful and responsible way, doing justice to their own normative views and experiences? A joint investigation of the values and normative considerations of all parties involved may provide a basis for a dialogical exploration of experiences and dilemmas around a patient's wish to die, which may result in new ways of dealing with individual patients and new institutional arrangements.

References

Abma, T. A., Molewijk, A. C., and Widdershoven, G. A. M. (2009). Good care in ongoing dialogue. Improving the quality of care through moral deliberation and responsive evaluation. *Health Care Analysis*, **17**, 217–235.

Battin, M. P. (1994). A dozen caveats concerning the discussion of euthanasia in the Netherlands. In: M. P. Battin (ed.), *The Least Worst Death. Essays in Bioethics and the End of Life*, pp. 130–144. Oxford: Oxford University Press.

Berghmans, R. L. P. (2010). Dementia and end-of-life decisions: ethical issues—A perspective from the Netherlands. In: H. Helmchen and N. Sartorius (eds), *Ethics in Psychiatry*, pp. 401–420. Dordrecht: Springer.

Cohen-Almagor, R. (2004). *Euthanasia in the Netherlands. The Policy and Practice of Mercy Killing*. Dordrecht: Kluwer Academic Publishers.

van der Dam, S., Abma, T. A., Molewijk, A. C., Kardol, M. J. M., Schols, J. M. G. A., and Widdershoven, G. A. M. (2011). Organising moral case deliberation in mixed groups: experiences in two Dutch nursing homes. *Nursing Ethics*, **18**, 327–340.

van Delden, J. J. M. (1999). Slippery slopes in flat countries—a response. *Journal of Medical Ethics*, **25**, 22–24.

van Dijk, G., and van Wijlick, E. (2010). Zorgvuldige euthanasie. [Careful euthanasia] *Medisch Contact*, **65**, 1612–1615.

Gill, M. B. (2009). Is the legalization of physician-assisted suicide compatible with good end-of-life care? *Journal of Applied Philosophy*, **26**, 27–45.

Griffiths, J., Bood, A., and Weyers, H. (1998). *Euthanasia and Law in the Netherlands*. Amsterdam: Amsterdam University Press.

ten Have, H. A. M. J. (2010). Expanding the scope of palliative care. In: R. B. Purtilo and H. A. M. J. ten Have (eds), *Ethical Foundations of Palliative Care for Alzheimer Disease*, pp. 61–79. Baltimore: Johns Hopkins University Press.

Hendin, H. (2002), The Dutch experience. *Issues in Law and Medicine*, **17**, 223–246.

Janssens, R., van Delden, J. J., and Widdershoven, G. A. M. (2012). Palliative sedation: not just normal medical practice. Ethical reflections on the Royal Dutch Medical Association's guideline on palliative sedation. *Journal of Medical Ethics*, **38**, 664–668.

Kennedy, J. (2002). *Een Weloverwogen Dood [A Well-considered Death]*. Amsterdam: Bert Bakker.

Keown, J. (ed.) (1995). *Euthanasia Examined*. Cambridge: Cambridge University Press.

Molewijk, A. C., Abma, T. A., Stolper, M., and Widdershoven, G. A. M. (2008). Teaching ethics in the clinic. Theory and practice of moral case deliberation. *Journal of Medical Ethics*, **34**, 120–124.

Olde-Rikkert, M. G. M., and Rigaud, A.-S. (2010). Hospital-based palliative care and dementia, or what do we treat patients for and how do we do it? In: R. B. Purtilo and H. A. M. J. ten Have (eds), *Ethical Foundations of Palliative Care for Alzheimer Disease*, pp. 80–96. Baltimore: Johns Hopkins University Press.

Onwuteaka-Philipsen, B. D., Brinkman-Stoppelenburg, A., Penning, C., de Jong-Krul, G. W. F., van Delden, J. J. F., and van der Heide, A. (2012). Trends in end-of-life decisions before and after the enactment of the euthanasia law in the Netherlands from 1990 to 2010: a repeated cross-sectional survey. *Lancet*, **380**, 908–915.

Steinkamp, N. and Gordijn, B. (2003). Ethical case deliberation on the ward. A comparison of four models. *Medicine, Health Care and Philosophy*, **6**, 235–246.

Steinkamp, N. and Gordijn, B. (2004). *Ethik in der Klinik. Ein Arbeitsbuch [Ethics in the Clinic. A Workbook]*. Cologne: Springer-Verlag.

Verkerk, M., Lindemann, H., Maeckelberghe, E., Feenstra, E., Harttough, R., and de Bree, M. (2004) Enhancing reflection: an interpersonal exercise in ethics education. *Hastings Center Report*, **34**, 31–38.

Widdershoven, G. A. M. and Molewijk, B. (2010). Philosophical foundations of clinical ethics. A hermeneutic perspective. In: J. Schildmann, J.-S.Gordon, and J. Vollmann (eds), *Clinical Ethics Consultation. Theories and Methods, Implementation, Evaluation*, pp. 37–52. Farnham: Ashgate.

WTLVHZ [Wet Toetsing Levensbeëindiging op Verzoek en Hulp bij Zelfdoding] (2014). Wet Toetsing Levensbeëindiging op Verzoek en Hulp bij Zelfdoding. URL: <http://wetten.over-heid.nl/BWBR0012410/geldigheidsdatum_24-06-2014>

Chapter 15

End-of-life ethics from the perspectives of patients' wishes

Christoph Rehmann-Sutter

Introduction to end-of-life ethics

The literature on end-of-life ethics mostly discusses the moral issues that arise from the perspective of those who offer—or could offer—treatment to patients. Healthcare professionals and regulators are supposed to put the patient's perspective, her or his needs and wishes, at the centre of their decision-making about what they offer: this is a prerequisite for a 'good death' (Woods 2013). What should they offer to those patients who wish to hasten death? What should they be allowed to offer? What ethical considerations are pivotal when deciding how to respond to patients' wishes? Where should the lines be drawn? There are many questions of this sort that all need careful attention. Here I want to look at these issues from the other side—from the perspectives of patients themselves. I shall discuss the ethical implications of patients' wishes from the ethical perspective of the people making these wishes, and who, through their wishing, participate in end-of-life decision-making.

Patients' perspectives on the end of life are also moral perspectives, because wishes in general and wishes to die in particular are existentially relevant expressions of their moral self. For somebody who wishes such important things as life or death, the phenomenology of wishing is multilayered and complex. Part of that is due to the special circumstances of suffering at the end of life that can contain elements that make life become deeply ambivalent, or even undesirable. If somebody is in the situation of not wanting to live 'this way' any longer, because it would mean 'too much suffering', she or he may prefer to die—but without desiring to die in the first place. If these conditions were to change, life might become desirable once again. But how much is 'too much'? Wishes to die are responses to a situation that can be differently interpreted but only partially influenced.

In order to discuss the ethical perspective of patients, I adopt a primarily descriptive and non-judgemental attitude, i.e. my aim here is not to sort wishes into those that are ethically 'right' and 'wrong'. I am not in a position to tell patients what they should ethically wish for. My approach is rather to reflect on the moral hermeneutics that is embodied in wishing. In wishing, a person interprets a situation and makes (partial) sense in a situation that may be disintegrating. I will use three patients' explanations and narratives to illustrate my point.

Wishing in a moral sense

When I describe what is going on in my mind when I wish, I begin by stating that to wish something is a kind of thinking. With Paul Ricoeur (1950), I believe that a wish is an *act of thinking*, in which I relate myself to this 'something', which is other than myself: the object of the wish. As we have pointed out in Chapter 1, wishes can be regarded as a part of human agency, which is characterized by own-ness, anticipation, and hope. In wishing, one has the sense of being the author of one's own thoughts, ideas, and imaginings. In wishing, one anticipates the content of an imagining to become or to be real. And the imaginative content of the wish is hoped to be or to become real. Some wishes are more actively formed and re-formed, others are more simply felt to be there. There is more or less activity in their formation, and more or less passivity. They are not static but dynamic—they are interactive. And they are accessible to reflection.

In this sense, wishes are elements of what Hannah Arendt has described as 'the life of the mind' (Arendt 1979). A wish can be questioned, can be left ambiguous and arbitrarily unclear, or can be made more precise. It can be communicated or kept secret. And by re-focusing the attention and the vision that a wish contains, it can be transformed within the patient's reflective agential mind. Harry Frankfurt's term of 'second-order volitions' (Frankfurt 1988) also applies to wishes. Second-order volitions include wishes that are directed to one's own wishes. Somebody can wish, for example, to have a wish to live. We are in a constant inner dialogue with ourselves (Archer 2000) about what we really wish, what we want ourselves to wish, and sometimes even what we ought to wish right now. In this reflexive way, wishes (first and second order) influence our actual choices, and they are influenced by others' wishes. And some wishes function just as wishes; they are not meant to form a will and be executed. This is the view I now want to explain.

The patient's situation at the end of life

Most patients who are confronted with inevitable death in the near future experience a situation that is existentially challenging. But exactly what is challenging, and how, depends on many factors that belong to the particular circumstances of an individual's biography. When we talk about the ethics of wishing from the perspective of patients it is important for us to try to imagine these patients' situations. The inevitability of death itself is part of the human condition. The circumstances of dying and the meanings that these circumstances carry can, however, be manifold, even in highly standardized clinical settings where many aspects of end-of-life care are routine. The fact of finitude, which is general, gains concrete significance and practical meaning only within the relationships and the particularities of an individual life. This of course affects the decisions that need to be taken and the attitudes that seem morally justified.

An end-of-life situation carries general characteristics that gain individual meanings in terms of the patient's particular biography, medical condition, and specific local circumstances:

1 Death is *unavoidable*. It may be possible to postpone it, but in the end it will come. The patient cannot live forever.

2 The time at which the end actually arrives is *unforeseeable*. This can remain so even in situations near death, when the dying person knows for certain that death

is close. Closeness is not measurable. Nobody knows exactly whether this will be within the next few minutes, within the next hour, or only after a few more nights.

3 Uncertainty about death can have *meanings* while also being *absurd*, showing the breakdown of meaning. For some, life's ending may be the final defeat of life by death; for them, it is uncertain when that battle will finally be lost. For others it may be a point at which they move on into another, transcendent, state of being, and the uncertainty is about when God calls. For some it may be a point when finally everything becomes quiet and the end is a release from struggle. Uncertainty then has to do with the balance of forces that collide in this struggle. Dying itself need not be seen as meaningful. It may be experienced as a loss or as a breakdown of meanings.

4 Since these meanings concern an existentially crucial event in life (its very end), patients are very *serious* about what they believe. Meanings are not products of stories that could be easily replaced or compensated for by other stories. They make up part of a person's identity.

5 If time is consciously experienced, a more acute awareness of *duration* may develop. Time becomes short, but it gains in intensity. Therefore, for some, time is felt to proceed more slowly; important aspects of the past are again present; loved ones want to say goodbye.

6 The dying person depends on *other people* in the course of her or his dying. They are important not only for the services they provide or refuse, for their capabilities and limits, but in a very existential way as essential others whose presence (or absence) matters.

7 For the person who is dying, death is not only a void, an unknown, but it can also be like a *mirror* in which they see an image of their past. What was important? What is important now? This 'mirror' can reveal things to the dying person that were less obvious before.

8 Dying means leaving behind a life with all that was important: other people, relationships, habits, hopes, ambitions, etc. This is a process of *letting go and holding on*, of accepting death and struggling for life, a shifting disequilibrium. The question arises of how much of each is necessary. Up to what point would letting go and accepting death be inappropriate or irresponsible? This also affects medical decisions, for example agreeing to another operation, or accepting life-prolonging treatments such as medications or tube feeding.

9 The end-of-life situation for the person who experiences it is *new*. The person who dies has never died before and hence cannot rely on experience or on learning. The experience of watching other people dying can help, but it is still not the same. What adds to its novelty is that the situation, depending on many contingent factors, may be rapidly changing.

10 Only a part of the development of the situation can be controlled. Death is essentially an experience of *loss of control*. The person is dependent on caregivers and natural processes, such as the progress of a disease. They take over and tend to dissolve the very capabilities of control and decision-making.

More characteristics could be added of course, and they could be described in other words with different emphases. I will use them here as a rough framework to explain why I believe that a description of the situation at the end of life as one of approaching disappearance would be much too simple. Death, for the dying, is more than 'only posthumous nonexistence' (Kamm 1993, p. 13), because the last phase of life in the expectation of death contains so many existential and moral challenges. Therefore the moral situation for patients who face unavoidable death, in other words questions of what is good and bad in death, are considerably more complex than what is sometimes caricatured as an 'Epicurean' view, which consists in not fearing death because nonexistence implies not having experiences at all, and therefore no bad experiences either. The 'wish to die' belongs to life, not to death. It is a formula that can capture some of this moral complexity.

A wish to die as a practical space

Seen from a remote and abstract perspective, the situation at the end of life may be considered under the expectation of a shrinking radius of activity and a foreseeable loss of all practical options. What this view suggests is that if death comes we have nothing about which to make choices. It does not, however, represent the experience of those actually living this situation. In the oncology part of the Basel wish-to-die study (see Chapter 8) we met 30 cancer patients in palliative care who knew about their terminal condition. In systematic qualitative interviews they told us their stories about decisions and choices that were important in the current, final phase of their lives. Cases 1–3 are three examples from the stories they told us.

Case 1: 'Yes, if it does not count as suicide' [patient 12]

Wilhelm, a 77-year-old male cancer patient suffering from bronchial carcinoma, gave us an interview in the palliative care ward of a general hospital 12 days before his death. A few years ago he had lost his wife, who had suffered from multiple sclerosis for 35 years and eventually died of it, and for 3 years he had lived in a new relationship. He said that it was only for his new partner that he agreed to undergo chemotherapy ('without her great love I would not have done chemo'). He said that he was no churchgoer but had always felt some direct connection to God. Now he wished that God would make the passage easy for him, and he hoped that death would come soon. He said that he believed that it is not up to humans to interfere with it, but confirmed that he was waiting for something to make that death come more quickly and easily, hopefully something that allowed him to 'sleep over', how he imagined palliative sedation, but only if it did not fall under the category of suicide ('Yes if this does not count as suicide'). Earlier in the interview he told us that he has lost his two sons, one from cancer, the other who had become unemployed and committed suicide by shooting himself just after Christmas, which was a major trauma in his family. Suicide and everything that falls into the same category was therefore absolutely impossible for him.

Case 2: 'Have I done enough? Did I suffer enough?' [patient 21]

Alette, a 57-year-old teacher of religious studies, looked back over a very long cancer history, with several operations, radiation treatments, and chemotherapies over the last 7 years. She was very tired when she gave us the interview in the hospice where she otherwise felt at ease. Her most acute concern was uncertainty as to how much time she still had. She said that she considered herself to be a natural fighter ('Well, I am a fighter. I have really done battle.'), but at a certain point she felt she had suffered enough and was ready to die. While still in the university hospital she felt the right moment had come ('Then I said: No, no! Just no more! Now it's enough. That was the moment.'). Alette then refused life-sustaining support (such as food or treatment) with the intention of hastening her death.

Case 3: Fine-tuning the wishes in regard to dying [patient 9]

Marie, a 81-year-old woman suffering from pancreatic cancer, was interviewed in the hospice 19 days before she died. She refused all chemotherapy and operations and only wanted painkillers. Over three pages of the transcript we find a dense passage where she gives a finely tuned description of her wishes. She said that: (1) she did not want to commit suicide; that (2) she had lived enough; that (3) she did not cling to life and could let go ('but men in general; they want to hold on to life.'); that (4) if somebody offered her the means for more quality time, she would probably take it; that (5) she did not wish to die 'now', but she was ready to accept death when it comes. Assisted suicide for her (6) would be a suicide, which she refused for moral reasons, and therefore it was not an option for her. (7) Palliative sedation (continuous sleep until death) would however not be suicide and would be desirable for her if the situation were to worsen ('I would opt for it if the situation becomes unbearable; I mean this is not taking one's own life'). She also said that she considered herself an independent person, but in regard to the disease she trusted the doctors on what would be best to do ('If somebody else knows more than I do, then they should decide.').

Wilhelm (Case 1) decided that curative treatments should be discontinued (no further chemotherapy), that 'sleeping over' would be desirable and make sense, but only if it were not suicide, because of his traumatic experience with the suicide of his son. Alette (Case 2), after a long battle against cancer that caused a lot of suffering, found that 'now' the right time to die had come. She had fought and suffered 'enough'. This was obviously a judgement that involved values as well as the experience of no longer being able to withstand the rigours of the treatment. Marie (Case 3) decided against curative treatments and against suicide and assisted suicide, and came to an acceptance of death in the foreseeable future. But she did not want her life to end, as long as she continued to enjoy it, and would even accept treatments for this. And she critically evaluated her own decision-making capacities and the role of experts who knew more, in these decisions. All these patients made up their minds in regard to what sort of wish to live or to die they had in their present situation. This present situation is an 'ethical situation' in the sense that George Herbert Mead (1938, p. 464) has suggested: they brought different values 'into a field of possibility' and evaluated the things they were going to do in terms of the things they could not do. They were 'weighing' the different good things against each other.

In order to describe this situation and the role of all these complex lines of thinking, which are sometimes in tension with each other but, taken together, can be seen as 'the patient's wish to die', it was necessary to see the patients' wishes as something extended: a practical space, a space expanded and worked through by the patients' agency. This was the emerging explanatory concept that enabled us (the authors of the study) to interpret patients' subjectivity (Ohnsorge et al. 2014a,b). To wish to die is a rich active–passive experience that involves the person who wishes as a thinking and reflecting subject, who is the author of her or his wishes, decisions, and attitudes. The wish extends in time and involves other important people in essential roles. The reflexivity involved is relational and dialogical (cf. Cunliffe and Easterley-Smith 2004). These other people who played a role in reflection can be living and closely present; they can, however, also be absent, or, in the case of Wilhelm's sons, even dead, but still important as references. They are present in the patient's mind as memories and they appear as figures in the patient's narratives.

Ethics of wishing

Why wishes matter ethically

Wishes to die belong to a category of wishes to which an ethical dimension is *intrinsic*, since they concern the life of the person who wishes. And since existence as a person is also in many ways interwoven with the life of others with whom one is involved, a wish to die, individual as it is, also concerns the lives of these others. For the person who wishes, a wish to die is not just a 'preference' like other preferences, since it is a wish to end the capacity to have preferences. And this ending is irreversible. Therefore wishes to die matter ethically for the person who wishes.

There is more about wishes to die than the identification and comparison of preferences, since the wisher may ask: Is it really *my* wish? (Does it belong to me, to what I consider as my true self?) Do I *trust* myself in this wish? (Is it an 'easy way out' of a difficulty in my life that demands another solution?) Does it *authentically* belong to me, or is it based on what I believe that others expect from me? Is it *dependent* on a situation that could be changed? Is it *strong* enough, compared with other wishes that I may also have, which are inconsistent with the wish to die?

For patients in certain situations it may be *unclear* what they really wish, or they can experience their situation as intrinsically ambivalent. Some patients whom we saw in our study, for example, wished to carry on living and *at the same time* they wished to die soon (Ohnsorge et al. 2012). Patients tell about disrupted, even chaotic or absurd, experiences that might be uncomfortable to hear (for caregivers too), and (for the patient) difficult to understand. To know what one should wish under such circumstances is an achievement that may not come easily. Wishes are therefore intentional mental processes, we could say 'practical spaces', in which the wisher comes to terms with a situation that she or he might perceive as chaotic or contradictory and difficult to understand. To shape a wish is to attempt to *respond* in a deep existential way to the 'meaning' of this challenging life situation. Responding is an activity, and at the same time is a form of perception.

What biomedical ethics traditionally discusses as the 'autonomy' of a patient is therefore founded in an open space of deliberative reflexivity. This space lies underneath the expressed wish that contains the lived reality of autonomy: its process, its thinking. Autonomy literally means living by one's own laws or rules. The subject embodies the time that thinking needs before the rules are found, and its autonomy comes to terms with the situation. The self must deliberate before it knows what wishes should guide it. The inner, subjective space–time that is contained in a wish is included when we speak of 'agency', which is the capacity to act in a way that the agent is the author.

Normativity in the context of wishes

When commentators who are not directly affected 'do' ethics at the end of life, they need to claim a discursive space for this deliberation, with criteria that make arguments rational and stringent. In these discussions they deal with the moral implications of end-of-life decisions, such as those about entering palliative sedation, about stopping therapies, or about providing assistance to die on request. Among the criteria for rationality and stringency one is particularly prominent: the question as to whether a certain moral claim can hold for everybody who is in a similar situation. As Kant suggested, and others have confirmed (Korsgard 1996), the universality of a moral claim establishes its normative authority. Kant suggested that we should ask: can I wish that the claim in question is a universal prescription? This is a safeguard against the arbitrariness of moral claims. We need to distinguish between moral claims which truly have a prescriptive authority, and which therefore guide our own practice, and moral claims that only re-formulate the idiosyncratic preferences or interests of those who claim them. But is such a view of normativity applicable to the goals and values involved in the wishes of patients?

Patients' reflections—local, particular, and situated as they are—are also related to what they see as their guiding principles, which help to make sense for them in their difficult situation. These principles may not be as universal in their scope as the principles that must compete in the marketplace of arguments. But as patients try to understand and communicate their own wishes, they must *make sense*, at least for themselves. This fragile normativity rests on the necessity that wishes must be understandable for those that hold them, and possibly also for others. A reflected wish to die, due to its existential weight, is more than an accidental viewpoint. Wishes are therefore serious in an important way, and as such they contain normative elements. The best way to explain this normativity is, I believe, that the wisher's self identifies with the wish. The wisher would probably not claim that everybody ought to wish the same if she or he were in a similar situation. But the wish must be coherent for the one who wishes, and that means that it needs to make sense in a life story that is essentially related to important others.

Are wishes to die self-annihilating?

Hannah Arendt has suggested that a wish to die is self-annihilating: 'Anybody who says "I'd rather not exist than be unhappy" cannot be trusted, since while he is saying it he is still alive' (Arendt 1979, Vol. 2, p. 91). However, I do not think that this argument holds for patients' wishes to die at the end of their life. The wishing subject, in order to have meaningful wishes that are always directed to the future in some way, does not assume by implication to continue to exist infinitely in time. It is possible to wish that even the faculty of wishing might come to an end at some point, since wishing is an expression of our embodied life. To wish that one's life may end now, that death may come sooner, even the wish to do something that hastens death, or to stop doing something that hinders the arrival of death, can, in certain situations, prove to be precisely the wish with which this embodied self, after reflection, can identify. If this is the case, this wish to die is self-vindicating rather than self-annihilating.

Wishing not to be a burden to others

Among the motives given by patients as being behind their wish to die, one in particular is relatively frequent and yet at the same time ethically challenging: wishing to die because one does not want to be a burden to others. One patient (patient 4) in our study said: 'I am burdened myself, I am such a burden to others; I want to end this' (see Ohnsorge et al. 2014b). Some might say: 'A slight burden is ok, but I should not be too much of a burden, only a burden I find acceptable to impose on them.'

This kind of wish to die relates to the moral issues of dependency, which are abundant in care relationships (Kittay 1999). The person who wishes not to be a burden to others anticipates the perspective of the others who may find caregiving burdensome. The two perspectives can be—to use Ronald Laing's language—knotted into each other in many ways: A thinks that B thinks A is a burden to her. B fears that A thinks that B thinks A is a burden to her. Or: A does not want B to think that A is a burden to her. Or: A does not want B to have to think that she should not find A a burden to her; etc. (cf. Laing 1970). It is therefore very difficult, if not impossible, to separate these two perspectives. The person who thinks they will be an unacceptable burden to others presumes these others' perspectives in some way. The assumption is that existence *is* a burden to them. The real others would possibly say that this is not the case. Their perception of being burdened need not correspond to how the patient imagines them to be burdened. Caregivers and healthcare professionals may have other, more important values, for instance the value of caring, of not leaving the patient alone, that outweigh the burden. They will optimize the way they treat the person, considering that she/he should not feel they are too great a burden, since this might be unacceptable for her or him. The psychology and morality of the feeling of being a burden to others is therefore very intricate.

As such, a wish to unburden others of oneself need not be illegitimate. But the person who wishes can nonetheless find that a certain wish not to be a burden to others should not exist, because this wish does not fit with her moral expectations of herself as a person who is capable of accepting nursing and others caring and helping, i.e. with her concept of being a virtuous person.

The language of duties is difficult here. There is no moral obligation to find being a burden to others acceptable. I cannot see a reason why such an obligation should exist. If there is no such obligation to find being a burden to others acceptable, then it is no breach of duty to wish not to be a burden any more, even if this implies no longer existing. It is each person's right to judge individually how heavily being this kind of burden to others might weigh in moral terms. But there are legitimate concerns as to whether a wish to cease to be a burden to others, and therefore to die, should be accepted from the perspective of those who are supposed to *carry* this burden. They might ask themselves: did we give reasons to suggest that we find her/him a burden? Did we signal that to her or him? They will then try to prevent this feeling of being a burden to them from becoming too obvious. The wish to die may then fade away, but one cannot be sure that this will happen. To disqualify a wish to die as illegitimate is not the best answer, since this disregards the experience of a patient who feels she or he is a burden to others, and who might feel that this is unacceptable with regard to her or his idea of virtue: of what kind of person she or he wants to be.

It is ethically problematic if society (or a family) is structured in such a way that those who are no longer useful start feeling they are nothing but a burden. This is ethically problematic because it does not treat these people as beings with inherent moral worth. Their worth is seen as being conditional on the services they could provide to society. There are many different ways a society can be structured such that patients who need care feel themselves to be an unacceptable burden: the distribution of healthcare costs, the cultural attitude towards ageing, assistance to die offers that are too readily accessible, a too individualistic model of social justice, and so forth. What can be said generally is that it is important to be attentive in order not to let this happen. The development of more positive images of old age would help too, images that explain why the oldest generation in human society is important and helpful for younger people, even if they must be cared for.

Wishing as dialogue

Hannah Arendt has interpreted the human condition of 'natality' in a way that is also applicable to humans at the end of their lives. We are born creatures, and not only born into finitude. Since we are born creatures, we are capable of making a beginning in our lives. 'Because they are initium, newcomers and beginners by virtue of birth, men take initiative, are prompted into action' (Arendt 1958, p. 177). A serious wish is an initiative, since it can effect a course of actions. It can be seen as a beginning even if the wish, under the circumstances of illness and dying, is directed towards life's end. Natality means seeing a person before death as a person who can be *initium*.

To see the wish to die as a beginning raises the question: a beginning of *what*? This question, which re-formulates the ethical question of end-of-life care, covers the perspective of the one who formulates the wish and the perspective of the others who are responding to the wish and are involved in the courses of action that the wish sets in motion. Between these perspectives there is a dialogical connection. The person who wishes to die (in a particular sense) is referring to others who should respond. And the others who can respond are involved as partners in a caring relationship, and as such they are responsible for the way they respond. For the patient the question is: what can or should he or she expect from others in response to his or her wish?

An automatic response is not really what a patient can wish for. If the other fulfilled every wish without even thinking about what the wish is, what it means, and how it came about, the reaction would not be a response in a dialogue, but a reflex. The wish would be heard not as a wish but as an instruction. The wish, which is a structure of hope, would go into the void. If the wisher expected others just to execute what the wish implies, he or she would not be entering into a responsive dialogue. He or she would not meet the others in their caring capacities. The same would be true if the others rejected every wish to die without a second thought. The others are expected to respond to the wishes in a qualified and loving way. This includes being concerned to perceive and understand the wish, in its background and its precise character. And it also includes respecting the wish.

References

Archer, M. (2000). *Being Human. The Problem of Agency*. Cambridge: Cambridge University Press.

Arendt, H. (1958). *The Human Condition*. Chicago: University of Chicago Press.

Arendt, H. (1979). *The Life of the Mind*. San Diego: Harcourt.

Cunliffe, A. L. and Easterley-Smith, M. (2004). From reflection to practical reflexivity: Experiential learning as lived experience. In: M. Reynolds and R. Vince (eds), *Organizing Reflection*, pp. 30–46. Aldershot: Ashgate.

Frankfurt, H. (1988). *The Importance of What We Care About*. Cambridge: Cambridge University Press.

Kamm, F. M. (1993). *Morality, Mortality. Vol. I: Death and Whom to Save from It*. New York: Oxford University Press.

Kittay, E. F. (1999). *Love's Labor. Essays on Women, Equality, and Dependency*. New York: Routledge.

Korsgard, C. M. (1996). *The Sources of Normativity*. Cambridge: Cambridge University Press.

Laing, R. D. (1970). *Knots*. London: Penguin.

Mead, G. H. (1938). *The Philosophy of the Act*. Chicago: University of Chicago Press.

Ohnsorge, K., Gudat, H. R., Widdershoven, G. A. M., and Rehmann-Sutter, C. (2012). 'Ambivalence' at the end of life: How to understand patients' wishes ethically. *Nursing Ethics*, **19**, 629–641.

Ohnsorge, K., Gudat, H., and Rehmann-Sutter, C. (2014a). Intentions in wishes to die: analysis and a typology. A report of 30 qualitative case studies of terminally ill cancer patients in palliative care. *Psycho-Oncology*, **23**, 1021–1026.

Ohnsorge, K., Gudat, H., and Rehmann-Sutter, C. (2014b). What a wish to die can mean. Reasons, meanings and functions of wishes to die, reported from 30 qualitative case studies of terminally ill cancer patients. *BMC Palliative Care*, **13**, 38.

Ricoeur, P. (1950). *Le Volontaire et l'Involontaire. Philosophie de la Volonté I*. Paris: Aubier.

Woods, S. (2013). The 'good death', palliative care and end of life ethics. In: L. Hagger and S. Woods (eds), *A Good Death? Law and Ethics in Practice*, pp. 103–121. Farnham: Ashgate.

Chapter 16

Dialogue intermezzo: II

KATHRIN OHNSORGE: We face many culturally or individually situated ideas about dying. Approaches towards the wish to die that cultivate responsiveness and attentiveness to other people's moral understandings, while being critically aware of not imposing one's own moral assumptions on the other, seem to be the most appropriate. Speaking provocatively, with these ideals in mind, do we still have grounds to challenge a wish to die?

LARS JOHAN MATERSTVEDT: When the patient is competent, we certainly do. First, in matters of life and death it is going to be difficult for any doctor somehow to 'conceal' his or her views. Second, I believe that trying to do so is in itself questionable, as it can be seen as not taking the patient seriously; it can, in certain instances, amount to disrespect for patient autonomy. If I were that patient and learned that my doctor did not want to discuss the issue with me 'for my own good', I would have rejected such paternalism. Third, engaging in a discussion like this is not tantamount to 'imposing' one's views on the patient; it's a matter of speaking one's mind out of both concern and respect for the patient. Hence the patient is not forced or coerced into thinking or acting in a particular way. And last but not least, a wish to die raises in the most fundamental way possible the issue of whether or not people are the 'best judges of their own interest'. I explore this issue in Chapter 12, and argue that this idea is surprisingly problematic even in those who aren't sick, and significantly more so in the seriously ill. So there are several well-founded reasons for critically challenging a wish to die.

CHRISTOPH REHMANN-SUTTER: I agree. For me it depends on what we mean by 'challenging a wish to die'. Lars Johan has interpreted it as not concealing one's own views, but rather entering in an engaged but respectful discussion with the patient. Yes, definitely, we are justified in doing so. This is a situation where respect can be expressed by saying both emotionally and with the best possible arguments: 'No, I want you to live! I don't accept your wish to die, because you are important to us, important to me.' Where I would be critical, however, is when caregivers condemn the other's wish in a moral way and say (or let the patient feel) something like: 'Shame on you! Nobody has the right to seriously wish to die. You are a morally weak person when you tell me a thing like that.' This would not be respectful. And it might even fail to challenge the wish to die. Therefore, challenging should mean something like fighting with the other for her or his own good, by respecting the other in her or his own right, by struggling with her or him. This can only work if we are quite clear about our own moral beliefs, and clear also that challenging the other's views does not mean imposing our own views. I am struggling with the analogy of fighting here, but it tells me something.

GUY WIDDERSHOVEN: From a hermeneutic perspective, the most important task is to try and understand the wish to die. This means trying to see the perspective of the patient who expresses this wish. What matters for him or her in the given situation? What does he or she value? We should acknowledge that, in our pluralist society, the answer is different for each patient. Patients have individual views on life and death, and individual perspectives on how to deal with suffering. From a hermeneutic point of view, understanding does not simply mean putting oneself in the shoes of the other and doing away with one's own perspective. Trying to understand the patient's wish to die implies investigating what the wish means to oneself. This means that one cannot take recourse to a relativist position, and say that it is fully up to the patient to determine whether or not his or her wish to die is valid. The wish asks for a response, which should go beyond merely indicating that one has noticed what the patient wants. This is especially, but not only, relevant for the physician. He or she has to respond to the patient's wish, and try to come to a joint conclusion with the patient about what is good in the specific situation. The Dutch euthanasia law underlines the importance of this process. It stipulates that euthanasia is only allowed if the physician and the patient have examined the situation, and have reached the conclusion together that there are no other reasonable solutions. This implies an active role for the physician, of questioning the patient's wish to die. Thus, the wish to die is not taken for granted, but is regarded as a starting point for a dialogue between the physician and the patient, in which both the patient's perspective and that of the physician are important, and neither of them is taken for granted.

MARIAN VERKERK: Recognizing another person as who she or he is also means challenging one's wishes and preferences, including the wish to die. I don't think that respecting another person as the person he is implies taking every wish at face (moral) value. Respecting someone's moral agency implies inviting her to account for what she prefers or wishes. We respect each other exactly by engaging in a dialogue about each other's deep convictions, especially when it comes to this kind of important decisions about life and death. This dialogue does not prevent deeply felt differences of opinion from remaining.

And so in a situation in which a person expresses her wish to die, the doctor has to become engaged in questioning the reasons for this wish. But there are conditions for this dialogue: the dialogue should be—as I write in Chapter 13—epistemically justified. Both need to be responsive and attentive towards each other.

BERT MOLEWIJK: I also think critically challenging the patient's wish to die is a hermeneutic requirement for understanding the wish, and for letting the patient understand her/his wish too. Furthermore, I think it is a sign of respect for the other when you respectfully and constructively (i.e. with the aim of understanding and finding a joint way to deal with the situation) challenge the wish to die. You are making the effort to understand the other. When challenging the wish to die, we, or healthcare professionals, should also inform the patient about *why* you are challenging her/his wish to die (we often forget this additional explanation about what we are trying to communicate), so that it is understandable to the patient why we are challenging his/her wish. However, at the same time we should also not forget about emotional support, independent of the moral reaction to the expressed wish. Finally, I think it is a professional duty of the healthcare professional, certainly when it involves a request for euthanasia or physician-assisted suicide: such a moral request deserves to be seriously scrutinized before it is actually carried out.

CHRISTOPH REHMANN-SUTTER: We seem to have quite a broad common ground: challenging a wish to die is not the same as failing to respect the wish. Challenging, you have said, may even be a necessary step in understanding, and it establishes a relationship of care and responsibility. This is particularly important when the wish is about assistance in dying.

But a next question would then be: What is the good caregiver's attitude in those other cases when the wish is only for death to come sooner, without wanting to hasten it, or when it is a hypothetical wish, which is formulated as an exit path in case the situation becomes much worse? We can see a whole range of variations in this intention in wishes to die. Hastening is the intention in only one group. And to have this wish to die might have a consoling effect for the patient now, it might make it easier to cope with the situation, or the wish itself may be a coping strategy. But this would not work if the wish were not meant seriously. And describing the wish to die in some situations as a coping strategy is, I believe, no reason not to take it seriously and respect it.

Part IV

Practice

Chapter 17

Issues of palliative medicine in end-of-life care

H. Christof Müller-Busch

If one is truly to succeed in leading a person to a specific place, one must first and foremost take care to find him, where he is and begin there . . . In order truly to help someone else, I must understand more than he— but certainly first and foremost understand what he understands . . . all true helping begins with a humbling. The helper must first humble himself under the person he wants to help and thereby understand that to help is not to dominate but to serve.

Kierkegaard (1859). Reproduced from Søren Kierkegaard,
The Point of View, p. 45, Princeton University Press,
Princeton, Copyright, © 1998, Princeton University Press,
with permission.

Principles and aims of palliative care

Since the opening of St Christopher's Hospice by Dame Cicely Saunders nearly 50 years ago some important changes have taken place in the palliative care approach. While it first concentrated mainly on the reduction of suffering for patients with life-limiting terminal diseases, mainly cancer, the palliative care approach has become increasingly important for medical and ethical treatment decisions at different stages in the course of chronic progressive diseases. This has been shown not only for patients with cancer (Temel et al. 2007) but also for those with degenerative neurological disorders, chronic progressive cardiac and pulmonary diseases, and dementia (Glare 2013). The idea behind the early integration of palliative aspects into treatment that still attempts to cure is that it can prevent suffering at the end of life, can ease the terminal and dying phase, and can contribute to a 'death with dignity'. With this aim in mind it is important to reflect on the basic principles of palliative care, not only in oncology but in many other disciplines of medical care as well.

Although the integration of palliative care and palliative medicine worldwide is recognized as an important medical, social, and ethical challenge, there are great differences in the acceptance and implementation of principles, service structures, and their promotion, especially between the highly industrialized Western world and the poorer less-developed countries which have a great number of patients in need of palliative care at the end of life. Although it can seem that palliative care is a privilege of the modern world, the World Health Organization (WHO) includes the principles and goal of reducing suffering in its comprehensive definition of palliative care, with a global call for better end-of-life care and its early application, in combination with life-prolonging treatment. The WHO (2002) defines palliative care as an approach that:

- provides relief from pain and other distressing symptoms;
- affirms life, and regards dying as a normal process;
- intends neither to hasten nor to postpone death;
- integrates the psychological and spiritual aspects of patient care;
- offers a support system to help patients live as actively as possible until death;
- offers a support system to help the family cope during the patient's illness and in their own bereavement;
- uses a team approach to address the needs of patients and their families, including bereavement counselling, if indicated;
- will enhance quality of life, and may also positively influence the course of illness;
- is applicable early in the course of illness, in conjunction with a range of other therapies that are intended to prolong life, such as chemotherapy and radiation therapy, and includes those investigations needed to better understand and manage distressing clinical complications.

(Reproduced from WHO definition of palliative care © 2002, World Health Organization.)

The aim of palliative care is to provide the best possible quality of life for people approaching the end of their life and for their families and carers. It is a holistic approach to care and support, and takes into account emotional, psychological, and spiritual as well as physical needs. In the WHO concept of palliative care, pain and symptom control is a central aim. Freedom from pain allows people to come to terms with their approaching death and enables them to make arrangements for the future of others who depend on them, as well as to live as fully as possible for as long as possible (Lucas 2002). Inadequate symptom control and the fear of pain are important factors in people's wishes to hasten or postpone death.

From terminal care to early intervention

Since 1973, when the term 'palliative care' was introduced into modern medicine by the Canadian urologist Balfour Mount, it has undergone a series of transformations in terms of defining tasks and goals. Although no consensus has been reached on the target groups and structures for the provision of palliative care, on tasks, or the kind of expertise needed (with particular conflict over the time at which to begin palliative care,

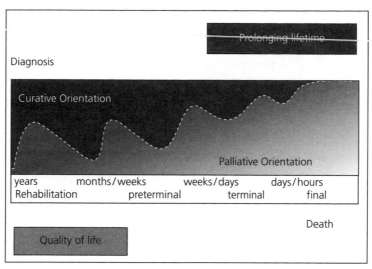

Fig. 17.1 Curative and palliative orientation in the course of life-limiting disease.

the definition of target groups, and the relationship to curative approaches), consistent and uniformly found common goals were the relief and prevention of suffering and the improvement of quality of life (Pastrana et al. 2008) (Fig. 17.1).

The pioneering work of Cicely Saunders drew attention to the physical, social, psychological, and spiritual needs of patients with advanced malignant and neurological life-limiting diseases in end-of-life care. The reduction of suffering, the amelioration of burdensome symptoms in the terminal phase of life, and 'letting people die' was a provocative message that irritated the highly technological medical world that strove to do everything to prolong and save life by any means. Although the holistic caring aspect of 'palliative care' has a long medical tradition, care of the dying had been excluded from modern medicine. However, in Great Britain and many other highly industrialized Western countries, there has been a dynamic development of palliative medicine or palliative care as a new specialized professional service in modern medicine, with an increasing number of multiprofessional palliative care services which were developed in many settings but were first closely related to oncology (Clark 2007). Meanwhile, palliative care aspects have been integrated into other medical disciplines in which patients with life-limiting illness are treated, and attention to the quality of the end of life and not just the prolongation of life is an accepted goal in modern Western medicine. But alongside the evolution of palliative care, indeed almost at the same time, a controversial debate arose among the public on patients' rights, self-determination, euthanasia, and assisted suicide. Related to the changes in mortality, morbidity, and disease trajectories associated with the capacity of modern medicine to prolong life, an increasing number of people were asking, 'How do I want to die?' thus raising the question of what a good death is. A hundred years ago death occurred mainly at home as a natural consequence of an incurable disease—the leading causes of death were infections, accidents, heart disease, and childbirth. By contrast we now have the situation in which dying occurs much later, after a long life and following a long and intensive treatment process in confrontation with chronic diseases. With the advanced capacity of medicine to cure diseases or to limit their progress, and the use of technical methods to support and substitute organs and body parts that are failing or loosing their function to prolong life artificially. Death 'happens' in hospitals or nursing homes as a consequence of medical and ethical decisions to limit treatment options that may have the potential to prolong life. This means that not only the time, but also the kind of death and the place of dying depend less on the natural course of a disease than on decisions about limiting these treatment options. The German term *Therapiezieländerung* [change in therapy objectives] implies that the goal 'to let a person die' is a therapeutic challenge for the provision of palliative care; but this means not only care to increase comfort through optimal symptom control, but also accepting responsibility for effective communication and thoughtful decision-making (Hutton 2005). This needs professional experience, responsibility, empathy, communication skills, ethical orientation, and respect for autonomy.

Illness trajectories and stages of palliative care

When it is accepted that palliative care is not just end-of-life support for the terminally ill and their families but an approach which should be related to the special needs of the ill person rather than diagnoses and medical findings, it then becomes important to integrate the needs-orientated palliative approach early in the care of patients with a chronic life-limiting disease. Here it is important and helpful to differentiate various stages of palliative care: the rehabilitative, the pre-terminal, the terminal, and the final stage (Jonen-Thielemann 2006) (Table 17.1). Integration and the implementation of palliative care aspects in the early stages is an important step to facilitate effective communication, advance care planning, and thoughtful decision-making.

Certainly, decisions about the restriction of treatment in progressive courses of life-limiting disease and in frail people are accepted as important and challenging, and must take into account the values, individual life expectations, and wishes of the

Table 17.1 Stages in palliative care

	Duration	**Mobility**	**Palliative intentions**	**Principles**
Rehabilitative	Months to years	Free	Restore autonomy by optimal symptom control	Aggressive interventions indicated
Pre-terminal	Weeks to months	Limited	Aim for best living with help of others	Social support necessary
Terminal	Days to weeks	Mostly bedbound	Achieve optimal comfort	Reduce strain—realistic goals
Final	Hours to days	Essentially bedbound	Human care for the dying	Value, acknowledge, accept, alleviate

Adapted from I. Jonen Thielemann, Sterbephasen in der Palliativmedizin, in A. E. Nauck and L. Radbruch (eds), *Lehrbuch der Palliativmedizin*, pp. 1019–1028, Schattauer Verlag, Stuttgart, Copyright © 2006, Schattauer Verlag.

patient as much as the medical aspects. The objectives of treatment must be defined and adapted to the individual situation. Prognostic uncertainty in any particular case and the confrontation with ambivalence make it difficult to determine the patient's wishes, which can change in progressive disease. Not only patients and relatives but physicians too are often led by unrealistic expectations and the belief that a highly unlikely outcome can be reached through risky and burdensome aggressive interventions. This is especially true when complications occur in situations in intensive care or in the terminal stages of patients with cancer, but also in old age with dementia, where direct communication is difficult and patients are unable to express their actual wishes in an informed and competent way. Advance directives and testimonies in which a prior will has been expressed are helpful instruments for communication and for a trusting dialogue with patients, their proxies, or surrogates, but they cannot free the medical carers from their responsibility to determine the indication and targets of treatment for the benefit of the patient in each individual case, taking into account the patient's values and wishes. Difficult discussions with patients and relatives about the aims of care and decision-making about restricting potentially life-prolonging medical treatment 'to let the patient die' are often avoided or at least postponed by the medical staff. Discussions in that field need expertise and communication skills. Reasons for avoidance include vulnerabilities of the patient and uncertainties about defining the 'point of no return', which signifies the stage when care is concentrated exclusively on comfort and on the palliative principle of not to prevent or prolong the dying phase. In fact, the avoidance of discussions about prognosis at all stages of palliative care causes more harm. It has been shown that early talks on prognosis in cancer patients, which must always take into account the inherent uncertainty in any individual case, are associated with less aggressive care and reduced symptom burden in the final phase and with better bereavement adjustment, without reducing time of survival (Wright et al. 2008). Moral concerns about lack of expertise in deciding on the withholding or withdrawing of potentially life-prolonging treatment, the fear of personal failure, and also worries about legal prosecution and sanctions if life is actively shortened are the main reasons for inappropriate medical 'actionism' or symbolic activity in end-of-life care. Inappropriate medical actionism in end-of-life situations concentrates on isolated aspects like laboratory parameters in an attempt to change pathological findings, but without influencing the palliative situation as a whole in an appropriate manner. Symbolic activity is the performance of measures that are not medically indicated to lull patients and their relatives into a false sense of security, disregarding the futility of the action. Both inappropriate actionism and symbolic activity are forms of medical activity commonly found in end-of-life situations.

With regard to the relevance of decision-making as a disease progresses, it is important to know the different courses and end-of-life trajectories of the main chronic diseases that finally lead to death. In relation to functional states, quality of life, and final decline, three typical illness trajectories have been described for patients with the most frequently diagnosed progressive chronic illnesses: (1) a trajectory with steady progression and usually a clear terminal phase, as in most cancers, (2) a trajectory as in the end stages of chronic heart disease and obstructive pulmonary disease, with ups and downs and often critical episodes of deterioration in functional health, associated with frequent admissions to hospital and intensive treatment, and (3) trajectories of slowly progressing disability, increasing general deterioration of multiple body systems due to older age or neurological disease with frailty and cerebral dysfunction such as in Alzheimer's or other form of dementia.

Being aware of these trajectories and patients' varying physical, social, psychological, and spiritual needs may help clinicians to plan care that better meets their patients' multidimensional needs and helps patients and family members or relatives to cope with their situation.

According to the kind of disease trajectory and the stage of palliative care, different approaches may be necessary to reflect patients' different experiences (Murray et al. 2005). Although the intentions behind interventions in different stages of palliative care might be different, the aim of the potential activity must be clear and should be discussed with the patient and family. This is especially important in situations in which patients express a wish to die, which has to be considered in the process of effective communication and thoughtful decision-making.

A recent survey on end-of-life practices in palliative care amongst physician members of the German Society for Palliative Medicine showed that in nearly 70% of cases limitation of potentially life sustaining treatment 'to let the terminally ill patient die' preceded death. In 78% of cases it was reported that the treatment intentions were characterized by an intensification of symptom alleviation in the terminal situation even if that entailed a potentially life-shortening side effect (Schildmann et al. 2010), and in only 1% of cases was it reported that death occurred after an active life-shortening intervention.

Challenges and aims of care in progressive disease and the four core questions

Despite reservations about the staging of patients and the inaccuracy of predicting lifespan, it is both practically and scientifically relevant to adapt and relate the intentions and principles of palliative care, especially the communication and decision-making process, to give a realistic answer to the first important question: 'Where can the patient be seen in relation to his or her biography and the burden of illness?'

In addition to the treatment of physical and psychological problems, many patients in palliative care need support with existential issues such as the settlement of disputes, inheritance arrangements, management of living conditions, and spiritual matters. If patients and relatives raise questions about the meaning of life when confronted with a shortened time span and lack of hope, this may indicate that they are considering a possible hastening of death. While in most clinical settings in Germany discussions about hastening death are still taboo, in palliative care those thoughts are expressed more often and more openly. Sensitive and empathic listening is needed to understand the meaning and the message behind the words. Therefore a meaning-centred approach is an integral part of a needs-adapted therapeutic relationship in palliative care (Breitbart and Heller 2002). Following this, the second important question in determining the aims of care and treatment goals is 'What does the patient want?' The third question should reflect in a critical way the needs of the patient in relation to the commitment of carers and their professional skills: 'What can we do, what can I do?' The fourth important question to be considered regarding palliative needs is concerned with the personal, cultural, and professional values in a relationship of care, finding the balance between respect for autonomy and the ethics of care: 'What should not be done?' The assessment and reassessment of the needs and possibilities of care using these four core questions is a basic person-centred strategy which can be helpful for communication and decision-making at all stages.

In the rehabilitation stage, in addition to the restoration of functional autonomy by optimal symptom control, the meaning-centred approach of palliative care is focused on the goal of finding meaning in the patient's remaining time. In the pre-terminal stage, in addition to optimal social support, it is important to find the meaning of relationships during the time of leave-taking. In the terminal and final stage, the palliative strategy is focused on ensuring comfort and preventing stress. Nothing should burden the process of dying. From the point of view of palliative care, questions about hastening death in the terminal and final stages can often be dealt with by ensuring that the patient is comfortable through medical interventions to reduce intolerable suffering and relaxation techniques to improve sleep. Besides the alleviation of suffering, the meaning-centred approach should explain, respect, and accept individual dying as an existential experience which remains in the memories and shapes the mourning of the bereaved relatives and carers. Rituals can also help to find a way. When patients ask for death to be hastened in the rehabilitative and pre-terminal stages of palliative care the person involved should respectfully try to understand why: what is the reason behind the request? Psychological interventions like dignity therapy (Chochinov et al. 2011) or narrative therapy (Stanley and Hurst 2011) may help to make the situation more understandable. Early and sensitive psychological interventions in a multiprofessional team approach should focus on making the leave-taking tolerable and finding a 'sense of coherence' (Antonovsky and Sagy 1986).

What is a 'good death'?

Up until the 1970s the issue of dying and death was not a topic for discussion among healthcare professionals. Scepticism about the ability of physicians and medical care to solve the problems of longevity and the burdens of artificially prolonged life increased the fear that aggressive and senseless interventions in the final stages of life, for example in intensive care, would lead to loss of dignity and death under conditions of intolerable suffering. This led to societal debate about the question of 'dying with dignity' and a 'good death'. These are philosophical themes with concrete legal and practical consequences, depending on the perspective taken. As a consequence of this, the debate on legal instruments to allow more control of the management of dying and the organization of death attracted widespread public attention, while focusing on different core themes. The discussion of patients' rights, living wills, advance directives, and healthcare proxies in the United States began in 1969 when the first living will was presented (Kutner 1969), while in Great Britain at almost the same time the modern hospice movement began. In the Netherlands in 1973 the legal case brought against Dr Gertrude Postma, a physician who injected her terminally ill mother with a lethal dose of barbiturates, attracted great public attention. The debate about this case launched the euthanasia movement in several countries, leading to changes in the law in the Netherlands and Belgium in 2002 such that euthanasia, performed by physicians under defined circumstances of intolerable suffering, and physician-assisted suicide became a possibility within medical care. In Switzerland in 1982, after a debate on the problem of 'Sterbehilfe', the organization EXIT was founded to support self-determination at the end of life and assisted suicide by non-medical personnel on the basis of a law dating from 1941 permitting altruistic help for severely ill people to perform suicide. The pragmatic Swiss situation led to an intense moral debate about medically assisted suicide and the direct or indirect role of physicians in assisting patients in the voluntary termination of their life by the administration of a lethal substance. The ethical debate on euthanasia and physician-assisted suicide, and its legalization in several countries, was accompanied by the evolution of palliative care showing an alternative approach to dealing with end-of-life problems and conflicts. After a debate on euthanasia in the European Parliament, a first position paper was formulated which clearly rejected euthanasia and physician-assisted suicide (Roy et al. 1994). This position paper was clarified in 2003 by a task force of the European Association for Palliative Care (EAPC) with the statement 'The provision of euthanasia and physician-assisted suicide should not be part of the responsibility of palliative care' (Materstvedt et al. 2003); since then this has been the guideline for moral and practical approaches for dealing with the problems and conflicts that arise when patients in palliative care request a hastened death. The clear statement on the incompatibility of the aims of palliative care with the aims of euthanasia and physician-assisted suicide in the EAPC position paper was controversial, but gave an orientation for ethical guidelines. It was adopted by the German Medical Association in the most recent version of the *Grundsätze zur ärztlichen Sterbebegleitung*, where the obligations of physicians in caring for severely ill and dying patients are outlined (Bundesärztekammer 2011).

Meanwhile, comprehensive care for the severely ill and the dying has become one of the great challenges for modern health care. Besides optimal medical care, the recognition of patients' perspectives and rights and 'respect for autonomy' are core principles in the debate on a 'good death'. To enable a 'good death' (Smith 2000) is certainly one of the main objectives of palliative care. It is interesting to note that with the development of transplantation medicine the term 'brain death' was revised when the need arose to find a definition for death that would allow the removal of organs from a dead person to be donated and live on in another body. In this context the term 'medicalization of dying' was introduced by Ivan Illich in the early 1970s (Illich 1981). It has been described by David Clark (2002) as:

> [1] a loss of the capacity to accept death and suffering as meaningful aspects of life, [2] a sense of being in a state of 'total war' against death at all stages of the life cycle, [3] a crippling of personal and family care, [4] a devaluing of traditional rituals surrounding dying and death, and [5] a form of social control in which a rejection of 'patienthood' by dying or bereaved people is labelled as a form of deviance.

In relation to the problems associated with brain death one could argue similarly for terminal situations. 'Since we do not know the exact borderline between life and death, nothing less than the maximum definition of death will do—brain death plus heart death plus any other indication that may be pertinent—before final violence is allowed to be done' (Jonas 1974). Although the concept of a good death is central to end-of-life palliative care, the criteria for a good death depend not only on the subjective views of the patient but also on the views of those who have to live on after experiencing their loved one's death. This consideration is especially important when the question of hastening death is raised in palliative care (Hendry et al. 2013). Even though there is no general definition of a good death one could say that, from a palliative care point of view, a 'good death' is a dying situation which is inherently consistent and can be tolerated and accepted by all involved. A good death is not just the final moment of life. Quality in end-of-life care and also in death is a dynamic process that is negotiated and renegotiated between patients, families, and healthcare professionals.

Conflicting situations—to be confronted with explicit requests for hastened death in palliative care

Although explicit requests for euthanasia and assisted suicide are rare, and much depend on the setting, many patients with progressive terminal disease raise the question of hastened death—although their motivation may not be clear. A national cross-sectional multicentred study of 789 palliative care organizations in France, a country which has not legalized euthanasia, found that 783 patients had made a request for euthanasia or assisted suicide (Ferrand et al. 2012). Although the figures from this study do not show the prevalence of wishes for euthanasia or suicidal ideas in palliative patients in the care of these organizations, they do give hints as to the underlying reasons: most of them were cancer patients in a terminal stage who had difficulties in feeding (65%), moving (54%), excretion (49%), or were cachectic (39%). In addition 31% were considered to be anxious or depressed, 79% did not give physical reasons for their request, 37% of the requests were constant, and 24% fluctuated, despite provision of regular follow-up by a palliative care team. Of the 783 patients who were reported to have made a request to hasten death, 68% died within a month (Ferrand et al. 2012). In Oregon, most requests for physician-assisted suicide are made by patients enrolled in hospice care and by people with higher levels of education. In 2013 the three most frequently mentioned end-of-life concerns were loss of autonomy (93%), decreasing ability to participate in activities that made life enjoyable (89%), and loss of dignity (73%). Inadequate pain control, or concern about it, was given as a reason by only 28%. Although the number of legal prescriptions for life-ending drugs has been increasing slowly over the years, the number of patients who did not take the prescribed medication but died from other causes also rose in parallel. The reports from Oregon show that latent psychosocial and sociocultural concerns in severely ill people with higher education seem to have a greater impact on suicidal ideas than somatic problems (Oregon Death with Dignity Act 2013).

Although exact figures are not known, my own personal experience over 15 years in palliative care supports the idea that some small percentage of patients, despite the best palliative care available, believe that their suffering is intolerable and request hastened death by euthanasia or assisted suicide. Then the question arises what the moral attitude towards these requests should be and which solutions can be offered.

The confrontation with a patient asking for hastened death in palliative care is a moral as well as a medical challenge; it might be seen as provocative but also as a chance to reflect personal values. Requests for euthanasia and assisted suicide must be acknowledged with respect and in a sensitive manner. The inclusion of somebody else in the planned ending of one's own life is a sign of great trust and confidence. The handling of requests for hastening death in palliative care depends very much on the stage at which the patient is (see Box 17.1). This should be addressed in an empathic way in dialogue with the patient and, if necessary, the family. In later stages of palliative care the focus in most cases is on ensuring that the patient is comfortable and unstressed. In earlier stages the psychosocial and existential problems behind the conceptualization of assisted suicide and euthanasia should be addressed sensitively and support should be offered to solve the underlying problems in another way. When it is possible to address the reasons behind the expressed wish, a solution may be found. In most of the cases in which I was confronted with requests for assisted suicide or euthanasia it was possible to refer to the underlying problem. When a situation can be identified as a conflict then ways to end the conflict should be sought. Often it is the need to end a conflict, and not the intention to solve the underlying existential problem, which drives patients in such intractable situations. There is no other kind of death that leaves such strong marks of dismay, shame, and guilt on the bereaved as a suicide. In palliative and hospice care, patient suicides can affect clinicians both personally and professionally (Fairman et al. 2014).

Even in palliative care, not every health problem can be solved. But at least in the rehabilitative and pre-terminal stages, the points at which concrete requests for euthanasia and assisted suicide are expressed most often in palliative care, it is important to create a problem-based deliberative patient–physician relationship which respects the other but also includes awareness of one's own ethical viewpoint (Box 17.1). The ethical principles of palliative care have been clearly outlined and should be the basis for a caring relationship involving mutual trust and respect for autonomy. It is always possible to talk in a structured manner about the hopelessness and the problems behind a suicidal plan, but also about the meaning of such an action for others. The concept of integrating euthanasia and assisted suicide into palliative care (Bernheim et al. 2008) is misleading, while from an epistemological viewpoint the benefit of death as a therapeutic goal cannot be justified on a normative basis or assumed by empirical experience or scientific results. The therapeutic goals in palliative care are always concerned with problems in life—even when death is accepted and respected as an inevitable fact, but not as a therapeutic goal.

The tasks and duties of the healthcare professional in palliative care depend on the stage of the patient, and can be broadly listed as:

Box 17.1 When patients ask for hastened death—aims and options in different stages of palliative medicine

Rehabilitative

◆ optimise symptom control
◆ try to understand
◆ respect different viewpoints
◆ problem-based deliberative patient–physician relationship
◆ concentrate on responsibility and care

Pre-terminal

◆ optimize symptom control
◆ try to understand
◆ respect different viewpoints, discover ambivalence
◆ problem-based deliberative patient-physician relationship
◆ concentrate on social support, communication, and existential issues

Terminal

◆ optimize comfort, respect
◆ calm and care
◆ prepare for dying, consider sedation to relieve suffering
◆ help the helpers

Final

◆ optimize comfort and atmosphere
◆ let the patient die
◆ concentrate on peace, informative elucidation, and grief

In the terminal and final stages, requests for hastened death may indicate a need for medical care and comfort to be improved. Information on 'what is happening' through effective communication with the patient and the family will in most cases help to reduce stress. In situations of extreme stress, for example patients with agitation, extreme breathlessness, or in total pain, palliative sedation and rarely even continuous deep sedation up to the point of death can be indicated. Various procedural and ethical guidelines have been established for palliative sedation, but there is currently no universally accepted standard of practice (Papavasiliou et al. 2013). The separation from euthanasia sometimes seems difficult, but palliative or terminal sedation can be clearly distinguished by its aims and intentions. Palliative sedation is a medical method with the goal of relieving unbearable suffering by reducing consciousness, while in euthanasia the goal is death through the application of life-ending medication. With regard to the difficulties in prognosis and the diagnosis of the beginning of the terminal or final phase, in our clinic the use of palliative sedation in patients with progressive incurable diseases was possible when, as a result of the underlying disease or some other event, death within the next 48 hours could be medically and ethically accepted—though not necessarily foreseen (Müller-Busch et al. 2003).

A final comment on effective communication and ethics

Effective communication and thoughtful decision-making in combination with optimal symptom control and transparency are core elements in palliative care. When faced with a patient who demands professional help to hasten death, problems can arise which conflict with the ethical principles of palliative care as well as with personal and societal values. With reference to what is probably the most prominent approach in bioethics worldwide, the four principles elaborated by Beauchamp and Childress, the overall obligation in end-of-life situations has been identified by Materstvedt as to do no harm, which precedes the principle of beneficence (Materstvedt 2013). The balance between potential benefit and foreseen harm in palliative settings is sometimes difficult to find. Though all actions must consider the awareness of approaching death, the principal goal of palliative care in assisted dying is the effective prevention and relief of suffering while respecting autonomy, but not the elimination of the sufferer. Therefore early integration of palliative care with committed communication is essential to prevent and reduce suffering in the terminal and final stages. In the later stages of palliative care in particular, physicians and the care team should be prepared to acknowledge their responsibility to provide a sense of coherence in the confrontation with dying, death, and grief. Experiences of dying leave behind traces. The memories of the experience of dying and death influence the life values of the bereaved.

References

Antonovsky, H. and Sagy, S. (1986). The development of a sense of coherence and its impact on responses to stress situations. *Journal of Social Psychology*, **126**, 213–225.

Bernheim, J. L., Deschepper, R., Distelmans, W., Mullie, A., Bilsen, J., and Deliens, L. (2008). Development of palliative care and legalisation of euthanasia: antagonism or synergy? *British Medical Journal*, **336**, 864–867.

Breitbart, W. and Heller, K. S. (2002). Reframing hope: meaning-centered care for patients near the end of life. *Journal of Palliative Medicine*, **6**, 979–988.

Bundesärztekammer (2011). Grundsätze der Bundesärztekammer zur ärztlichen Sterbebegleitung. *Deutsches Ärzteblatt*, **108**, A346–A348.

Chochinov, H. M., Kristjanson, L. J., Breitbart, W., et al. (2011). Effect of dignity therapy on distress and end-of-life experience in terminally ill patients: a randomized controlled trial. *Lancet Oncology*, **12**, 753–762.

Clark, D. (2002). Between hope and acceptance: the medicalisation of dying. *British Medical Journal*, **324**, 905–907.

Clark, D. (2007). From margins to centre: a review of the history of palliative care in cancer. *Lancet Oncology*, **8**, 430–438.

Fairman, N., Montross Thomas, L. P., Whitmore, S., Meier, E. A., and Irwin, S. A. (2014). What did I miss? A qualitative assessment of the impact of patient suicide on hospice clinical staff. *Palliative Medicine*, **17**, 832–836.

Ferrand, E., Dreyfus, J. F., Chastrusse, M., Ellien, F., Lemaire, F., and Fischler, M. (2012). Evolution of requests to hasten death among patients managed by palliative care teams in France: a multicentre cross-sectional survey. *European Journal of Cancer*, **48**, 368–376.

Glare, P. A. (2013). Early implementation of palliative care can improve patient outcomes. *Journal of the National Comprehensive Cancer Network*, **11**, 3–9.

Hendry, M., Pasterfield, D., Lewis, R., Carter, B., Hodgson, D., and Wilkinson, C. (2013). Why do we want the right to die? A systematic review of the international literature on the views of patients, carers and the public on assisted dying. *Palliative Medicine*, **27**, 13–26.

Hutton, N. (2005). Palliative care, time, and core values. *Patient Education and Counseling*, **56**, 255–256.

Illich, I. (1981). *Die Nemesis der Medizin. Von den Grenzen des Gesundheitswesens*. Hamburg: Rowohlt.

Jonas, H. (1974). *Philosophical Essays: From Ancient Creed to Technological Man*, p. 130. Englewood Cliffs, NJ: Prentice-Hall.

Jonen-Thielemann, I. (2006). Sterbephasen in der Palliativmedizin. In: A. E. Nauck and L. Radbruch (eds), *Lehrbuch der Palliativmedizin*, pp. 1019–1028. Stuttgart: Schattauer Verlag.

Kutner, L. (1969). The living will: a proposal. *Indiana Law Journal*, **44**, 539–554.

Lucas, S. (2002). *Palliative Care: Issues and Challenges*. URL: <http://www.who.int/3by5/en/palliativecare_en.pdf> (accessed 5 November 2013).

Materstvedt, L. J. (2013). Palliative care ethics: the problems of combining palliation and assisted dying. *Progress in Palliative Care*, **21**, 158–164.

Materstvedt, L. J., Clark, D., Ellershaw, J., et al. (2003). EAPC Ethics Task Force. Euthanasia and physician-assisted suicide: a view from an EAPC Ethics Task Force. *Palliative Medicine*, **17**, 97–101 [discussion 102–179].

Müller-Busch, H. C., Andres, I., and Jehser, T. (2003). Sedation in palliative care—a critical analysis of 7 years experience. *BMC Palliative Care*, **2**, 2.

Murray, S. A., Kendall, M., Boyd, K., and Sheikh, A. (2005). Illness trajectories and palliative care. *British Medical Journal*, **330**, 1007–1011.

Oregon Death with Dignity Act (2013). *Oregon Death with Dignity Act 2013 report*. URL: <https://public.health.oregon.gov/providerpartnerresources/evaluationresearch/deathwithdignityact/documents/year16.pdf>

Papavasiliou, E. S., Brearley, S. G., Seymour, J. E., Brown, J., and Payne, S. (2013). From sedation to continuous sedation until death: How has the conceptual basis of sedation in end-of-life care changed over time? *Journal of Pain and Symptom Management*, **46**, 691–706.

Pastrana, T., Jünger, S., Elsner, F., and Radbruch, L. (2008). A matter of definition—key elements identified in a discourse analysis of definitions of palliative care. *Palliative Medicine*, **22**, 222–232.

Roy, D. J., Rapin, C. H., and the EAPC Board of Directors (1994). Regarding euthanasia. *European Journal of Palliative Care*, **1**, 57–59.

Schildmann, J., Hötzel, J., Müller-Busch, C., and Vollmann, J. (2010). End-of-life practices in palliative care: a cross sectional survey of physician members of the German Society for Palliative Medicine. *Palliative Medicine*, **24**, 820–827.

Smith, R. (2000). A good death. *British Medical Journal*, **320**, 129–130.

Stanley, P. and Hurst, M. (2011). Narrative palliative care: a method for building empathy. *Journal of Social Work in End-of-Life and Palliative Care*, **7**, 39–55.

Temel, J. S., Jackson, V. A., Billings, J. A., et al. (2007). Phase II study: integrated palliative care in newly diagnosed advanced non-small-cell lung cancer patients. *Journal of Clinical Oncology*, **25**, 2377–2382.

WHO (2002). WHO definition of palliative care. URL: <http://www.who.int/cancer/palliative/definition/en/> (accessed 4 November 2013).

Wright, A. A., Zhang, B., Ray, A., et al. (2008). Associations between end-of-life discussions, patient mental health, medical care near death, and caregiver bereavement adjustment. *Journal of the American Medical Association*, **300**, 1665–1673.

Chapter 18

Spirituality at the bedside: negotiating the meaning of dying

Settimio Monteverde

People work much in order to secure their future,
I gave my mind much work and trouble,
Trying to secure the past.

> *Isaak Dinesen (1885–1962)* Shadows on the Grass

Henrietta's question

'When a patient is dead, is the corpse sick or healthy?' Henrietta, a first-semester student of nursing science, asked this question in a tutorial following a lecture on health and disease. She was astonished by the reaction of her fellow students: after a moment of perplexity, some of them began to laugh. One student said: 'Of course it is sick, why else would the patient have died?' Visibly unsettled, Henrietta replied: 'But a corpse is a corpse and not a person any more. So why should it be sick, why could it not also be healthy?' As the group's tutor I was grateful for this unexpected teaching moment and for the opportunity it gave us to speak about the boundaries between curing, caring, and healing in the nurse–patient encounter. I also wondered what experiences this young woman might have in mind that gave rise to her question. But we ran out of time and the bell rang. Awkwardly I closed the tutorial by saying: 'Well, we will keep Henrietta's question in mind. It is a very important one. When we speak about health and disease, we usually think of living beings that can be born, fall ill, recover, and die. If we use these terms in thinking of a corpse, we are presumably already using them in a metaphorical way.' I had not finished the last sentence when the first students began to stand up and proceed to the next lecture. Henrietta was still taking notes. Then she checked her emails and left the classroom in a hurry, leaving me convinced that I had missed the teaching moment. But I was grateful for this insight into the students' reasoning, knowing that death and dying will be constant companions in their future professional lives. Henrietta's question, although theoretical at the moment, will sooner or later re-emerge at the bedside, with patients or relatives who are faced with imminent death or bereavement and who try—in Isak Dinesen's words—to *secure* their past, to understand and enshrine their stories in order to retell them to future generations.

Spirituality and the caring professions

Following broad definitions of spirituality (Puchalski et al. 2014), securing the past and acknowledging life's achievements and experiences in the context of caring relationships can be considered a formal, non-technical circumscription of spirituality at the end of life. Since the pioneering work of Cicely Saunders, Elisabeth Kübler-Ross, and Balfour Mount, the pivotal importance of meeting spiritual needs in providing effective palliative care has been repeatedly claimed and corroborated by empirical research (e.g. Cobb et al. 2012). Influential notions of 'total pain', 'spiritual pain' (as a component of the former; Clark 1999), and 'existential suffering' (Boston et al. 2011) have been proposed to translate the centrality of spirituality into the clinical realm. The most visible and sustainable manifestation of this process is the definition of palliative care itself provided by the World Health Organization (Sepúlveda et al. 2002; WHO 2013), which mentions spirituality twice. First, the definition addresses spiritual issues in the context of symptom management by stressing the importance of '. . . the prevention and relief of suffering by means of early identification and impeccable assessment and treatment of pain and other problems, physical, psychosocial and spiritual' (WHO 2013). Second, it lists the integration of '. . . psychological and spiritual patient care' among the core principles that distinguish palliative care. At first glance, the prominence of spirituality in the context of palliative care can be seen as a characteristic feature of this novel approach and an expression of its leitmotiv to overcome a perceived marginalization of dying in modern medicine (see Brooksbank 2009). Today, spiritual issues have been successfully integrated into professional education for generic and specialist palliative care (Puchalski et al. 2014). In recent decades, the professions acting in palliative care have increasingly gathered empirical evidence about the interconnectedness of spirituality, health, and quality of life (e.g. Draper 2012; Mount 2013; for a critique see Sloan et al. 2001). Through the different phases of the institutionalization of palliative care—first as an 'approach', later as a discipline, and nowadays as a medical, nursing, psychological, pastoral, and other therapeutic specialization—spirituality has been progressively explored from different disciplinary perspectives. It is hardly surprising that the study of spirituality has proved to be a source of friction between the informal and the formal providers of spiritual care. Two groups can be identified among these providers: whereas 'transcendentalists' criticize the trend towards operationalizing spiritual issues within the provision of health care (Mann 2006; McCulloch 2010), 'immanentists' depart from the salience of religious and spiritual phenomena in the context of health and the importance of describing and understanding them (Gordon and Mitchell 2004; Watts and Psaila 2010). As an expression of the same tension, the Canadian medical sociologist Arthur W. Frank deplores a problematic trend towards the medicalization of spirituality. He contends that, conversely, efforts should be directed towards a spiritualization of medicine: 'The contemporary conjunction of spirituality and medicine fills me with equal measures of hope and aversion. My question is whether these two forces can be kept in balance with each other or whether one will dominate. Current indications are that the volition for a medicalized spirituality is stronger than the possibility of a spiritualized medicine' (Frank 2005, p. 142). Although reflecting opposite (world) views, both transcendentalism and immanentism offer important understandings of the dynamics of spirituality within medicine. They can be seen as windows to the same spiritual phenomena witnessed by patients who are confronted with death and suffering, and who express a wish to die. Importantly, neither a view of spirituality as fully detached from medicine (as expression of a radical transcendentalism) nor a complete assimilation of spirituality by medicine (as expression of a radical immanentism) fully covers the dynamics of spirituality within medicine. In order to overcome both reductionisms, Frank's notion of 'spiritualized medicine' offers a useful intermediate position that acknowledges the value of both approaches. In the context of patients expressing wishes to die, 'spiritualized medicine' acknowledges the value of different sources of spirituality that shape human thinking, but it also addresses physical and psychosocial needs that emerge in the clinical encounter. In this chapter these dynamics are described as the connection of metanarration and narration. This connection is presented as an essential feature of 'spiritualized medicine' at the end of life. It sets a framework that also enables caregivers adequately to address patients' wishes to die at their life's end.

The 'spiritual turn' and its critics

Providing spiritual care and assisting patients in the quest for meaning are indispensable elements of a holistic practice, particularly in palliative care. However, spiritual care is not unique to palliative care. As the history of modern medicine shows, the spiritual turn first originated in a much broader movement outside medicine before it became a major concern within it.

As for the *outside* stimulus for the spiritual turn, in the second half of the twentieth century threats to the ecological balance inherent to the industrialization progress gradually became public knowledge. In the United States they gave rise to a major discussion about sustainable development and how to contain an uncontrolled exploitation of the natural environment. The biochemist Van Rennselaer Potter (1911–2001) presented the neologism 'bioethics' as the new science of survival for an endangered ecosystem. It brought the humanities and the natural sciences together in a common discourse about the values that should guide them in view of the preservation of the foundations of life (Potter 1971). On the basis of this understanding, Peter Whitehouse established the link between Potter's bioethics as 'science of survival' and medicine. He modelled some kind of evolutionary medicine inspired by a 'deep bioethics' and moving towards the spiritual dimension:

> I believe that exploring the depths of deep bioethics will be essential, for without the spiritual, human life is meaningless. Survival enhancing human culture is based on shared beliefs and purposes. The co-evolution of human beings as biological and social entities in community needs to be better understood. The study of evolutionary medicine will likely contribute to an understanding of how health and values changed over time in response to different environments.

Reproduced from The rebirth of bioethics: extending the original formulations of Van Rennselaer Potter, Peter J. Whitehouse, *The American Journal of Bioethics*, 3(4), pp. 26–31, doi: 10.1162/152651603322614751 Copyright © 2003, Taylor & Francis. Reprinted by permission of the publisher (Taylor & Francis Ltd, <http://www.tandfonline.com>).

Simultaneously, breath-taking innovations and discoveries *within* medicine successively transformed hospital wards in many developed countries: the possibility of diagnosing death early by neurological criteria, substituting functions of vital organs after failure (e.g. lung, kidney, heart), or transplanting vital organs from a dead to a severely ill patient, demanded a thorough reflection on the goals and limits of medicine (Hanson 1999). This took place in the light of recurrent reports of medical treatment provided under questionable or futile conditions, but also in the light of growing disparities in people's *access* to health care and the relative scarcity of resources resulting from a mismatch between supply and demand for available medical treatment (Newton 2013). As long as there was no consensus about where doctors' duty to treat ended, cases were often settled by the courts. With the emergence of biomedical ethics as a 'second-order discipline' (Kopelman 2013), the successive implementation of clinical ethics structures, and the theoretical reflection on 'applying' or 'doing' ethics within the clinical realm (Stevens 2000; Magill 2014), the actors within health care began to take a more active role in discussing the goals of medicine, the boundaries of treatment, and the transitions between *cure* and *care*. Where cure was no longer possible, the pioneers of palliative care contended that the healthcare and allied professions still had much to offer in terms of presence, knowledge, skills, and attitudes. The dynamic tension of cure between a challenging present and a better future, between surrender and hope, was not simply set aside when patients faced an incurable disease and imminent separation from their beloved. It was still preserved and transferred into a metaphorical use of cure in terms of *healing* by addressing the spiritual dimension and the resources of patients and families in the quest for meaning. The multidisciplinary dialogue between medicine and the human and social sciences was intensified.

As vividly depicted in the writings of Cicely Saunders, this patient orientation contributed to a veritable 'social turn' within medicine (e.g. Saunders 1959, 1996). At the same time, catalogues of *patients' rights* were formulated. It was claimed that respecting these rights in healthcare contexts was a fundamental legal and moral prerequisite for professionals if they needed to intervene in a patient's physical and mental integrity. This shift towards *patient centredness* later gained pivotal importance for the core principle of palliative care, *following the patient*, in not only a spatial sense but also a spiritual one, i.e. in the patient's quest for meaning within the vicissitudes of life (see Haugen et al. 2011). Patient centredness was not just a synecdoche for medicine or a meaningless slogan—it highlighted the importance of public accountability of healthcare actors, especially with the first signs of scarcity of health resources, recurring cases of malpractice, and abuse in research (Friedman 2014). Finally, in parallel with the spiritual and social turn within the culture of medicine, there was an *epistemological* turn aimed at overcoming the dichotomous relationship between disease and health. As an alternative to the dominant pathogenic model, a biopsychosocial model was proposed (Engel 1977) and extended to a biopsychosocio-*spiritual* model (Sulmasy 2002) that addresses these four constitutive and interdependent dimensions of human existence. The global turn towards bioethics as a 'science of survival' was accompanied by a social and epistemological turn within medicine. In both, spirituality had acquired a prominent place.

Sceptics of this upcoming 'spiritual turn' viewed spirituality in the proper or customary sense as having lost its specificity and—through operationalization in the form of spiritual *care*, *assessment*, and *interventions*—suggested manageability of the otherwise non-manageable *human condition*. In this line of argument, Draper and McSherry argued that issues characterized as spiritual care '. . . are all aspects of care that are integrated and not separated within the provision of holistic care. However, we argue that it is unnecessary and potentially harmful to place this activity under the umbrella of spirituality and spiritual care' (Draper and McSherry 2002, p. 2). Likewise, the 'natural propensity' of nursing and the caring sciences in general to spirituality, and the place of spiritual care within health care, were also questioned. Departing from the difficulties of definition, the danger of dissipation of the term was soon recognized by covering virtually all dimensions of medical practice. In addition, the availability of different assessment tools gave rise to questions of validity of assessment and reliability of measurement. Spirituality was therefore considered an 'elastic term' (Bash 2004) that 'moves beyond clarity' (Swinton and Pattison 2010). As to radical transcendentalism, critics argued that the notion of spirituality suffers from 'metaphysical backwater' (Kevern 2013) and 'obscurantism' (Paley 2008). In addition to the critics addressing conceptual and practical issues, more philosophical and ideological aspects were also brought forward that called into question the historical and cultural underpinnings of the 'spiritual turn'. First, a perceived tendency towards 'reductionism' (Paley 2008, 2010). Secondly, the Judeo-Christian origins that shape spiritual thinking in Western healthcare practice, and the question of whether they can be representative for societies that are increasingly pluralistic and secularized. Thirdly, the issue of specific actors of spiritual care and the relationship between formal and informal spiritual caregivers. Last but not least, the inherent risk that spiritual assessments and interventions will 'standardize' patterns of dying and exercise social control over the dying process, patients, and families by imposing—albeit benevolently—patterns of successful spiritual coping and good death or by distinguishing 'orthodox' from 'deviant' ways of dealing with illness and dying (e.g. Hart et al. 1998). However justifiable these different lines of argument may be, the actual consequences of such criticisms for the practice of palliative care remain vague. The growing body of empirical evidence of the met and unmet spiritual needs of patients receiving palliative care (e.g. Cobb et al. 2012) awaits a humane, professional and interdisciplinary response, which is still best captured by the term 'spiritual care'.

In sum, developments within and outside medicine have marked a deepened awareness of the spiritual dimension of curing and caring. As a consequence, it has been natural for the palliative care approach to address spiritual issues from the beginning, but also to refine its conceptual, empirical, and interdisciplinary basis. Although addressing spiritual issues is an indispensable component of a holistic palliative care approach, the critic reminds its actors and protagonists that the way spiritual care is conceived and performed deserves the highest possible attention. Patients finding themselves in institutional settings with the existential task of facing their own end of life are in a condition of *spiritual vulnerability* in the sense that salient features of spirituality (convictions, beliefs, and hopes) are called into question, or are in a process of being 'worked out' that takes place within the interaction with caregivers, healthcare chaplains, families, and significant others. Patients at the end of life who are spiritually vulnerable navigate between hope and anxiety, resistance and acceptance, the love of life and the wish to die, telling their stories to others in order to understand them.

Death, dying, and its metaphors

The question of whether the corpse is sick or healthy is presumably of no interest from a narrow biological viewpoint. But the possibility that healing may not be reducible to biological functioning and may even transcend the event of death stands for the search for meaning, which characterizes human thinking. As Henrietta's question suggests, addressing spiritual issues is much more than simply responding to the needs of a particular population being cared for: it is also about the carers themselves working with patients and families who face existential concerns about dying and loss (Kalish 2012). Her question, about whether a corpse is healthy or ill, is *trans*empirical by its very nature. It cannot be answered by merely referring to empirical facts, but by relating it to the construction of meaning in the context of the transformative social, physical, and spiritual processes that precede and follow death (Allmon et al. 2013). And here, it reveals its metaphoric potential. Metaphors are creative phenomena of language that transport meanings between different life worlds. The metaphorical method is essential for understanding medicine, whose meanings '. . . are generated by a constant stream of metaphors' (Maier and Shibles 2011, p. 2). As Henrietta's question shows, metaphors generate 'category mistakes' (Maier and Shibles 2011, p. 2) that open up interpretive spaces, for example by connecting nature and culture when a patient is said to be 'strong as a tree' or 'willing to fight the cancer'. By using metaphors, meaning is not only *transferred* in a literal sense (fighting against an enemy and fighting against cancer) but also *expanded* in a figurative sense (the heroic attitude of a patient who does not surrender to the disease). As the Swiss artist Ferdinand Hodler (1853–1918) expresses in his famous painting of his dying girlfriend Valentine Godé-Darel (1915), in the final course of a terminal illness the body itself becomes a living metaphor of the illness.

When metaphors—as stated by Maier and Shibles—can be considered as 'carriers' of meaning between different life worlds, they can also be seen as windows to spirituality. They are generated within the lived experience of dying and they transcend this experience by putting it into a wider frame, becoming part of the patient's stories of hope and despair, courage and cowardice. In addition, wishes to die are seldom expressed in an unequivocal, 'digital' language (like the time on a digital clock), but are interwoven in metaphors. Mr Schneider, a patient with advanced amyotrophic lateral sclerosis, sat in a wheelchair and stared for hours over the pond in the hospice garden and the fir trees on the horizon. As a healthcare chaplain, I asked him what he was thinking when looking out of the window. 'You know', he answered, 'I am not afraid of dying, but I am tired of living. When I am dead, I will be part of that nature over there, like one of those trees.' In the next room, Mrs Rossini, a woman with a pancreatic tumour told me, 'I am ready to die, I am longing to see my dead husband again. Since he went, I miss him every day. The only thing I am afraid of is suffering pain.' On the upper floor, Mrs Tanner, an elderly woman with a brain tumour said, 'I am old and I should be prepared to die. Nevertheless I am afraid of dying. But my faith is strong. I ask God every day to help me endure.'

As these narratives show, metaphors are interwoven into patients' narrations as horizontal constructs in the axis of time. By creating and using them, patients and carers try to secure their past in the face of death, make sense of the lived experience, connect present and past experience, and envisage the future. And even after death, metaphors continue to unfold their significance: answering Henrietta's question in the affirmative could mean proposing the *healthy corpse* as a metaphor for death as an act of *healing* from an incurable disease, for overcoming the disease through death. Conversely, speaking of a *sick corpse* could be related to the Heideggerian notion of being-toward-death as a characteristic of the *human condition* (Heidegger et al. 2008), which therefore cannot be fought, but only accepted. Importantly, both answers to Henrietta's question are situated at a metaphorical level and use figurative language in order to weave narration, and by doing so construct meaning (see Maier and Shibles 2011, p. 2).

At this point, a clarification is needed. Creating metaphors and evoking them in the face of imminent death and bereavement gives no information about which construction is meaningful or, in Aaron Antonovsky's (1923–1994) terms, promotes a salutogenic *sense of coherence* (Antonovsky 1987). With tears in her eyes and keeping a rosary firmly in her hands, Mrs Lang, a patient with advanced ovarian cancer, asked the healthcare chaplain: 'Why can nobody help me? I hope for cure, I pray every day for it, but God does not hear me. Does anybody hear me? Nobody believes that I can be cured. Do *you* at least believe that I can be cured?' As this example shows, spiritual care at the end of life cannot be provided without a minimal 'spiritual diagnosis'. Simply assessing religious beliefs, personal convictions, or formal religious membership without asking whether the construction of the patient is coherent or a source of suffering brings the validity of spiritual assessment into question (e.g. McSherry and Ross 2002). Therefore, caregivers and healthcare chaplains have the difficult task of addressing metaphors and narrations that have the potential to be 'pathogenic' in the literal sense of generating suffering instead of helping the patient to cope with it (Draper 2012). This point also demarcates the boundary between informal and formal spiritual caregiving and underlines the need to recognize the limits of competence of informal spiritual caregivers. Referrals to healthcare chaplains, psychologists, or psychiatrists can be essential for enabling the patient to use metaphors in a salutogenic manner on his or her path of constructing meaning.

From narration to metanarration

Metaphors are never built in a cultural vacuum. As components of narration, many of them are inspired by religious accounts of sin, grace and redemption, guilt or expiation. Others draw from 'naturalistic' accounts of the 'inspirited' nature and humans as part of it. Other accounts finally follow humanistic traditions that depart from the ability of humans to *think* their death and the subsequent duty of them to *prepare* for it. This web of meaning, in which patients' narrations are situated, is the *metanarration* that informs, inspires, and shapes narration. These metanarrations become manifest in patients who share explicit religious beliefs or specific worldviews, belong to religious communities, and follow their practices. Therefore, patients' wishes to die in terms of readiness, willingness, and inner preparedness are also interwoven with metaphors that draw from narration as well as metanarration. Mrs Bauer, a patient belonging to the Buddhist community, was asked about her experience of being in a hospice. She answered, 'You know, we are born to learn. And we will be measured by what we have learned. I ask myself every night: what did I learn today? Not living or dying matters, but learning.' It is the metanarration of 'living for learning', taken from the Buddhist worldview on the meaning of life, that offered her an interpretive lens for the narration of her illness. This led her to take progressive bodily decay not as threat to her integrity but as an opportunity to understand, value, and accept this experience.

The connection of narration and metanarration frames the lived experience and the metaphors we forge in a wider context in order to make it *ours*, to confirm our social, religious, philosophical, and cultural identity in the face of death and dying. Enhancing this connection can be seen as the proper task of spiritual care at the end of life. It explores the patient's resources, enhances constructs that are salutogenic, incorporates and makes sense of experience. The shift from narration to metanarration and back offers a thin, rather formal conceptual framework for providing spiritual care which departs from patients' experiences, captures their metaphors, and is responsive to their narrations and metanarrations. It fully takes into account the *dangers at the bedside* inherent to the 'spiritual turn' within medicine and nursing as expressed by its critics and the need to circumnavigate the extremes of radical transcendentalism and radical immanentism. But it also underlines the need to address the spiritual needs of patients and caregivers. This thin framework of narration and metanarration allows a differentiation between 'generic' and 'specialist' spiritual caregiving without evoking a rivalry or hegemony among the members of the multidisciplinary team. The principle of patient centredness, described earlier as a core element within the provision of palliative care, means in this context that it is up to the patient to 'choose' among possible spiritual caregivers—if choice is possible. In addition to patient choice, the decision as to *who* actually provides spiritual care cannot be planned in advance. It should be guided by situational adequacy, spontaneity, personal experience, and 'attached neutrality' by exploring the salutogenic character of the patient's construct. It makes sense to address frailty in the context of physiotherapy or to discuss the changes in the perception of the body during wound care, but also to talk about problems within family relationships during pastoral conversations. As in the situation of Mrs Lang, existential struggle with metanarrative issues, guilt, and death anxiety may be an indication for a referral to a healthcare chaplain and experts within medicine and psychology, whereas the dimension of narration requires active listening, authenticity, and responsiveness, skills that are expected to be a general part of a holistic palliative care practice (Mann 2006).

The wish to die as an expression of spiritual labour

The 'spiritual turn' within medicine—as documented in the context of palliative care—has proved to be essential for the self-understanding of medicine as a holistic practice. However, within evidence-based medicine the question arises as to *what* type of evidence can be expected within the provision of spiritual care. Going beyond the assessment of needs brings not only challenges concerning external validity but also the risk of the commodification of spirituality. In Arthur W. Frank's words, this would increase the risk of a medicalization of spirituality (Frank 2005, p. 142) that would go as far as *prescribing* prayers and *measuring* their effects on hope, health, or other 'dependent variables'. But 'spiritual interventions' are means and not ends in themselves.

By contrast, *spiritualized medicine* (Frank 2005, p. 142) chooses the harder task of searching the evidence in patients, relatives, and caregivers' narration, aligned with their metanarration.

The constructive tension between narration and metanarration offers a framework for locating patients' wish to die at the end of life. As Ohnsorge et al. (2012, p. 636) conclude: '. . . a close reading of the patients' narratives shows that their statements about dying are embedded in more general frameworks of meaning within their personal narratives and how these wishes or expectations contribute to or conflict with the patients' sense of identity.' Knowing that the patient wants to live or wishes to die is not static knowledge. Within the dynamics of narration and metanarration, meaning is not deduced top-down, but constructed bottom-up and aligned with the great metanarratives of living and dying that shape human thinking. In such a framework, meaning is never static, but is dynamic and negotiable until the patient's narration and metanarration 'fit' together. This spiritual labour is common to patients, relatives, and healthcare professionals. And it persists after death, as Henrietta's question highlights. The only normative claim of this framework is the *salutogenic character* of this construct: it helps the patient to *secure the past*, but also to deal with the present and be open to the future. The knowledge, skills, and attitudes that are needed to reach this goal are the essence of spiritual care.

References

Allmon, A. L., Tallman, B. A., and Altmaier, E. M. (2013). Spiritual growth and decline among patients with cancer. *Oncology Nursing Forum*, **40**, 559–565.

Antonovsky, A. (1987). *Unraveling the Mystery of Health. How People Manage Stress and Stay Well*, 1st edn. San Francisco: Jossey-Bass.

Bash, A. (2004). Spirituality: the emperor's new clothes? *Journal of Clinical Nursing*, **3**, 11–16.

Boston, P., Bruce, A., and Schreiber, R. (2011). Existential suffering in the palliative care setting: an integrated literature review. *Journal of Pain and Symptom Management*, **41**, 604–618.

Brooksbank, M. (2009). Palliative care: where have we come from and where are we going? *Pain*, **144**, 233–235.

Clark, D. (1999). 'Total pain', disciplinary power and the body in the work of Cicely Saunders, 1958–1967. *Social Science and Medicine*, **49**, 727–736.

Cobb, M., Dowrick, C., and Lloyd-Williams, M. (2012). What can we learn about the spiritual needs of palliative care patients from the research literature? *Journal of Pain and Symptom Management*, **43**, 1105–1119.

Dinesen, I. (1984). *Shadows on the Grass*. London: Penguin Books.

Draper, P. (2012). An integrative review of spiritual assessment: implications for nursing management. *Journal of Nursing Management*, **20**, 970–980.

Draper, P. and McSherry, W. (2002). A critical view of spirituality and spiritual assessment. *Journal of Advanced Nursing*, **39**, 1–2.

Engel, G. L. (1977). The need for a new medical model: a challenge for biomedicine. *Science*, **196**, 129–136.

Frank, A. W. (2005). You can't use plywood: the perilous success of spirituality and medicine. *EXPLORE: The Journal of Science and Healing*, **1**, 142–143.

Friedman, A. S. (2014). A primer on medical malpractice. In: F. Kavaler and R. S. Alexander (eds), *Risk Management in Healthcare Institutions. Limiting Liability and Enhancing Care*, 3rd edn, pp. 243–277. Burlington, MA: Jones & Bartlett Learning.

Gordon, T. and Mitchell, D. (2004). A competency model for the assessment and delivery of spiritual care. *Palliative Medicine*, **18**, 646–651.

Hanson, M. J. (1999). *The Goals of Medicine. The Forgotten Issue in Health Care Reform*. Washington, DC: Georgetown University Press.

Hart, B., Sainsbury, P., and Short, S. (1998). Whose dying? A sociological critique of the 'good death'. *Mortality*, **3**, 65–77.

Haugen, D. F., Nauck, F., and Caraceni, A. (2011). The core team and the extended team. In: G. Hanks, N. I. Cherny, N. A. Christakis, M. Fallon, S. Kaasa, and R. K. Portenoy (eds), *Oxford Textbook of Palliative Medicine*, 4th edn, pp. 167–176. Oxford: Oxford University Press.

Heidegger, M., Macquarrie, J., and Robinson, E. (2008). *Being and Time*. New York: Harper-Perennial/Modern Thought.

Kalish, N. (2012). Evidence-based spiritual care. *Current Opinion in Supportive and Palliative Care*, **6**, 242–246.

Kevern, P. (2013). Can cognitive science rescue 'spiritual care' from a metaphysical backwater? *Journal for the Study of Spirituality*, **3**, 8–17.

Kopelman, L. M. (2013). The growth of bioethics as a second-order discipline. In: J. R. Garrett, F. Jotterand, and D. C. Ralston (eds), *The Development of Bioethics in the United States*, pp. 137–160. Dordrecht: Springer.

Magill, G. (2014). USA. In: H. A. M. J. ten Have and B. Gordijn (eds), *Handbook of Global Bioethics*, pp. 1625–1642. Dordrecht: Springer.

Maier, B. and Shibles, W. A. (2011). *The Philosophy and Practice of Medicine and Bioethics. A Naturalistic-Humanistic Approach*. Dordrecht: Springer.

Mann, S. (2006). On sacred ground—the role of chaplains in the care of the dying. A partnership between the religious community and the healthcare community. In: C. M. Puchalski (ed.), *A Time for Listening and Caring. Spirituality and the Care of the Chronically Ill and Dying*, pp. 115–128. Oxford, New York: Oxford University Press.

McCulloch, A. (2010). Comment: why spiritual care is best left to a chaplain. *European Journal of Palliative Care*, **17**, 109.

McSherry, W. and Ross, L. (2002). Dilemmas of spiritual assessment: considerations for nursing practice. *Journal of Advanced Nursing*, **38**, 479–488.

Mount, B. (2013). Healing, quality of life, and the need for a paradigm shift in health care. *Journal of Palliative Care*, **29**, 45–48.

Newton, L. (2013). *The American Experience in Bioethics*. Heidelberg: Springer.

Ohnsorge, K., Gudat Keller, H., Widdershoven, G. A., and Rehmann-Sutter, C. (2012). 'Ambivalence' at the end of life: How to understand patients' wishes ethically. *Nursing Ethics*, **19**, 629–641.

Paley, J. (2008). Spirituality and nursing: a reductionist approach. *Nursing Philosophy*, **9**, 3–18.

Paley, J. (2010). Spirituality and reductionism: three replies. *Nursing Philosophy*, **11**, 178–190.

Potter, V. R. (1971). *Bioethics: Bridge to the Future*. Englewood Cliffs, NJ: Prentice-Hall.

Puchalski, C. M., Blatt, B., Kogan, M., and Butler, A. (2014). Spirituality and health: the development of a field. *Academic Medicine*, **89**, 10–16.

Saunders, C. (1959). Telling the cancer patient. *British Medical Journal*, **2**, 580.

Saunders, C. (1996). A personal therapeutic journey. *British Medical Journal*, **313**, 1599–1601.

Sepúlveda, C., Mariin, A., Yoshida, T., and Ullrich, A. (2002). Palliative care: the World Health Organization's global perspective. *Journal of Pain and Symptom Management*, **24**, 91–96.

Sloan, R. P., Bagiella, E., and Powell, T. (2001). Without a prayer: methodological problems, ethical challenges, and misrepresentations in the study of religion, spirituality, and medicine. In: T. G. Plante and A. C. Sherman (eds), *Faith and Health. Psychological Perspectives*, pp. 339–354. New York: Guilford Press.

Stevens, M. L. T. (2000). *Bioethics in America. Origins and Cultural Politics*. Baltimore: Johns Hopkins University Press.

Sulmasy, D. P. (2002). A biopsychosocial-spiritual model for the care of patients at the end of life. *The Gerontologist*, **42**(Supplement 3), 24–33.

Swinton, J. and Pattison, S. (2010). Moving beyond clarity: towards a thin, vague, and useful understanding of spirituality in nursing care. *Nursing Philosophy*, **11**, 226–237.

Watts, J. H. and Psaila, C. (2010). Spiritual care in the end of life: whose job is it? *European Journal of Palliative Care*, **17**, 126–129.

Whitehouse, P. J. (2003). The rebirth of bioethics: extending the original formulations of Van Rensselaer Potter. *American Journal of Bioethics*, **3**, 26–31.

WHO (2013). WHO definition of palliative care. URL: <http://www.who.int/cancer/palliative/definition/en/>

Chapter 19

Communication of wishes to die

Heike Gudat, Christoph Rehmann-Sutter, and Kathrin Ohnsorge

An everyday story

While working on this book project the story of a good friend reached us. She is herself working in the palliative care field. Her life partner had 'bad news'. He had an advanced tumour but had recently been in remission. A routine MRI examination found 'suspicious changes'. The oncologist promised to get back to him as soon as possible to discuss the findings. However, after a week he had still not been in touch. It was therefore clear to the patient and his partner that this was the dreaded recurrence. Now neither chemotherapy nor an operation was possible. They talked about death, where this should take place, about things that had to be arranged, they grieved.

This example could have happened anywhere. It demonstrates the truth of Paul Watzlawick's first axiom: 'One cannot not communicate' (Watzlawick 1967). Superficially, the oncologist had simply neglected to do something. Perhaps it was out of carelessness, or because the MRI findings were not significant; perhaps because other events had intervened; or perhaps it was deliberate. We cannot know. But from the patient's perspective, this negligence was actually a type of communication, which in the circumstances sent a very clear message: *There was nothing more to say.* Nothing more except what they already knew or dreaded. The oncologist had lost interest in the two of them as he could no longer help them. They assumed the worst, because this fear had been a constant companion at the 'table of dialogue', and inevitably influenced their interpretation.

There are numerous theories and models that describe the act of communication from various perspectives. In this chapter we wish to concentrate on the special aspects that we encounter in discussions with people who are confronted with the end of their life, particularly with people who in some form harbour a wish to die. We are assuming that a wish (to die) is not an isolated incident of volitional practice, but appears in meaningful and narratively accessible connections and is difficult to jettison (Mattingly 2010). We would like to examine the conditions in which discussion partners open up to each other; the roles the discussion partners play in relation to each other and the difficulties that may be experienced; how anchored the conversation must be in reality for something to 'happen'; the tension between professional distance and engagement; the limits to communication in our practical everyday life; and the opportunities for action that arise from what is said.

Disparity between discussion partners

Communication is an intersubjective interaction that involves not only an exchange of verbal information but also opens a space where demanding work on relationships is done by people with different biographies and visions. In communication, participants are assigned particular roles and, in order to stabilize this complex and dynamic process, much is ritualized. Every communication is also linked to an inner conversation (Archer 2003), which takes place partly verbally and partly non-verbally, and which contributes to the emotional work of the subjects who are in communication.

All these aspects are put to the test in the difficult conversations about uncertain prognoses, dying, death, and death wishes. One important reason is the disparity between the discussion partners: a person who is most likely not affected in the same way by illness speaks to an ill person, whose biography has been ruptured due to health impairment, losses, and abandonment; a medical expert conceptualizes and describes illness in rational terms to a patient who is confronted with his or her own dying and death existentially; a medical expert meets a person who wants to preserve his or her own existence, which is why he or she submits to treatments that might increasingly take away his or her agency. The opinion and actions of the physicians are held in high regard. Patients, however, have an undeniable privilege in connection with their illness and prospects: knowledge deriving from experience. They are the ones affected and should therefore be heard first on grounds of their practical–experiential competence.

The value of biography and narration

Anyone who sits opposite someone with an advanced or terminal illness encounters a person with a whole life story. As Yasmin Gunaratnam describes in detail in Chapter 2, the work associated with biography—narratology—fulfils three important purposes for seriously ill people and their families.

1   Healthcare professionals hear patients' stories and see how they are affected.

2   While patients are telling their stories, they can sort, remodel, and find a creative space to experience more control over their personal stories.

3   Narration, understanding and reflecting together enhances mutual trust and improves the relationship between patients and their healthcare professionals.

Getting to know the patient's biography

Getting to know the patient's biography and environment is not only a mark of respect; it is just not possible to understand the other person's attitudes and decisions without knowing the important cornerstones of his or her life. When things are told, related parts of the personal history (the 'biography', as the patient understands it) always resonate. Telling the story of all of this, about how the patient experienced what happened, explains, assesses, and sorts these experiences narratively, shows the listener the patient's moral understandings, attitudes, needs, hopes, and aims, and indicates the meaning that he or she is able to give to what he or she experiences.

Those who wish to get to know the thoughts of these particularly vulnerable patients about their dying, their death, and their spirituality, have to 'take care to find them, where they are' (Kierkegaard 1998) in their story and understanding of their illness. It is, by analogy with Kierkegaard, the prerequisite to offer care and advice. Open questions help to fathom the situation from the patient's point of view, as suggested by Baile (Baile et al. 2000; see also Chapter 17):

- Where are you in the course of your illness?
- What does your illness mean to you?
- Can you describe what sort of a person you are—today and in the past?
- What are your wishes for the future?
- What do you want from me/us?
- What do you *not* want?

Patient-centred diagnosis includes knowledge of the patient's treatment preferences. A 'preference misdiagnosis is a silent misdiagnosis' (Mulley et al. 2012). Such a preference misdiagnosis is not only unprofessional (Mulley et al. 2012), but also unethical, since good care must first of all include the patient's wishes and needs (Reader 2007).

Recounting and sorting their story

Recounting and sorting their story can help people affected by serious illness to reclaim a sense of agency and responsibility. Although it can be burdensome to look back over their own story, patients generally experience guided story-telling as being supportive and giving value. Loss of autonomy and control caused by illness are often given as important reasons for a sense of hopelessness and a wish to die. If biographical work helps patients to win back control over their own stories, to rediscover the thread, and to find resources, this may counteract hopelessness and might help them re-evaluate their wish to die.

With their narrations, patients remodel what they see as their 'biography', or the many storylines that might count as such. Through stories they explain and interpret moral feelings of guilt and shame, risky behaviour (for example smoking as the cause of their lung cancer), failed relationships, or difficult decisions related to their present illness. Most patients want to be treated as competent people capable of making their own decisions. They want to have 'done the right thing' at the end, despite all their mistakes, detours, doubts, and forbidden wishes. The same applies to relatives who have to endure so much without being able to help (although it is precisely through enduring and standing by that they do help), or who are hard on themselves because they feel they have not done everything possible for the person who is ill.

Affirmation from carers is particularly important, especially when patients feel that, because of their wishes and decisions, they have not fulfilled the expectations of others. With a terminal illness, this may be the case if wishes turn against carrying on living, for example wishes for a premature termination of treatment or the wish to die. Although the physician will carefully put into perspective unrealizable wishes to extend one's life, these wishes are nevertheless approved of because the main task of medicine continues to be to preserve life, and medicine affirms itself through a wish to go on living. Saying no to curative medicine, does not conform to the system. Modern medicine often struggles to support these people in a caring way.

Conversations about dying

Conversations about dying, death, death wishes, and questions of meaning require trust. Through their experiences, ill people in particular, and their relatives, develop fine antennae for moments where they can really open up. Trust can only be built if the conversation partner shows willingness to engage with what is important to the other.

As conversational partners, healthcare professionals must find the right combination of distance, authenticity, and empathy (Derksen et al. 2013). They have to become involved and accept that it will require emotional work—not least because it makes one think about one's own mortality. Professionals' own life experiences are also required, as patients expect them to respond to their existential questions.

Stabilizing while allowing emotion

When the partners in a challenging dialogue do not know each other well, they should tread carefully. The dialogue could be compared with a dance: you smarten yourself up, look for a partner, leave behind normal interpersonal distances, approach each other, touch each other, get a sense of each other, and dance to the same music. Leading and letting ourselves be led is a subtle art. You can become one with the music, or you can step on your partner's toes. You perspire, you need to be fit. And despite all your intuition—you have to practise.

As in a dance, the success of a conversation depends on various factors: the time, place, partner, and atmosphere have to be just right. There must be a willingness to talk. Communication with patients and their relatives follows important rules, such as patient autonomy, shared decision-making, and truth telling at the bedside. The question is not only *whether* but most importantly *how* to speak to the patient and his or her relatives. When faced with a serious illness the art is to find the right balance between stabilizing the emotions and allowing thoughts about the harsh reality. Stabilizing can mean reassuring, giving confidence, but also nourishing thoughts of hope, repressing reality, or even encouraging futile therapeutic activism. On the other hand, addressing reality and openly providing information allows the patient to deal with reality and play an active role, and thus contributes to patient empowerment. However, if the truth about reality is too hard to internalize, then destabilization, hopelessness, and fatalism can gain the upper hand.

The right balance between stabilization and confrontation differs between individuals and may change over time, as priorities change. Coping with illness is a process. Patients, however, find that the quality of the patient–doctor relationship improves if the physician engages with their critical questions about the end of life: the prognostic expectations, what the final phase will be like and how it can be organized, what dying is like, whether they will have to suffer, what options are available, and which end-of-life scenarios are possible.

Handling a wish to die

People with incurable and advanced disease are confronted early on with the prospect of death. When cancer is diagnosed it still has a stigma as a fatal illness that causes great suffering, tears people out of their life, and drives them into the mills of modern medicine:

Yes, I'd believe it [that someone would have a need to take their own life]. I too left the university hospital following diagnosis [of cancer] and thought, this is how someone feels who commits suicide. [patient 21 with jaw carcinoma from the study 'Terminally ill patients' wish to die']

Patients are challenged to deal with questions of life and death, to evaluate and to explore different paths, in order to find the best solution to this difficult situation. In this complex and dynamic process it is understandable that different wishes can coexist—including the wish to die. The patient may feel ambivalence (Ohnsorge et al. 2012).

The first and most important task of the healthcare professional is to acknowledge patients' wishes to die and to understand them. Acknowledgement means conceding that patients have a wish to die and that they are *allowed* to have this wish, because wishing is always allowed. At the same time, healthcare professionals may have another perspective on things, such as their own moral beliefs or doubts which they cannot hide (they are not 'neutral'). It is fair for them to express their own point of view and they might even engage in a sensitive dialogue about that, but it is of utmost importance not to devalue or judge what patients express. However, experience has shown that healthcare professionals tend to feel verbally and non-verbally overwhelmed or inexperienced if questioned on subjects about which they feel unsure (Ahluwalia et al. 2012, 2013).

In practice it has been found useful for healthcare professionals to consider the following questions (see also Gastmans et al. 2004):

◆ Why is there a wish to die? What does it mean for the patient? Get them explain it. Does the wish to die fit into the patient's story?

◆ Is the wish to die hypothetical, for the future?

◆ Have you been able to dispel specific fears, such as the fear of pain or choking?

◆ Is palliative care fully put into operation? Do you need the support of a palliative specialist?

◆ What do the relatives say? Have you welcomed them?

◆ Do you feel uncomfortable or unsure of yourself? Have you been able to speak, for example with your colleagues, in a discussion group or an interdisciplinary board?

◆ Do you know the relevant laws?

Many healthcare professionals feel unable to talk about spirituality. They feel that spiritual ideas are a private matter, which may be in tension with their own spirituality, and would prefer to leave such discussions to a chaplain (Post et al. 2000; Vermandere et al. 2011). Patients often register their discussion partner's lack of a 'spiritual language', and this might lead to their reaching silent and mutual agreement to avoid the topic. Patients have different reasons for intuitively avoiding topics that could cause dissonance between them and their healthcare professionals—out of fear, shame, dependency, their own loss for words, because they do not have an opportunity, or because they feel they are not on the same wavelength as their counterpart (Frank 1995).

Although conversations about spirituality require cautious dialogue and the subject does not seem at first glance to be 'objectifiable', structured assessments can help to get the conversation flowing. The HOPE guideline, developed by general practitioners (GPs), is one such aid (H, sources of hope, meaning, comfort, strength, peace, love, and connection; O, organized religion; P, personal spirituality and practices; E, Effects on medical care and end-of-life issues) (Anandarajah and Hight 2001). This guideline asks about hope, meaning, and the associated resources within the current life situation. FACIT-sp, FICA, and others function similarly (Puchalski 2002; Canada et al. 2008).

Many countries now have their own guidelines and recommendations on the ethics of dealing with a wish to die and with wishes for suicide or assisted death. Gastmans et al. (2004) and Hudson et al. (2006) have published detailed and helpful clinical practice guides.

Limits of communication

Daily life in hospital is busy. Conversations are often carried out under time constraints or pressure to make a decision. The same applies to conversations about the final phase of life. They are too rarely anticipated and cannot therefore take place when all is quiet—more often during a routine appointment that was actually intended for something else, or just in the context of a crisis. Healthcare professionals shy away because of lack of time, not wanting to ask questions that will require long answers. But they should be more courageous. The time invested is a gain for the future. When they are open to listening and ask the right questions, most patients get to the heart of the matter quickly. They have after all thought about it again and again. Patients keep conversations on difficult subjects short as they are emotionally stressful.

Another challenge in palliative and end-of-life care is that many patients are unable (or able only for brief periods) to make their own decisions. They are often confused, delirious, tired, forgetful, or otherwise cognitively impaired. Dementia is increasingly a primary or secondary diagnosis. This situation is difficult as patients are intellectually no longer able to develop new, helpful strategies for coping with the death and dying. Information given to patients then should concentrate on the here and now. The team should have a concerted approach, as cognitively impaired patients react more sensitively than other patients to conflicting or overwhelming information.

Even patients with cognitive impairments can express a wish to die. Their experience should be taken very seriously and they should be given plenty of support. It is a difficult task for healthcare professionals to judge how far the patient can appreciate the consequences of what he or she asks for. At this point, the healthcare professional should negotiate with the patient, while respecting her or his autonomy: sensitively and with care, they need to weigh the demands of autonomy against the harm that can be caused by burdensome or overwhelming information. These situations are very delicate. Decision-making procedures should not be shortened and a paternalistic approach should not be used automatically, even if everything is being done in the (assumed) best interests of the patient.

The right to autonomy and full information is a key ethical principle of Western medicine. This was not always the case. Many older patients are still marked by the paternalistic medicine of earlier decades. At the same time, people from other cultural backgrounds who may have different social values and moral ideas are encountered. Patients and their relatives reflect this heterogeneity and these changes in values. They have various ideas about autonomy and illness and their decision-making processes follow multiple pathways. Some make their decisions alone. For others, it is important that their families determine or support their decisions, and still others expect their physician to make specific suggestions as to how they should proceed and give them then moral approval (Blackhall et al. 1995; Loge et al. 1997; Moazam 2000; O'Kelly et al. 2011; Gilbar 2012). In our pluralistic society it is therefore of utmost importance to clarify the personal concepts of illness and the coping strategies of patients and their families.

Autonomy includes the 'right not to know'. Patients and their relatives do not have to talk about things they do not want to. They are allowed to ignore their situation even if it concerns the end of their or their relative's life. Patients are allowed to believe in miracles and to use repression to stabilize themselves in an unstable, threatening situation. On the other hand, this can prevent relatives from talking about a patient's impending death, to sort things out, and to mourn (together). How should healthcare providers deal with this? What is the task? Whose well-being has priority? For example, it is problematic for a young child to play along with a parent when the sick parent ignores or represses the severity of the situation and continues to live as if everything was normal. The child's needs are different; it would perhaps be important for her or him to be more open. How will the patient deal emotionally with the truth when death can no longer be avoided and an avoidance strategy no longer helps? What responsibility do healthcare professionals have to prevent ineffective treatment and its associated suffering and costs?

Sometimes silence is the expression of profound speechlessness. The existential threat is overwhelming; there are no words that could express what is at stake or felt. Some patients have never learnt to frame their wishes or feelings in words. Patients can have wishes to die, and can suffer from them without finding a way to express them. In daily hospital life, this speechlessness—if acknowledged—is a great challenge. Sometimes patients find expression though touch and nursing, through relaxation, movement or art therapy, in nature or in contact with animals. But often the internal speechlessness remains and then it is important to maintain the relationship, and to endure this speechlessness.

If patients are unable to open up at all, it is important, time and again, to assess what responsibility healthcare professionals have regarding patient autonomy, the needs of the relatives, and society. In particular situations it is necessary to determine whether the rights of particularly vulnerable relatives such as young children should be given more weight than those of a patient under real existential threat. These decisions require courage.

Experience has shown that in practice a conversation where nothing is 'said', nothing is understood, and no inner feelings have been expressed—thus there has been no emotional friction for the patient—does not achieve anything. Emotional work is inescapable. If healthcare professionals bracket out the difficult truths or even avail themselves of a 'compassionate lie', then they deny patients and their relatives the opportunity to have a clear picture of their reality and to deal with it—always assuming that the patient actually does want to be informed. It is sometimes easier for healthcare professionals to engage in activity rather than to deal with difficult feelings such as hopelessness, grief, anger, and ambivalence. At the end of the day, the patients who would actually have wanted to know, and the relatives who remain, are the ones who pay the price.

Physicians' handling of communication about end-of-life care issues

Breaking bad news is something that healthcare professionals need to do frequently, but are often very poorly trained in. This applies also to nursing staff, but particularly to physicians. During professional life, a physician with 40 years of experience and about 10 patient appointments a day (which is a low estimation) will have about 100,000 conversations, part of them about the end-of-life.

GPs look after the majority of people in palliative and end-of-life care. They support chronic and terminally ill patients and their families over years throughout their whole illness. The biopsychosocial model is an integral part of family-centred medicine. GPs see it as one of their core tasks to accompany the patient and his or her relatives, to give attention and continuity of care, and thereby also to talk about spiritual themes (Borgsteede et al. 2006).

In an interview study of 20 terminally ill patients, their relatives, and their GPs, Grant et al. (2004) found that 'patients' spiritual needs centred around their loss of roles, their self-identity and their fear of dying'. Most patients wished that their treating physicians would approach the difficult topics of dying and death of their own accord. Tierny et al. (2001) found that elderly patients with chronic illnesses were more satisfied with their GPs when end-of-life care measures were discussed and recorded by advance directives. The improvement in visit satisfaction was substantial and enduring.

However, according to the EAPC's *Atlas of Palliative Care in Europe 2013*, many countries do not have comprehensive undergraduate and post-graduate palliative care curricula for medical students (Centeno et al. 2013). In Chapter 21 Cristina Monforte-Royo and colleagues note that this is the same for nurses. Although most patients wish to spend the last weeks of their life at home being cared for by their GP, GPs in particular are insufficiently prepared to deliver high-quality palliative care (Mitchell 2002; Gomes et al. 2013). GPs for their part complain of a lack of formal training in palliative care during their training and continuing medical education (Pype et al. 2014). This also applies to communication on spiritual healthcare issues, where GPs feel a lack of specific knowledge, skills, and spiritual language (Vermandere et al. 2011). Empathic responsiveness is a further skill that can be taught, as it is a prerequisite for quality care and communication (Buckman et al. 2011). As Pollak et al. (2007) observed in video-taped consultations, specialists (oncologists) regularly confronted with end-of-life care issues indicated their own emotional discomfort when patients expressed difficult feelings, and responded to their patients' emotions in only 22% of about 200 such moments. In patients who do not have cancer, physicians often miss the opportunity to discuss advance care directives, although patients obviously expect them to prompt such discussions (Ahluwalia et al. 2012; Thomsen et al. 1993). Formal arrangements for GPs to work with specialized palliative care teams have been shown to improve patient satisfaction, functional outcomes, and effective use of resources (Mitchell 2002).

In Switzerland assisted suicide is permitted, under specific conditions. This means that physicians in Switzerland may need to enter a discussion about this if a patient wants to accelerate dying (see Chapter 9). It is noticeable that although there are large regional differences, physicians in Switzerland tend to treat the topic rather defensively (Fischer et al. 2005). This is in contrast to the assisted suicide organizations, which have a continual media presence on wishes to die, assisted dying, and even the topic of the end of life itself. What makes physicians defensive, and whether their attitude has anything to do with a tendency that the topic is monopolized in the media by assisted suicide organizations, can only be surmised (see Chapter 9). In any case, it is difficult for patients and their relatives if wishes to die are under discussion. During their training or continuing medical education, physicians are not adequately prepared to have these conversations and often start to talk about dying and death when it is too late. But poor or delayed communication might deny patients the opportunity for dialogue about their wish to die. This can contribute to an internalization or growth of these wishes and make patients who have to rely on themselves more receptive to offers from the assisted suicide organizations. Hence, physicians' reticence in communication about the wish to die and the liberalization of forms of assisted suicide together form a 'toxic mix' for the patient.

What can be done?

Empathic communication is a skill set that can be specified, taught, and learned (Buckman et al. 2011). All large palliative care organizations in Europe, the United States, Canada, and Australia have been demanding for some time, that communication skills should become an integral part of physicians' training and continuing medical education.

Education and practice cannot be separated. The effectiveness of undergraduate education is improved by clinical exposure, as it ensures appropriateness and consistency when delivering bad news (Merckaert et al. 2005; Pype et al. 2014). Conversely, postgraduate practice alone does not guarantee good-quality palliative care and communication (Choudhry et al. 2005).

Important curriculum components are interactive learning, lessons in small groups, self-reflection, and the experience of interdisciplinarity (von Fragstein et al. 2008; Jackson and Back 2011; Gamondi et al. 2013a,b). Learner-centred, skills-focused, and practice-oriented communication skills training programmes organized in small groups seem to be effective (Merckaert et al. 2005), although strong clinical outcome studies are still lacking (Barth and Lannen 2011; Moore et al. 2013). Mandatory and formation-linked programmes for healthcare professionals in non-oncological specialties need to be extended. Further, open learning models, such as I*CARE (MD Anderson Cancer Center 2013), should be developed. Standardized training and examinations are possible, for example using objective structured clinical examination (OSCE) stations (Harden and Gleeson 1979).

Healthcare professionals tend towards excessive optimism (Christakis 2001; Glare and Christakis 2003). Patients and their relatives tend to filter out positive messages from prognoses that are given. It is therefore all the more important to have conversations early on about a 'plan B'. Communication with foresight about possible problems helps the patient to keep an overview and control over what is happening. Patients and relatives expect healthcare professionals, and particularly physicians, to be proactive about approaching them with information (Mitka 2012). Advance care planning or advance directives are very valuable; however, the most important thing is the process of engagement with the topic, and the dialogue between patients, their healthcare professionals, and relatives.

We assume that many of these instruments are helpful, but if used only occasionally they are too static or selective for an ongoing dialogue about life and death. Wishes for the last period of life should be discussed much more as a matter of course, even in public life. Antenatal classes are offered everywhere. What about preparing for the last phase of life? The GP system could give the topic more space as part of the provision of basic medical care. This could include preventive discussions about how to organize the last period of life. Access to services and advice should be low-threshold, and earlier consultations and planning could be linked to incentives, such as protected access to palliative care, better support of end of life care by health insurance, and others. Public discussions, national campaigns, and media coverage could help raise public awareness of the issue. A good example of a media presence that works is the project *Du bist Radio* [You are radio] where people in particular life situations—including those with advanced illnesses—create their own radio programmes (Stutzki et al. 2013).

Relatives also need to be valued and supported more actively. Without the significant contribution of relatives to patient care, the healthcare system would probably collapse. Only recently has more attention been paid to the financial hardship of caregiving relatives, their own care-related health problems, their emotional distress, and the fact that they largely have to rely on themselves to deal with their own needs. In addition to associations for cancer, rheumatism, lung, or other diseases, many countries could benefit from associations for family carers, similar to those already developed in the United Kingdom (<http://www.nhs.uk/carersdirect/guide/bereavement/pages/overview.aspx>).

In Switzerland, the presence of assisted suicide organizations influences the advisory activities for people at the end of life. Palliative care, on the other hand, is something everyone has to seek out for him- or herself. While membership of EXIT is associated in public with a commitment to self-determination, people are often ill-informed about what palliative care actually is.

Conclusions

Caring with openness and respect for patients of any kind—palliative or not, those with or without a wish to die—requires a basic familiarity with the great questions at the edges of life. To achieve this in the professional area, a firm approach within the core areas of medicine is necessary, as Mitka (2012) states: 'Every physician who touches patients needs to have a fundamental grounding in palliative care, to have basic communication competency and listening competency. And that will require a revolution in medical school.'

Unfortunately, physicians and nurses often introduce conversations about dying and death too late in the course of patient care. Poor or delayed communication takes the opportunity for dialogue away from the patient, which in consequence might contribute to an internalization of the growth of a wish to die.

Instead, the final phase of life, and dying, should be accorded the same respect as being born. Patients' wishes to die should be treated with the utmost care and professionalism. And patients who express such a wish, and their relatives, should be supported and accompanied with the utmost openness and attention. This implies that healthcare professionals should talk to patients early on about the future, finding the words and the rhythm that patients and relatives need to be able to express themselves, becoming familiar with the narrative structure of their wishes and the moral understandings that lie behind them, acknowledging the possible ambivalence of their wishes, enduring contradiction and silence in order thereby to 'keep . . . moral spaces open' (Walker 1993) for patients to enter dialogue, if they so wish, about what is important to them in these situations.

References

Ahluwalia, S. C., Levin, J. R., and Gordon, H. S. (2013). 'There's no cure for this condition': how physicians discuss advance care planning in heart failure. *Patient Education and Counseling,* **91**, 200–205.

Ahluwalia, S. C., Levin, J. R., Lorenz, K. A., and Gordon, H. S. (2012). Missed opportunities for advance care planning communication during outpatient clinic visits. *Journal of General Internal Medicine,* **27**, 445–451.

Anandarajah, G. and Hight, E. (2001). Spiritual and medical practice. Using the HOPE questions as a practical tool for spiritual assessment. *American Family Physician,* **63**, 81–89.

Archer, M. S. (2003). *Structure, Agency, and the Internal Conversation.* Cambridge: Cambridge University Press.

Baile, W. F., Buckman, R., Lenzi, R., Glober, G., Beale, E. A., and Kudelka, A. P. (2000). SPIKES—a six-step protocol for delivering bad news: application to the patient with cancer. *Oncologist,* **5**, 302–311.

Barth, J. and Lannen, P. (2011). Efficacy of communication skills training courses in oncology: a systematic review and meta-analysis. *Annals of Oncology,* **22**, 1030–1040.

Blackhall, L. J., Murphy, S. T., Frank, G., Michel, V., and Azen, S. (1995). Ethnicity and attitudes to toward patient autonomy. *Journal of the American Medical Association,* **274**, 820–825.

Borgsteede, S., Graafland-Riedstra, C., Deliens, L., Francke, A., van Eijk, J., and Willems, D. (2006). Good end-of-life care according to patients and their GPs. *British Journal of General Practice*, **56**, 20–26.

Buckman, P., Tulsky, J. A., and Rodin, G. (2011). Empathic responses in clinical practice: Intuition or tuition? *Canadian Medical Association Journal*, **183**, 569–571.

Canada, A. L., Murphy, P. E., Fitchett, G., Peterman, A. H., and Schover, L. R. (2008). A 3-factor model for the FACIT-Sp. *Psycho-Oncology*, **17**, 908–916.

Centeno, C., Pons, J. J., Lynch, T., Donea, O., Rocafort, J., and Clark, D. (2013). *EAPC Atlas of Palliative Care in Europe 2013*. Milan: EAPC Press.

Choudhry, N., Fletcher, R., and Soumerai, S. (2005). Systematic review: the relationship between clinical experience and quality of health care. *Annals of Internal Medicine*, **142**, 260–273.

Christakis, N. A. (2001). *Death Foretold: Prophecy and Prognosis in Medical Care*. Chicago: University of Chicago Press.

Derksen, F., Bensing, J., and Lagro-Janssen, A. (2013). Effectiveness of empathy in general practice: a systematic review. *British Journal of General Practice*, **63**, e76–e84.

Fischer, S., Bossard, G., Faisst, K., et al. (2005). Swiss doctors' attitudes towards end-of-life-decisions and their determinants. *Swiss Medical Weekly*, **135**, 370–376.

von Fragstein, M., Silverman, J., Cushing, S., Quilligan, S., Salisbury, H., and Wiskin, C. (on behalf of the UK Council for Clinical Communication Skills Teaching in Undergraduate Medical Education) (2008). UK consensus statement on the content of communication curricula in undergraduate medical education. *Medical Education*, **42**, 1100–1107.

Frank, A. (1995). *The Wounded Storyteller. Body, Illness and Ethics*. London: University of Chicago Press.

Gamondi, C., Larkin, P., and Payne, S. (2013a). Core competencies in palliative care: an EAPC White Paper on palliative care education—part 1. *European Journal of Palliative Care*, **20**, 86–90.

Gamondi, C., Larkin, P., and Payne, S. (2013b). Core competencies in palliative care: an EAPC White Paper on palliative care education—part 2. *European Journal of Palliative Care*, **20**, 140–145.

Gastmans, C., Van Neste, F., and Schotsmans, P. (2004). Facing request for euthanasia: a clinical practice guideline. *Journal of Medical Ethics*, **30**, 212–217.

Gilbar, R. (2012). Asset or burden? Informed consent and the role of the family: law and practice. *Legal Studies*, **32**, 525–550.

Glare, P. and Christakis, N. (2003). A systematic review of physicians' survival predictions in terminally ill cancer patients. *British Medical Journal*, **327**, 195–198.

Gomes, B., Calanzani, N., Gysels, M., Hall, S., and Higginson, I. J. (2013). Heterogeneity and changes in preferences for dying at home: a systematic review. *BMC Palliative Care*, **12**, 7.

Grant, E., Murray, S., Kendall, M., Boyd, K., Tilley, S., and Ryan D. (2004). Spiritual issues and needs: Perspectives from patients with advanced cancer and nonmalignant disease. A qualitative study. *Palliative and Supportive Care*, **2**, 371–378.

Harden, R. M. and Gleeson, F. A. (1979). Assessment of clinical competence using an objective structured clinical examination (OSCE). *Medical Education*, **13**, 39–54.

Hudson, P. L., Schofield, P., Kelly, B., et al. (2006). Responding to desire to die statements from patients with advanced disease: recommendations for health professionals. *Palliative Medicine*, **20**, 703–710.

Jackson, V. A. and Back, A. L. (2011). Teaching communication skills using role-play: an experienced based guide for educators. *Palliative Medicine*, **14**, 775–780.

Kierkegaard, S. (1998). *The Point of View*, p. 45. Princeton, NJ: Princeton University Press.

Loge, J. H., Kaasa, S., and Hytten, K. (1997). Disclosing the cancer diagnosis: the patients' experiences. *European Journal of Cancer*, **33**, 878–882.

Mattingly, C. (2010). Moral willing as narrative re-envisioning. In: K. M. Murphy and C. J. Throop (eds), *Toward an Anthropology of the Will*, pp. 50–68. Stanford: Stanford University Press.

MD Anderson Cancer Center (2013). *Interpersonal Communication and Relationship Enhancement: I*CARE*. URL: <http://www.mdanderson.org/education-and-research/resources-for-professionals/professional-educational-resources/i-care/index.html>

Merckaert, I., Libert, Y., and Razavi, D. (2005). Communication skills training in cancer care: where are we and where are we going? *Current Opinion in Oncology*, **17**, 319–330.

Mitchell, G. K. (2002). How well do general practitioners deliver palliative care? A systematic review. *Palliative Medicine*, **16**, 457–464.

Mitka, M. (2012). Cancer experts recommend introducing palliative care at time of diagnosis. *Journal of the American Medical Association*, **307**, 1241–1242.

Moazam, F. (2000). Families, patients and physicians in medical decision making: a Pakistani perspective. *Hastings Center Report*, **30**, 28–37.

Moore, P. M., Rivera Mercado, S., Grez Artigues, M., and Lawrie, T. A. (2013). Communication skills training for healthcare professionals working with people who have cancer. *Cochrane Database of Systematic Reviews*, **28**, 3:CD003751.

Mulley, A. G., Trimble, C., and Elwyn, G. (2012). Stop the silent misdiagnosis: patients' preferences matter. *British Medical Journal*, **345**, e6572.

Ohnsorge, K., Gudat, H., Widdershoven, G., and Rehmann-Sutter, C. (2012). 'Ambivalence' at the end of life: How to understand patients' wishes ethically. *Nursing Ethics*, **19**, 629–641.

O'Kelly, C., Urch, C., and Brown, E. (2011). The impact of culture and religion on truth telling at the end of life. *Nephrology, Dialysis, Transplantation*, **26**, 3838–3842.

Pollak, K. I., Arnold, R. M., Jeffreys, A. S., et al. (2007). Oncologist communication about emotion during visits with patients with advanced cancer. *Journal of Clinical Oncology*, **25**, 5748–5752.

Post, S. G., Puchalski, C. M., and Larson, D. B. (2000). Physicians and patient spirituality: Professional boundaries, competency, and ethics. *Annals of Internal Medicine*, **132**, 578–583.

Puchalski, C. M. (2002). Spirituality and end-of-life care: a time for listening and caring. *Palliative Medicine*, **5**, 289–294.

Pype, P., Symons, L., Wens, J., Van den Eynden, B., Stes, A., and Deveugele, M. (2014). Health care professionals' perceptions towards lifelong learning in palliative care for general practitioners: a focus group study. *BMC Family Practice*, **15**, 36.

Reader, S. (2007). The other side of agency. *Philosophy*, **82**, 579–604.

Stutzki R., Weber, M., and Reiter-Theil, S. (2013). Finding their voices again: a media project offers a floor for vulnerable patients, clients and the socially deprived. *Medicine, Health Care and Philosophy*, **16**, 739–750.

Thomsen, O. O., Wulff, H. R., Martin, A., and Singer, P. A. (1993). What do gastroenterologists in Europe tell cancer patients? *Lancet*, **341**, 473–476.

Tierney, W. M., Dexter, P. R., Gramelspacher, G. P., Perkins, A. J., Zhou, X. H., and Wolinsky, F. D. (2001). The effect of discussions about advance directives on patients' satisfaction with primary care. *Journal of General Internal Medicine*, **16**, 32–40.

Vermandere, M., De Lepeleire, J., Smeets, L., et al. (2011). Spirituality in general practice: a qualitative evidence synthesis. *British Journal of General Practice*, **61**, e749–e760.

Walker, M. U. (1993). Keeping moral spaces open: new images of ethics consulting. *Hastings Centre Report*, **23**, 33–40.

Watzlawick, P. (1967). The impossibility of not communicating. In: P. Watzlawick, J. H. Beavin, and D. D. Jackson (eds), *Pragmatics of Human Communication: A Study of Interactional Patterns, Pathologies, and Paradoxes*, pp. 48–51. New York: W. W. Norton & Company.

Chapter 20

From understanding to patient-centred management: clinical pictures of a wish to die

Heike Gudat

Introduction: clinical pictures of a wish to die

Wishes to die in patients with incurable cancer seem to be very complex and surprisingly dynamic constructs. I have selected two out of thirty case studies from a study on terminally ill cancer patients' wish to die (Ohnsorge et al. 2012, 2014a,b; see also Chapter 8) in order to demonstrate both their complexity and their dynamics. The in-depth case analyses of two study patients (patients 4 and 22), here given the pseudonyms Jane and Cyril, are examples that highlight the complex reality of wishes to die, their course over time, and how they were interpreted and handled in practice. All statements by Jane and Cyril have been extracted from qualitative interviews conducted as part of the study.

Jane, aged 76 years

Jane was 60 when she discovered the lump in her breast. She immediately suspected a malignant tumour, and decided to keep her discovery to herself for the time being.

Jane would describe herself as independent and carefree. She was married and could look back on a fulfilled life. Jane and her husband were both open-minded and had many friends, some of whom were politicians, artists, and philosophers. In the last few years their life had become quieter. Jane and her husband were on good terms with their two children, who lived close by.

Jane tended to place her family first and her own wishes second. When we interviewed her at the age of 76 she said:

Well, you do have a responsibility if you have relatives. I always think, if someone has no one, it's terribly sad, but they really are free to do whatever they want.

Jane felt grateful that life had been good to her. As a result she felt that she carried a certain responsibility. She had a physically disabled twin sister whom she loved dearly and who had had a much harder time in life. Throughout her life Jane had felt guilty of her twin sister's disability by 'taking up space and energy during pregnancy'. The sister was part of Jane's family and accompanied them everywhere. Jane's daughter said that her mother 'was actually married to two people'.

Jane concealed the growing lump, firstly to protect her sister. When her sister died a year afterwards Jane was devastated. The loss deeply affected her. Later she wanted to protect her husband from the 'breast cancer diagnosis'. As the skin over the big lump became ulcerated she did not want to shock her family with her situation. Then, as the ulcer became infected and started to smell she was ashamed and once again did not want to say anything.

She was not sure if the tumour was a punishment, justice, or destiny. She reflected back on her life. Later she mentioned that in a way she was prepared to die from the very first day. From the beginning she did not want to do anything about the tumour. She was afraid of getting onto the merry-go-round of burdensome and futile treatments.

Interviewer: What was going through your head at that time?

Jane: Well, I thought on numerous occasions that I should contact someone from EXIT [a right to die organization]. I even registered with Dignitas [another right to die organization] because I thought, if it got to the point where everyone had to run around looking after me, it would be unbearable and I would have to finish it all.

[. . .] You know I'm no saint. I have to tell you that I was quite friendly with several people who had breast cancer and they went through all the treatments and the nausea related to the chemotherapy and all this to no avail as the tumour returned. I thought to myself, what's the point? I was over 70 at this stage. Something was bound to come. It would be this or something else. You just never know.

As the tumour grew and the possibility of treatment diminished, she often thought she would just like to get it over with. The loss of her twin sister initiated a deep desire to die and to see her again. At that time she slowly began to cut herself off from social contacts.

She had been brought up in a strongly religious family but had lost contact with the church over the years. She associated her sense of shame and guilt with her religious upbringing. Her thoughts about life and death were closely related to nature. She saw herself as a part of the nature and its flux of creation and dissolution. She wanted to keep her freedom of choice.

. . . I said to my wonderful doctor, 'beggars can't be choosers'. You know, when you have the feeling that you can't stand it anymore, you think that at least with Dignitas it will be over quickly.

Six years after her own diagnosis Jane could not hide the tumour from her family any longer. Her husband tried to convince her to get help from oncology and surgery, but she refused and openly expressed her wish to die. Then nodular skin metastases developed and she had progressive difficulty breathing. Her general practitioner (GP) was alarmed, but proceeded carefully. She avoided putting pressure on Jane, and accepted that she was refusing any anticancer therapy. She was, able to convince Jane to accept treatment at the hospice, just 'for ulcer care'.

In the hospice, Jane's physical and psychological exhaustion became evident. Initially only one person was allowed to look after the superinfected and strongly smelling wound. Jane never left her room. She was too embarrassed by the smell and by her appearance. After a few weeks, Jane realized how her condition was improving. This change triggered a turning point. Jane discovered that even a palliative care situation could open a new space for agency.

Jane: [. . .] something like a hospice, I didn't know that. And then I simply noticed: even this phase can give you an unbelievable amount. Thanks, thanks, of course, to all the angels working there.

Step by step she began to leave her room and became friendly with another patient. This friendship lifted her spirits.

Jane mentioned, however, that the time in the hospice was a gift, but it was also time to die. It was not right to prolong her life at this stage. She wanted to be able to decide how and when it should end. On the other hand the burgeoning of nature in spring, she said, was a gift and she could not just throw her life away.

The death of her new friend, although expected, affected her deeply. Shortly afterwards she decided to leave the hospice and join her husband in a nursing home apartment. Now she felt that the hospice was 'like a waiting room'. Jane began hormonal therapy; the tumour receded, the ulcer healed, and the skin metastases disappeared totally. Four years later, her husband died. Jane held on her wish to live, experiencing a good quality of life.

Interpretation

Jane was a reflective woman who gave detailed insight into her thoughts and decision processes. Here, I analyse her wish according to a model that distinguishes between 'intentions', 'motivations', and constitutive 'social interactions' (Ohnsorge et al. 2014a,b).

At the time of her hospice admission Jane's 'intention' was to die as soon as possible, and so she renounced any treatment for the tumour. However, her intention toward life and death changed over time. At the point of her self-diagnosis Jane described a mere acceptance to die. She was convinced she had a malignant disease and accepted that she would die from it. Probably with the death of her twin sister 2 years afterwards, the acceptance of death was replaced by a wish that death might come or, temporally, that it should even come faster. The wish to die and to let the tumour proceed persisted over 4 years, before she was admitted to the hospice. Hastening death by suicide with collected drugs or assisted suicide with a right to die organization had been on her mind, but was rejected for moral reasons. Then, during the 4 months of her stay in the hospice, the wish to die became hypothetical. Simultaneously a wish to live became dominant. It prompted her to move into an apartment and to start antitumour treatment.

Jane's self-perception and values were shaped by her experiences and important sociocultural changes that occurred during her life. The 1968 generation and her political activities then had influenced her a lot. She adopted some modern ideas of feminism, and rejected others. She had strong family ties. She seemed to adhere to a more conservative image of a woman of her generation when she defined her role as being there for her family and not wanting to be a burden to others if she became dependent on their help. Besides her strong rationality, spirituality was an important resource to her. In her spiritual reflections she used images of nature, its beauty and power. She distanced herself from her constrictive religious upbringing, but was never really able to free herself from images and values of guilt, atonement, and punishment stemming from her youth.

The 'motivations' that led Jane to conceal her malignant disease can be interpreted in different ways. Jane explained her decision using her social role. Her sense of responsibility towards others combined with guilt related to her disabled sister motivated her to let the illness run its course, untreated. This self-perceived role helped her to cope with her self-diagnosis and the stigma of having cancer. We might interpret that veiling the disease was also a way to retain agency and control over the situation and decision-making. Her GP, however, retrospectively suspected depressive episodes due to the shock of diagnosis and later of her twin sister's death, since during that time Jane withdrew into herself and expressed strong feelings of sadness, hopelessness, and guilt. The wish for control belongs to the 'meanings', the depressive episodes around her sister's death to the 'reasons'.

Physical suffering was an important reason for the wish to hasten death, when Jane was admitted o the hospice. Jane defended her decision to reject therapy to reject therapy by her desire to be in control and her concern not to be a burden to her family. Her GP again realized that there were other, unspoken reasons why Jane was sticking to her strategy:

GP: In retrospect, it was probably less her wish to die and more the need for emergency care [that led to her admission to the hospice]. [. . .] She was also very ashamed, I think, that she hadn't shown it to anybody, because she actually knew in her head that a little something could have been done.

The most radical solution, assisted suicide, was not possible on moral grounds. As it became clear in the interview with Jane's daughter, Jane's husband and daughter had important reservations about suicide. They argued that the time of death is predetermined. However, the GP noticed that, as soon as Jane exposed her cancer, she felt she had a moral obligation to take the last logical step as well, which was to die as soon as possible.

GP: Well, she had never visited a doctor. And only when it broke open like that did she somehow have to admit to it. Then she thought—well, *this is her story*—if you admit it, that's when dying begins. So then she could say goodbye to the people in her life and then she could die. And yes that was . . . .

Interviewer: Could I just get back to that point, the moment she started to talk about it . . .?

GP: [. . .] where she revealed it, I mean told her family: I have an ulcerated tumour on my breast; that she admitted that and that she decided she wasn't going to do anything about it, then she could, when she sort of took her leave of the family, then she could die.

There are turning points. For 4 years Jane held tight to the idea that she wanted to die and then managed to make a complete turnabout during her hospice stay. Her GP had described her determination to die as 'cemented' and 'rigid'. The ulcerated tumour changed everything, as Jane could not hide it any more. Her stay in the hospice was supposed to be end-of-life care, where Jane could 'ease the way with morphine' (interview quote from her GP) and have as speedy a death as possible. Actually, it brought the unexpected. The place of death brought back her will to live. The main factors responsible for her new approach to life might have been her improved physical condition, putting her torn body back in order, continuing the antidepressant treatment initiated by the GP, and experiencing care without feelings of being forced or preached to. A further trigger point was the loss of her new companion. It led to a short flashback of the wish to die, but then the chance to make a fresh start outside the hospice prevailed. Jane said in the interview, which took place 3 months after being admitted to the hospice and 1 month before she left:

Interviewer: And in the course of your illness, was there a moment when you wished the illness would progress faster?

Jane: Yes, very often in fact.

Interviewer: Would you like to talk about this? Or could you describe this in more detail?

Jane: Yes, I just thought: it would be wonderful not to wake up in the morning. Yes, well it was a great longing for an end, yes.

Interviewer: And could you in hindsight . . . Has that changed now?

Jane: It has changed, actually. At the beginning I just thought: oh yes, if only it would just hurry up. But then afterwards there was the, the warmth of the people. Well, I do believe it's important what conditions your experience when you are at the end.

The GP added: And it also changed [her], that she was in the clinic [the hospice], and she says it was one of the most formative experiences in her life, and she wouldn't have wanted to change anything before. Well, because we sometimes talk about it: shouldn't she have taken this treatment, the hormone therapy, earlier after all? And she says, no, otherwise she would never have landed in the hospice.

Jane's adjustment and decision processes were not linear, and in the transitional periods sometimes led to feelings of ambivalence. But Jane always managed to steady herself. Her rational and spiritual introspection, family support, symptom management, and time and space in the hospice allowed her to find the common thread running through her life again. It helped her to get to know herself, to regain agency, and to be a person in control.

Cyril, aged 87 years

Cyril was 87 years old when he was found to have an advanced pulmonary tumour. He had felt well up to that point. He was single with no children, and had worked as a lawyer.

His start in life had been difficult. He was one of five children growing up in a harsh environment. His mother, to whom he was very attached, suffered from pulmonary tuberculosis. He only knew her ill. She died, when he started school. She had not been around for him much as she was often away for therapy in a sanatorium. Because of her severe pulmonary illness she was not in a position to give him the loving physical contact he desired.

Cyril: My poor mother, I think I was five, no, just when I started primary school, when she died. These terrible years because of her tuberculosis. At that time things were different, they just sent them to the mountains. Then she came back occasionally. I don't even know if my mother was even able [*hesitates, cries a little*] to hold me in her arms because of her severe tuberculosis.

Cyril's father married again, but Cyril never really got on with his stepmother. His childhood experiences taught him to take destiny into his own hands and that he was responsible for his own happiness. Cyril described it as follows:

Cyril: When I look back on my life: a lot went wrong. Our parents . . . No, let's put it like this: I grew up in an unhappy family. [. . .] That's why my first experience: you have to see for yourself how to organize your life. Expect help from outside, I'd rather not. And so the rest of my life passed off reasonably well.

His strong sense of responsibility and his own childhood experiences kept him from starting a family. It was enough of a job to look after himself. His philosophy was to live properly and modestly, and always to be able to look after himself. Being in control was very important to him; he therefore joined the right to die organization EXIT in 1982, the year it was founded. He did not want to suffer at the end of his life as his mother had. He did not want to be a burden to society either.

Interviewer: Cyril, what importance do independence and self-determination have for you?

Cyril: The utmost importance! Utmost importance, that I can do what I want. [. . .] Many people were surprised of course: Why are you with EXIT? I said: look it's a possibility if I just can't go on otherwise. And I want to hang on to this possibility regardless of the church, of my strict Catholic family, for almost two decades after all. It stayed with me. You can't just shed the church's influence, which is particularly strong in the Catholic Church.

Cyril bought his own apartment when he retired. He read a lot, was interested in world events, and kept in contact with a few people. Cyril did not pamper himself. He lived simply. We got to know him dressed in a khaki-coloured waistcoat from his time in the military (he had served in the Swiss army), with lots of small pockets containing only basic necessities such as tissues, a pencil, a Swiss army knife, and, surprisingly, an extravagantly decorated small box which was of no use—it contained nothing. He had purchased this little casket and showed it with great care to the interviewer.

Cyril: I once went to Zurich and said to myself: I want to buy something luxurious for once. [*laughs*] I couldn't do it, I just couldn't. I brought this little box home for 50 Swiss francs.

The diagnosis of the pulmonary tumour came unexpectedly. At diagnosis he already had malignancy in the bones and in both lungs. The puncture of extensive pleural effusions provoked a painful pneumothorax. Cyril refused further therapy. He just wanted palliative care and the best symptom control.

Over the following months, Cyril's strength decreased little by little and his breathing difficulties increased. Cyril adapted his activities. He completed final tasks and took stock. If the situation became unbearable he wanted to be able to rely on the possibility of an assisted suicide. Cyril explained that it was his responsibility not to become a burden to society. His GP of many years contemplated the situation. He saw that his patient still had a will to live and a good quality of life.

Five months following his first diagnosis, Cyril fell in his apartment and lay there weak on the floor for several hours. He was convinced that he was going to die there and under those circumstances. By chance a neighbour discovered him and contacted the GP. After giving him painkillers and fluids he discussed with Cyril what should be done. Cyril was really shaken by the whole experience. He wanted to end his life immediately by assisted suicide and with help from the right to die organization. But the GP had his doubts. As it was the weekend and it would take time to organize everything, he admitted him to the hospice.

At first, Cyril felt restricted by this admission and protested loudly as he moved in. He agreed with the care team that he would just spend the weekend in the hospice. As soon as possible, on Monday, they would get in contact with the right to die organization. This agreement allowed an open conversation about the situation. Cyril insisted to be kept informed of all decisions. His voice was loud and strong and his tone sharp and militant, but at least he was participating in the dialogue. The team was convinced that this intelligent, fully competent man, lawyer, EXIT member of over 30 years, would make use of assisted suicide after the weekend. The hospice team respected his wish. They could understand his reasoning, which appeared to be well thought through. The necessary procedures for managing his breathing difficulties were initiated.

On Sunday, the second day of his hospitalization, Cyril felt physically better. He could once again breathe more easily thanks to morphine. He felt well cared for and respected. He was able to accept help. He still wanted to stick to his decision because 'there is no sense to this situation'. Because of his wish to die he was asked to take part in the interview study 'Terminally ill cancer patients' wish to die'. He agreed immediately as he wanted to support science and to allow others to learn from his situation. The interview took place on the Monday, the day he had planned to have the right to die organization come.

On Monday, when the doctor visited, Cyril showed further physical improvement. He was grateful for the care he received and the chance to talk. He emphasized that it was time 'to end the situation when you have a serious illness and a lack of prospects'. He kept repeating that it was a 'reasonable solution'. He did not mention the right to die organization directly.

The study interview carried out on that same Monday went as follows:

Interviewer: So, the first question.

Cyril: Can I say something first?

Interviewer: Yes, of course.

Cyril: About this here.

Interviewer: Yes, then tell us about that first.

Cyril: [*Reads from a prepared text, with strong Swiss accent, somewhat stilted*] I hope that my mental capacity will remain better than my physical capability, which shows significant age-related weakness and which incapacitates me daily. As a result, I have to set a limit: I do not wish to bring death or even speed it up, but I hope that I can continue to live under good conditions here in the hospice until I simply die of old age.

Interviewer: Fine.

Cyril: And in particular I don't want to use the opportunity, which I have also mentioned or held in my thoughts, namely to anticipate death and kill myself or have myself killed. But the problem of assisted death still remains, as I am not sure how things will go and how my condition will change.

[And a little later]

Cyril: [. . .] I am in the fortunate situation that the critical illness itself doesn't impair me all that much. I am just very tired in the morning and also tired during the day, but people here help me and I get by like that. That's why this restriction, I don't wish to bring on death or to speed it up right at this moment, but I want to see how things develop. And I believe that the good care here can help me to die slowly, but not have to put an end to it all violently.

Over the following days Cyril ritually greeted the doctor with the words: 'See, I'm still here'. Then he confirmed his condition was still stable at the good level he had achieved over the first few days. Then he discussed his existence, that 'old people are an enormous expense to society', that he had been 'in the hospice long enough', and 'how important it was to be in control till the end' (interview citations). This discussion about being a burden to society was conducted calmly and without difficulty. Then he relaxed with long and animated discussions of other topics.

Seven days after his admission, Cyril and his doctor met to decide what he wanted from his treatment. Under symptom improvement and care Cyril did not longer intend to accelerate his death. He expressed his gratitude to his GP, whom he had not understood initially. He also expressed, however, that he did not want to extend 'his suffering'. For him, suffering was dependency and a fear that he would choke to death in the end. If he was to suffer physically, mentally, or otherwise, he wanted to receive deep palliative sedation. This treatment option gave him the security he needed.

Twelve days after his admission Cyril suddenly experienced a physical deterioration. His breathing difficulties were exacerbated, possibly related to a pulmonary embolism. Cyril was not able to communicate, but his limbs were restless. In line with his presumptive will, palliative sedation was started using midazolam. Together with the necessary morphine dose and other medications for symptom control, the signs of stress and restlessness calmed down. Cyril died quietly the same day through respiratory failure. Throughout this time he was accompanied by one of the nursing staff.

Interpretation

Again, I will discuss here the wish to die according to our three-dimensional model of 'intentions', 'motivations', and 'social interactions'. The intention is what Cyril wished concerning life and dying: hence his wish to die, wish to live, acceptance of dying, and how this changed over time. The 'motivations' are again differentiated into the 'reasons', the underlying 'meanings', and the 'functions' of a wish to die.

On his admission to the hospice, Cyril fully intended to commit assisted suicide. Only the office closure at the weekend kept him from calling the right to die organization. He accepted the hospice admission only to bridge the unwanted waiting time.

The acute wish to hasten death had been triggered by a serious incident, in which he lay on the floor without help from anybody. In our model, this crisis would be described as a 'reason' for the wish to die. The fall provoked further problems (also 'reasons'), which resonate with the 'biopsychosocial model' frequently used in palliative care practice (Engel 1977): Cyril felt persistent pain from the fall and from his uncomfortable position on the cold floor; he was short of breath, and associated his own difficulties of breathing with his mother's situation; he felt abandoned, hopeless, and vulnerable; and the helplessness caused by this dreadful situation exacerbated his fears.

Having an accident alone at home and being out of reach of help is a terrible experience. Cyril was also deeply traumatized by this episode and the associated loss of control. To stay in control was one of his core values. In our model, overcoming a loss of control would be described as an underlying 'meaning' for the acute wish to hasten death actively. By committing assisted suicide he himself wanted to define the moment of his own death.

Other important concerns underlying the wish for control were the right to express his free will, and his duty and responsibility toward society. These concerns legitimated Cyril to consider a wish to die or even to hasten death actively. His values were influenced by his difficult experiences during childhood and adolescence and led to his longstanding membership of a right to die organization. He deliberately wanted the option of putting an end to his life if conditions became unacceptable.

In the interview he associated the expectations for his future with the feelings of helplessness, sadness, and loss that he had experienced as a child watching his critically ill mother, who had also suffered from lung problems. Cyril's intention to hasten death changed over time. Years ago, it arose hypothetically to consider dying under certain circumstances, but without knowing what the future would bring. The onset of the malignant disease let the option of a hastened death become more concrete, but was still not something to be carried out. The crisis of lying on the floor without getting help triggered his decision to hasten death actively by assisted suicide. But under the supportive care in the hospice, the wish to die became vague, but did not disappear completely. It remained hypothetical in relation to feared symptoms in the future, since he was afraid that he would choke to death someday as his mother had.

This change of intention was astonishing after his vehement request—but only at first glance. The option of an assisted suicide was also a burden to Cyril. Many of his comments indicated that he would actually have liked to live, particularly in better and more manageable conditions. Assisted suicide was a 'last resort'. If there was unbearable suffering, i.e. pain or the dreaded breathing difficulties, then suicide would be the more acceptable option. It was noticeable in the interview that he distanced himself from any active wish to die, whereas he intended to hasten death, when he was admitted to the hospice. Instead, at the beginning of the interview he read his written explanation that he did not want to die. As the interview went on to show, his own death was a difficult idea, particularly if he had a hand in it. Even though he had been raised as a strict Catholic he was sceptical about life after death.

Astonishingly, the discussion around hastening death persisted. He felt he had a moral duty to fulfil for society. He felt that he was a burden; as a sick person but also as an elderly person who was not productive, but just a cost.

Death is a terrible thing! Death is a terrible thing, everything is snapped off. As I said: it's like a library that burns and only the ashes remain. Unfortunately, it's our fate that we have to die. But I could imagine it differently. I could imagine a kind of spiritual world where you can just keep living, reading thoughts without having to be a burden to others with all the high costs of ageing.

The tension between perceived obligations, options, and wishes probably explains the ritualized daily visits. The talk about becoming a burden became shorter and more formal as time went on. Cyril had to declare, 'I am still here', but he was glad when the doctor also felt it was right that he should be still there. The doctor represented medicine, and in his view handled the case medically and ethically in an appropriate and reasonable way. In this light, the wish to hasten death seemed to have what we call a 'function' in our model. Pronouncing a wish to die and checking the response was like a thermometer, a yardstick measuring and confirming his right to be there. The ritualized dialogues seemed to have had the function of reassuring him of his existence, and hence that he was welcome, although his disease and dependency proceeded. Perhaps he wanted to affirm that he would indeed be willing to put an end to his life, being aware of his moral obligations, but that his physician always confirmed that 'society' never demanded such a step from him.

Cyril was only a short time in the hospice. But he was grateful that his GP's intervention and the care in the hospice created conditions for a dignified and autonomous life. With his symptoms kept at a tolerable level, he regained control over decision-making and was sure of having a right to live.

Lessons for carers

Wishes to die are common among patients in palliative care situations (Chochinov et al. 1995; Johansen et al. 2005). Wishes may be for the present or for the future, some are raised overtly, some seem to be clear, others prompt a gut feeling that something does not match up, and in many patients the inclination toward life and death is different from what was thought before assessing the whole story.

Jane and Cyril engaged the care team in this matter. Both were intelligent and reflective, and had a long-lasting wish to die. Both were members of a right to die organization. The hospice team was convinced that both would stick to their wish to die, but in fact both dropped their idea.

Their cases show the multidimensionality of wishes to die, which can only be understood through the patient's biography and his or her own narration. They also demonstrate that the process needs time and space: time to listen and to understand the affected person. Conversely, patients need time and space to reflect, to develop, and to decide. This principle may be feasible in a hospice or at home, but is challenging in an emergency ward or an intensive care unit, where a substantial number of patients are in a palliative care situation and dying occurs every day. (Sprung et al. 2003; Cook and Rocker 2014). Careful multidimensional management of physical and emotional symptoms and of spiritual needs is a prerequisite for engaging in a dialogue about wishes to die and other existential questions.

This matters for two reasons. Symptom management is often suboptimal, especially when access to palliative care is late and when carers' knowledge and skills are poor, as is still the case in many primary-care and hospital-care settings for tumour and non-tumour patients (Curtis et al. 2001; Parikh et al. 2013). Second, physical and emotional symptoms, such as pain, breathing problems, nausea, anxiety, depression, and social problems such as loneliness, lack of resources, or financial constraints, are important factors that may contribute to a wish to die. In our model they are described as 'reasons', which corresponds to the "bio-psycho-social model" of palliative care. Reasons may be reversible, and better management may lead to a modification of a wish to die, as seen in the case of Cyril. Thus, it is necessary to identify any remediable underlying factors behind a wish to die. Gastmans et al. (2004) have suggested a 'palliative care filter' in their guidelines for patients requesting euthanasia.

On diagnosis, cancer patients start to reflect on the finiteness of their life, on death and dying. Carers have to be mindful of that. It counts not only for professional carers in palliative and end-of life-care settings, but is even more important for those who are involved in earlier stages of disease and who, in a modern medical approach, prepare individual, patient-oriented treatment plans.

At the hospice, Jane went through a transformative process. The moments of ambivalence caused great discussions among the care team. Looking back, support and medical care gave space and time and avoided pressure and helped in her case. But for how long can one just look on? How best do we deal with ambivalence? Ambivalence is a normal reaction in unstable or frightening situations. It enables us to choose the best from among various options for action (see Ohnsorge et al. 2012). Considering contradictory options can be associated with feelings of ambivalence, and not all patients experience this tension. When ambivalence has paralysing or burdensome effects, assistance should be considered.

Jane's story shows that even rigid and long-term wishes to die can change. The term 'long-term' is relative and probably misleading. The fact of whether or not a wish to die changes under new conditions is probably more crucial. On the other hand, a constant and reflected wish to die has to be respected. It is a permanent challenge to find the right balance between negotiating respectfully with a wish to die and reviewing it under changed conditions.

Spiritual ideas and values (Pétremand and Odier 2008) can give strength and sense in life crises but they can also be destructive. They are also part of the decision-making process in people who are not religious believers. As Jane's story shows, spirituality can act as a 'kit' to cope with extreme situations and to deal with the unavoidable. The spiritual ideas that had previously 'animated' her wish to die (naturalistic pictures of emergence and disappearance, of being reunited with her twin sister) later helped Jane to start afresh (the renewal of nature, being with her family). It is therefore important that carers are open to the 'spiritual language' of their patients.

Some patients with advanced illness argue that they feel like a burden. They worry about causing work for others, costing too much, and being an emotional strain to others. Jane, Cyril, and other patients in the study also mentioned this. The reasoning may be grounded in different ideas. It can be associated with the desire for autonomy (to remain independent, not to have to ask for help), but can also be an issue of self-assurance (only feeling valued if able to care for others, rather than be cared for); it can be understood as a moral obligation, a duty to the community or it can 'function' as a way of coming into contact with others. Feeling like a burden was sometimes abandoned when care and dialogue were intensified. In other patients the feeling of becoming a burden played such an important role in self-perception that it could not be dispelled despite the best palliative care approaches.

The argument also mirrors the willingness of a society to make the conditions available in which sick people can feel well and cared for. In practice, the signals are often conflicting. The lack of networks available to care for the patient, suboptimal palliative care, and constant discussions of costs can initiate in patients feelings of worthlessness and of being no more than a burden to society. The argument about being a burden seems to be a complex construct and should be investigated more thoroughly.

Wishes to die can exist in tension with wishes to live. As the example of Cyril shows, different and even contradictory wishes may coexist. While having an explicit wish to die, he wished to live the stages of life as they came. On the one hand he was afraid of the dying process, but on the other his severe symptoms and loss of control made death appear the lesser of two evils. In a way, he had to wish something that he did not actually desire. He suffered from his own wish. With better symptom control he distanced himself from his wish to die.

Conclusion: considerations for practice

Taking these aspects into account, the following considerations may help in practice when a wish to die has to be addressed:

- ◆ Let your patient tell his or her story. Listen actively: what do they say and what do they leave out; how does he or she interpret and reflect?

- ◆ Do not be afraid of 'wasting time' when listening to the narrative of your patient or his or her relatives. Your time is well invested. Patients may restrict dialogue time themselves, since they too find the topic exhausting. Important information is often collected in a very short time. Communication training can facilitate time and information management significantly.

- ◆ Patients and relatives are highly sensitive to the attitudes and mindfulness of others. They do not open themselves up if they sense resistance or unease from their dialogue partner.

- ◆ Analyse the wish to die. Which intentions, reasons, meanings, functions, or underlying sociocultural aspects do you find? Which triggering factors cause a wish to change over time and what is feared or hoped for the future?

- ◆ Do you see reversible factors? Did you implement the best possible palliative care?

- ◆ Does the wish to die provoke conflicts or tension (i.e. with the family, morally) or feelings of ambivalence?

- ◆ Discuss your findings and analysis with your team or with a colleague, especially when the strands of the argument 'do not fit together' or when you feel uneasy or uncomfortable.

- ◆ Reflect on your own attitudes and beliefs. Which feelings does the wish to die arouse in you?

- Did you acknowledge the perspective or opinion of the relatives, especially of vulnerable family members (young children still living in the household, others)?
- Document the entire process carefully.

The two patients from our interview study on terminally ill cancer patients illustrate that a wish to die is a multidimensional construct with a history, a time course, and an interpersonal and social dimension. It can be described by its intentions, motivations (reasons, meanings, and functions), and the underlying sociocultural factors. It is important to know these components of a concrete wish to die. It is crucial to identify triggering factors that can be tackled. Regaining control over them may lead to a relevant modification of the wish to die. This typically includes physical or emotional symptoms and social or economic factors that affect daily living. Other factors are strongly linked with a person's self-perception. To question them would destabilize the person overall. This may be the case for attitudes and beliefs, in our model described as underlying 'meanings' of a wish to die. The model of course is ideal-typical. In reality we found many overlaps, connected to individual situations and conditions. Astonishingly, important values such as moral beliefs and perceived obligations toward society were sometimes accessible to modification. Furthermore, some wishes had, at least in part, the 'function' of facilitating contact with others. On these occasions it would be a misunderstanding to interpret the information content verbatim. Different partial wishes can exist simultaneously, sometimes in tension with each other. A wish to die may even coexist with a firm wish to live. The 'co-wish' to die may be burdensome and also feared, but the patient considers it to be the only way out of an unbearable life situation.

Many (not all) patients want to discuss their thoughts about life, dying, and death. Although it may be sad and burdensome to the patient, early and active communication about these issues can help to clarify thoughts and to find coping strategies where there is incurable disease and an uncertain future. Being so vulnerable, many patients are particularly grateful to have someone to accompany them through the process. It is perhaps the best remedy we have.

References

Chochinov, H. M., Wilson, K. G., Enns, M., et al. (1995). Desire for death in the terminally ill. *American Journal of Psychiatry*, **152**, 1185–1191.

Cook, D. and Rocker, G. (2014). Dying with dignity in the intensive care unit. *New England Journal of Medicine*, **370**, 2506–2514.

Curtis, J. R., Wenrich, M. D., Carline, J. D., Shannon, S. E., Ambrozy, D.M., and Ramsey, P. G. (2001). Understanding physicians' skills at providing end-of-life care: perspectives of patients, families, and health care workers. *Journal of General Internal Medicine*, **16**, 41–49.

Engel, G. L. (1977). The need for a new medical model: a challenge for biomedicine. *Science*, **196**, 129–136.

Gastmans, C., Van Neste, F., and Schotsmans, P. (2004). Facing requests for euthanasia: A clinical practice guide. *Journal of Medical Ethics*, **30**, 212–217.

Johansen, S., Hølen, J. C., Kaasa, S., Loge, J. H., and Materstvedt, L. J. (2005). Attitudes towards, and wishes for, euthanasia in advanced cancer patients at a palliative medicine unit. *Palliative Medicine*, **19**, 454–460.

Ohnsorge, K., Gudat, H., Widdershoven, G. A. M., and Rehmann-Sutter, C. (2012). 'Ambivalence' at the end of life: How to understand patients' wishes ethically. *Nursing Ethics*, **19**, 629–641.

Ohnsorge, K., Gudat, H., and Rehmann-Sutter, C. (2014a). Intentions in wishes to die: analysis and a typology. A report of 30 qualitative case studies of terminally ill cancer patients in palliative care. *Psycho-Oncology*, **23**, 1021–1026.

Ohnsorge, K., Gudat, H., and Rehmann-Sutter, C. (2014b). What a wish to die can mean: reasons, meanings and functions of wishes to die, reported from 30 qualitative case studies of terminally ill cancer patients in palliative care. *BMC Palliative Care*, **13**, 38.

Parikh, R. B., Kirch, R. A., Smith, T. J., and Temel, J. S. (2013). Early specialty palliative care—translating data in oncology into practice. *New England Journal of Medicine*, **369**, 2347–2351.

Pétremand, D. and Odier, C. (eds) (2008). *Recommendations Soins Palliatifs et Soins Spirituels* [Best Practice Recommendations of the Swiss Society for Palliative Care]. URL: http://www.palliative.ch/fr/professionnels/groupes-de-travail-standards/best-practice/ (in French).

Sprung, C. L., Cohen, S. L., Sjokvist, P., et al. (2003). End-of-life practices in European intensive care units: the Ethicus Study. *Journal of the American Medical Association*, **290**, 790–797.

Chapter 21

What does the wish to hasten death mean for the palliative patient? Clinical implications

Cristina Monforte-Royo, Albert Balaguer, and Christian Villavicencio-Chávez

Introduction: what does the wish to hasten death mean for the palliative patient?

In recent decades clinicians and researchers have shown a growing interest in studying the wish to hasten death (WTHD) in the context of life-limiting illness. This phenomenon seems to affect a certain number of patients, especially those facing the end of life or advanced stages of disease. Given medical advances, increased life expectancy, and other social phenomena linked to economic development, situations involving the WTHD are likely to become more common.

Difficulties in studying the WTHD in patients with advanced disease

Conceptual definition of the WTHD

One of the main difficulties that researchers face concerns the lack of conceptual precision in the international literature on this phenomenon. In fact there is neither an explicit nor an implicit consensus regarding the definition of the WTHD, and consequently one finds the term being used (alongside other similar expressions such as 'wish to die', 'want to die', 'desire to die', or 'desire for early death') to refer to what may actually be distinct experiences. Indeed, terms such as these have been used to describe a variety of scenarios, ranging from a mere acceptance of imminent death or a vague desire to die but without the intention of hastening the event, to strong desires or intentions to end one's life, or even specific requests for euthanasia or assisted suicide. This lack of distinction between what, in our view, are very different realities hinders research into the WTHD and generally makes it impossible to compare results across studies (Breitbart et al. 2000; Rosenfeld 2000; Monforte-Royo et al. 2011).

A fluctuating phenomenon

The nature of the WTHD may vary enormously depending on the circumstances and the patient's condition at a given point in time. This adds to the difficulty of studying the phenomenon and of estimating its frequency. Numerous studies have highlighted this lack of temporal stability in the WTHD and have noted its relationship not only to changes in symptom management but also to psychosocial and spiritual factors, including the perception of care received and the patient's sense of his or her role in life (Chochinov et al. 1995, 1998, 1999; Filiberti et al. 2001; Tataryn and Chochinov 2002).

The importance of ruling out clinical depression

Depression is one of the factors that has been most widely analysed as a possible cause of the WTHD (Akechi et al. 2001; Bharucha et al. 2003; Arnold 2004; Albert et al. 2005; Battin et al. 2007). Moreover, it is recognized as one of the most common yet potentially treatable mental health problems among patients in end-of-life care (Wilson et al. 2000). A study by Breitbart et al. (2000) found that patients who expressed the WTHD were around four times more likely to suffer depression than those who did not wish to die or who had not considered such a possibility. However, it is thought that in these circumstances depression may easily go undiagnosed or not be adequately treated (Brown et al. 1986). Indeed, it can be difficult in clinical practice to distinguish clinical depression from the feelings of anxiety, hopelessness, or depressed mood that patients with advanced disease may present. Furthermore, many physical symptoms may be due to the underlying illness rather than to depression (Olden et al. 2009). Our experience in this regard suggests that there needs to be close collaboration among members of the psycho-oncology team so that possible depression in these patients can be ruled out on the basis of the criteria established by Endicott (1984).

Attempts to assess its epidemiology

Despite the limitations imposed by the above-mentioned points, several authors have sought to estimate the frequency of the WTHD and to provide epidemiological data by means of measurement scales. The first such scale to be used was the Desire to Die Rating Scale (DDRS), developed by Chochinov et al. (1995). Kelly et al. (2003) added an extra item to this scale and administered their modified version to a sample of 256 palliative care patients in Brisbane, Australia. Eighteen per cent of these patients said they had talked to relatives about their wish to die, while 14% said they had done so with a healthcare professional. The authors analysed the reliability and validity of the instrument and found that it showed adequate psychometric properties. Rosenfeld et al. (1999) designed a new instrument, the Schedule of Attitudes Toward Hastened Death (SAHD), and published the results obtained when it was administered to ambulatory HIV patients ($n = 148$) and terminally ill patients with AIDS who had been admitted to a facility for end-of-life care ($n = 47$). They reported that scores on the SAHD ranged from 0 to 20, with a mean of 3.05 (SD = 3.85). The scale showed adequate psychometric properties and has subsequently been widely used, not just in palliative populations (Rosenfeld et al. 2000; Mystakidou et al. 2004; Ransom et al. 2006) but also among patients in active cancer treatment (Jones et al. 2003; Rodin et al. 2007) and in those with amyotrophic lateral sclerosis (Rabkin et al. 2000).

Although such scales can be helpful in terms of quantifying and comparing the WTHD in different populations, a common problem is that the quantified construct is inevitably broad and imprecise. For example, a potential limitation of the SAHD, which has been acknowledged by the scale's authors, is that it may not distinguish clearly between the WTHD and an acceptance of death, and this hampers our understanding of the phenomenon. A further point to consider is the need to address the patient's emotional state when administering scales of this kind. In this regard, clinical experience is of key importance for achieving the delicate balance between obtaining the required information and managing the emotional distress that may emerge during the interview.

Quantitative approaches to the aetiology of the WTHD

Various quantitative clinical studies have sought to identify the factors associated with the WTHD. The factors that have been reported include unmanaged pain, the presence of depression, hopelessness (often as a precursor to depression), the feeling of being a burden, the loss of meaning in life (Willems et al. 2000; Ganzini et al. 2002; Morita et al. 2004b), a perceived loss of dignity, and a loss of autonomy. In general, clinical research supports a multifactorial aetiology for the WTHD. Interestingly, the emerging literature also suggests that factors related to spiritual and psychological dimensions are increasingly relevant to the WTHD, a finding that may be due to improvements in the treatment of pain and other physical symptoms. What limits these studies, however, is the difficulty of acquiring information in these contexts. Research to date has generally selected and assessed a limited range of factors potentially associated with the WTHD, such that our understanding of the phenomenon may be framed solely in terms of the small number of variables analysed (Monforte-Royo et al. 2011). Consequently, although these quantitative studies have documented interesting findings regarding the WTHD they are limited in their ability to capture in greater depth the lived experience of the patient who wishes to die.

Understanding the subjective experiences of patients requires a qualitative approach (Morse and Field 1995), and in this context studies that examine the wish to die from the patient's own perspective can provide key information.

The contribution of qualitative research

In order to explore the meaning of the WTHD and the reasons for its emergence in patients with advanced disease or chronic illness, we recently conducted a systematic interpretative review of qualitative studies in this area (Monforte-Royo et al. 2012). The initial procedure was the same as that used in any systematic review or meta-analysis. Specifically, we searched six electronic databases for qualitative studies reporting the perspective of patients with advanced disease regarding the WTHD. This search was supplemented by literature searches and through consultation with experts. A total of 191 publications were screened, leading to the selection of seven articles that met the pre-established inclusion criteria. The quality of the studies included was assessed using the Critical Appraisal Skills Programme (CASP), which was adapted and used to assess papers prior to the synthesis. Data were then extracted independently onto a standard form. The method chosen to analyse the studies was meta-ethnography, as developed by Noblit and Hare (1988). This method was applied in two stages: the first involved identifying the main themes that emerged across all the studies analysed, while in the second these themes were again compared in order to obtain a reconceptualization of the findings, thereby generating a new interpretation of the phenomenon and an explanatory model. This model explained the meaning of the WTHD as expressed by patients with advanced disease. Of the seven studies included in the final analysis, two were conducted in Canada (Lavery et al. 2001; Nissim et al. 2009), three in the United States (Coyle and Sculco 2004; Pearlman et al. 2005; Schroepfer 2006), one in Australia (Kelly et al. 2002), and one in China (Mak and Elwyn 2005). All the studies reported the experiences and perceptions of the WTHD from the point of view of patients with some form of advanced disease. Participants in all but two of the studies were cancer patients in palliative care: one of those two concerned older people with associated comorbidity (Schroepfer 2006) while the other involved HIV and AIDS patients at the end of the 1990s (Lavery et al. 2001), a point at which the process of this disease resembled that of an incurable cancer.

Meanings of the WTHD for the patient who expresses it

Considered globally, the WTHD appears to be a phenomenon that does not necessarily imply the wish to die, since among patients with advanced disease it emerges in response to suffering. Our systematic interpretative review identified six broad areas of meaning (or main themes): the WTHD as a response to physical/psychological/spiritual suffering; loss of self; fear; the WTHD as a way of ending suffering; the WTHD as a desire to live 'but not in this way'; and the WTHD as a way of exerting some control over one's life, like 'having an ace up one's sleeve'.

The first theme, *the wish to hasten death as a response to physical/psychological/ spiritual suffering*, explains how the WTHD emerges as a complex phenomenon with a multifactorial aetiology, one that is triggered by the exacerbation of physical and/ or psychological signs and symptoms, which in turn produces hopelessness in the patient and leads him or her to experience overwhelming emotional distress. All the patients interviewed in the seven studies presented physical, psychological, and spiritual suffering, and the WTHD appeared in response to this.

The second theme, *loss of self*, refers to a set of multiple losses: loss of function, of role, of control, and of meaning in life. The loss of bodily function was a common thread that linked all the participants and all the contexts. The disease process implies physical deterioration and a progressive loss of bodily function, which was described by all the patients as a negative experience, especially because of the dependence it produced. This dependence on others with regard to activities of daily living is linked to hopelessness and emotional distress. To compound matters, the loss of bodily function also leads to the loss of various roles that the person had previously had in life, the new role being one of a dependant. Furthermore, as the disease progresses and function is lost, so too is the sense of individual control. The latter is experienced in two ways: first, as a loss of control over the body as its functions become increasingly impaired, and secondly, as the feeling of no longer controlling one's own life and future. Dependence invariably leads patients to feel useless and that they are a burden on family and caregivers. Some

of the participants in the studies reviewed referred to this sense of burden and uselessness in terms of a feeling of lost dignity, although it should be noted that the term 'dignity' was understood by patients as 'not being able to do anything unaided', and losing it
is therefore closer to the idea of dependence. In a similar vein, they sometimes alluded
to the idea that life as they were living it was 'not dignified', stating that they *weren't like
this before* and that *they didn't want people to remember them in this way*, that is, as fragile and dependent. This perception led some patients to feel a '*loss of meaning*'. All these
aspects lead to a progressive undermining of how patients see and regard themselves,
and constitute what is referred to here as 'loss of self'.

The third theme was *fear*. When patients became aware of their prognosis they often
came to regard the ensuing physical deterioration as worse than death itself, and this
produced a *fear of the dying process*. Their previous experiences of pain and suffering
led all the patients to fear that they would again have to suffer. A *fear of imminent death*
also emerges when patients become aware of how near the end is. The acknowledgement of death's inevitability and of the suffering that it might involve was perceived as
being too overwhelming.

The WTHD *as a way of ending suffering* was the fourth theme identified. Patients
saw a hastened death as a way—perhaps the only way—of bringing their suffering to an
end. Death was thus regarded as a way out rather than as an objective in itself. For some
patients the thought of bringing their life to an end brought relief.

The fifth theme identified was the WTHD *as a desire to live 'but not in this way'*—the
WTHD as a sort of cry for help. Rather than manifesting as a genuine wish to die, the
WTHD paradoxically appeared as an expression of the wish to live, but not like this. It
also emerged as a cry for help in the face of suffering. Patients were aware of the precarious and extreme nature of their situation, experiencing it as unbearable and about
which something had to be done immediately. In this sense, the WTHD served as a
way of letting others know how painful life was and as a call for help in bearing this
situation. Behind each WTHD one finds hidden cries and desires for understanding
and for someone to accompany the person in his or her suffering and in the process of
mourning for what has been lost.

The final theme to emerge was the WTHD as *a kind of control, as 'having an ace up
one's sleeve'*. The majority of patients saw the possibility of choosing when to die as
being a way of exerting some control over their lives. This would be an extreme (or perhaps the sole) manifestation of the desire for control. When patients felt they had very
little left, and that they no longer controlled many aspects of their lives, the potential
to decide how and when to die was seen by some of them as being all that remained of
their autonomy. In general, those patients who had decided to hasten death as a way
of reaffirming their ability to make their own decisions reported feeling more able to
tolerate the pain of the present and the uncertainty of the future. The desire for control
was also expressed as a kind of safety net that was there 'just in case'. For these patients
the sense of control came from having a hypothetical escape plan, of having an ace up
their sleeve, since at the end of the day they did not act on it.

The explanatory model derived from this synthesis of qualitative research reveals the
WTHD to be a reactive phenomenon, a response to the presence of multidimensional
suffering. According to this model the factors that lead patients with advanced disease

to experience the WTHD are total suffering, loss of self, and fear, which together produce overwhelming emotional distress. In this context the WTHD constitutes an escape route, a way out (often the only one), since the person no longer wishes to live in this way (i.e. to go on suffering) and a hastened death is seen as a way of exerting some control over the situation. This model therefore suggests new meanings for the WTHD and highlights the factors that are associated with it or that may trigger its emergence.

Implications for patient care

Within the health sciences the wish to die has traditionally been regarded as something negative or even pathological, it being stressed that a depressive state or illness must be ruled out in those individuals who express such a wish or who present suicidal ideation. However, the emergence of a transitory or vague wish to die in response to a particular mood or spiritual state may lack this kind of negative connotation. In fact, such a wish may not be linked to a process of suffering at all, but rather be a sign of a person's preparedness to die, or of faith in a better life ahead. Although in cases such as these there may be some kind of wish to die, the person who experiences it does not intend to take any practical steps towards this goal.

By contrast, the kind of WTHD that we have discussed throughout this chapter is linked to extreme suffering, and it can therefore be distinguished from a transitory wish to die in that the person concerned *does* intend to hasten his or her death, even if, in many cases, such an intention does not actually materialize. If we accept that in these patients with advanced illness the WTHD is a reaction to suffering (Monforte-Royo et al. 2012), then its expression by a patient should always be cause for concern. However, the evidence suggests that such a wish does not necessarily imply a genuine wish to bring one's life to an end, and consequently it should not be interpreted as a request for euthanasia or assisted suicide. Given the multifactorial origin of the WTHD, and the fact that it may have different meanings, its expression by a patient should lead us to explore the six broad categories of meaning already described. This could help to identify the root or roots of the wish in a specific patient.

Some of the areas identified may be amenable to specific therapy. Of course, whenever we are faced with patients who are suffering to such an extent we should always ensure that they are treated with warmth and sensitivity, and that everything possible is done to relieve their suffering, not only with regard to physical symptoms but also in relation to psychological, social, and spiritual matters. An example of what might be done in this context is the psychotherapeutic intervention developed by Breitbart et al. (2004). These authors designed a group-based approach that focused on meaning in life, and which was based on the logotherapy of Viktor Frankl; this intervention can be offered individually in those patients who are too weak or impaired to participate in group work. Breitbart and colleagues described how they used this intervention in patients with advanced cancer as a way of improving their quality of life and reducing their distress, anxiety, and depression. Another example is the approach known as dignity therapy, developed by Chochinov et al. (2005). In this therapy, patients are invited to discuss those aspects of their life and illness that matter the most. They are thus able to address grief-related issues, to offer comfort to their soon-to-be bereft loved ones, or to give instructions to friends and family. Mention should also be made of the study by Morita et al. (2004a), who identified three factors (loss of autonomy, lowered self-esteem, and hopelessness) that were associated with existential distress. Interestingly, a theme common to these three factors was 'meaninglessness in one's present life', suggesting a conceptual conflation between hopelessness and lack of meaning. Based on their findings these authors designed a training programme for palliative care nurses that aimed to improve their skills in relieving meaninglessness in terminally ill cancer patients (Morita et al. 2007). Although several studies have reported that emotional distress can be reduced through psychotherapeutic interventions that target meaning in life, only two studies to date have implemented such an intervention with palliative care patients (Breitbart et al. 2010, 2012). Further research is therefore required in order to explore the potential benefits of this approach.

Although some patients spontaneously express the WTHD, in other individuals with advanced or severe disease such a wish may be present but unexpressed. Consequently, tactful and sensitive enquiries should be made with such patients so as to explore their views and feelings about the end of life. When considering the possibility of a WTHD it is important, however, that this is properly distinguished from the mere acceptance of impending death. Those patients who feel they can die in peace as they are satisfied with the life they have lived may accept that the end is approaching, but this does not mean that they wish to hasten their death.

A further point to consider is that palliative care implies addressing the needs not only of the patient but also of his or her family. On occasions it may be family members who ask for the process to be brought to a close, and such a request can also be understood as a response to the suffering that both they and their relative, the patient, are experiencing. In these cases it is important to explain to all concerned the care and information that the patient will receive. Our experience suggests that relatives find it easier to cope once they understand that the goal of the palliative care team is to alleviate the patient's suffering, and that palliative sedation can be administered in the event that symptoms become refractory.

Possible implications for research

Efforts are needed to tighten up the concept of the WTHD, and both clinicians and researchers would benefit from greater consensus regarding its operational definition. Research should also explore how healthcare professionals interpret and respond to the expression of a WTHD among their patients, and examine the impact it may have on their attitudes and behaviour.

The instruments available for assessing the WTHD have proved to be extremely useful for research purposes, but they have serious limitations when it comes to the healthcare context, not least because they are unable to distinguish clearly between the WTHD and the mere acceptance that death is near. In this regard, the availability of simple instruments for detecting and assessing the WTHD would enable early intervention, including in those patients who are less disposed to express their innermost feelings.

Finally, a better understanding of the WTHD should also imply the development of comprehensive care plans that could help prevent and address this phenomenon when it appears. It is also necessary to develop specific therapeutic strategies that could be targeted at those areas that are most relevant to a given patient.

Implications for training

Suffering and death are inherent features of the work of doctors, nurses, and other health-care professionals, and these people may all be affected by their experiences. As the role of nurses brings them into close daily contact with patients it is vital that they learn to deal with this complex reality (Gray 2009). Indeed, Ferrell (2006) argued that being able to cope with the suffering of patients who are reaching the end of their life is a basic skill that all nurses need to acquire, and this issue should be addressed as part of continuing education programmes for all health professionals (Hirai et al. 2003; Edo-Gual et al. 2011).

Social implications

Although patients should be respected as autonomous individuals, some of the findings from clinical research call into question the advisability of actively facilitating euthanasia or of physician-assisted suicide. First, the WTHD appears to vary over time and to depend on both intrinsic and extrinsic factors. Obviously, however, once a patient's wish to die has been acted on it cannot then be revoked. Second, the need to rule out a comorbid depressive illness in patients who express the WTHD is an argument in favour of the need for appropriate diagnosis and treatment, not the promotion of irreversible measures. Finally, if the WTHD is indeed best understood as a response to multidimensional suffering, this would reinforce the need for adequate care, rather than support the idea that such wishes are merely the affirmation of personal autonomy.

Final considerations

In summary, in patients with advanced disease the WTHD is a reactive phenomenon, a response to multidimensional suffering. A synthesis of the research findings suggests that such a wish has different meanings, and that it does not necessarily imply a genuine wish to die. These meanings can be grouped into six categories: a response to physical/psychological/spiritual suffering, loss of self (including loss of function, of control, and of meaning), fear of dying, a way of ending suffering, a desire to live but not in this way (a sort of 'cry for help'), and a kind of control over one's life (described as 'having an ace up one's sleeve just in case'). These meanings bear a causal relationship to the WTHD.

This way of understanding the WTHD has specific implications not only for research but also for the training of healthcare professionals, and efforts are needed to ensure that it leads to better patient care. The findings discussed are also relevant to the public debate on euthanasia and assisted suicide.

References

Akechi, T., Okamura, H., Yamawaki, S., and Uchitomi, Y. (2001). Why do some cancer patients with depression desire an early death and others do not? *Psychosomatics*, **42**, 141–145.

Albert, S. M., Rabkin, J. G., Del Bene, M. L., et al. (2005). Wish to die in end-stage ALS. *Neurology*, **65**, 68–74.

Arnold, E. M. (2004). Factors that influence consideration of hastening death among people with life-threatening illnesses. *Health and Social Work*, **29**, 17–26.

Battin, M. P., van der Heide, A., Ganzini, L., van der Wal, G., and Onwuteaka-Philipsen, B. D. (2007). Legal physician-assisted dying in Oregon and the Netherlands: evidence concerning the impact on patients in 'vulnerable' groups. *Journal of Medical Ethics*, **33**, 591–597.

Bharucha, A. J., Pearlman, R. A., Back, A. L., Gordon, J. R., Starks, H., and Hsu, C. (2003). The pursuit of physician-assisted suicide: role of psychiatric factors. *Journal of Palliative Medicine*, **6**, 873–883.

Breitbart, W., Rosenfeld, B., Pessin, H., et al. (2000). Depression, hopelessness, and desire for hastened death in terminally ill patients with cancer. *Journal of the American Medicine Association*, **284**, 2907–2911.

Breitbart, W., Gibson, C., Poppito, S. R., and Berg, A. (2004). Psychotherapeutic interventions at the end of life: a focus on meaning and spirituality. *Canadian Journal of Psychiatry*, **49**, 366–372.

Breitbart, W., Rosenfeld, B., Gibson, C., et al. (2010). Meaning-centered group psychotherapy for patients with advanced cancer: a pilot randomized controlled trial. *Psychooncology*, **19**, 21–28.

Breitbart, W., Poppito, S., Rosenfeld, B., et al. (2012). Pilot randomized controlled trial of individual meaning centered psychotherapy for patients with advanced cancer. *Journal of Clinical Oncology*, **30**, 1304–1309.

Brown, J. H., Henteleff, P., Barakat, S., and Rowe, C. J. (1986). Is it normal for terminally ill patients to desire death? *American Journal of Psychiatry*, **143**, 208–211.

Chochinov, H. M., Wilson, K. G., Enns, M., and Mowchun, N. (1995). Desire for death in the terminally ill. *American Journal of Psychiatry*, **152**, 1185–1191.

Chochinov, H. M., Wilson, K. G., Enns, M., and Lander, S. (1998). Depression, hopelessness, and suicidal ideation in the terminally ill. *Psychosomatics*, **39**, 366–370.

Chochinov, H. M., Tataryn, D., Clinch, J. J., and Dudgeon, D. (1999). Will to live in the terminally ill. *Lancet*, **354**, 816–819.

Chochinov, H. M., Hack, T., Hassard, T., Kristjanson, L. J., McClement, S., and Harlos, M. (2005). Dignity therapy: a novel psychotherapeutic intervention for patients near the end of life. *Journal of Clinical Oncology*, **23**, 5520–5525.

Coyle, N. and Sculco, L. (2004). Expressed desire for hastened death in seven patients living with advanced cancer: a phenomenologic inquiry. *Oncology Nursing Forum*, **31**, 699–709.

Edo-Gual, M., Tomás-Sábado, J., and Aradilla-Herrero, A. (2011). Miedo a la muerte en estudiantes de enfermería. [Fear of death among nursing students]. *Enfermería Clínica*, **21**, 129–135.

Endicott, J. (1984). Measurement of depression in patients with cancer. *Cancer*, **53**, 2243–2249.

Ferrell, B. R. (2006). Understanding the moral distress of nurses witnessing medically futile care. *Oncology Nursing Forum*, **33**, 922–930.

Filiberti, A., Ripamonti, C., Totis, A., et al. (2001). Characteristics of terminal cancer patients who committed suicide during a home palliative care program. *Journal of Pain and Symptom Management*, **22**, 544–553.

Ganzini, L., Silveira, M. J., and Johnston, W. S. (2002). Predictors and correlates of interest in assisted suicide in the final month of life among ALS patients in Oregon and Washington. *Journal of Pain and Symptom Management*, **24**, 312–317.

Gray, B. (2009). The emotional labour of nursing. Defining an managing emotions in nursing work. *Nurse Education Today*, **29**, 168–175.

Hirai, K., Morita, T., and Kashiwagi, T. (2003). Professionally perceived effectiveness of psychosocial interventions for existential suffering of terminally ill cancer patients. *Palliative Medicine*, **17**, 688–694.

Jones, J. M., Huggins, M. A., Rydall, A. C., and Rodin, G. M. (2003). Symptomatic distress, hopelessness, and the desire for hastened death in hospitalized cancer patients. *Journal of Psychosomatic Research*, **55**, 411–418.

Kelly, B., Burnett, P., Pelusi, D., Badger, S., Varghese, F., and Robertson, M. (2002). Terminally ill cancer patients wish to hasten death. *Palliative Medicine*, **16**, 339–345.

Kelly, B., Burnett, P., Pelusi, D., Badger, S., Varghese, F., and Robertson, M. (2003). Factors associated with the wish to hasten death: a study of patients with terminal illness. *Psychological Medicine*, **33**, 75–81.

Lavery, J. V., Boyle, J., Dickens, B. M., Maclean, H., and Singer, P. A. (2001). Origins of the desire for euthanasia and assisted suicide in people with HIV-1 or AIDS: a qualitative study. *Lancet*, **358**, 362–367.

Mak, Y. Y. and Elwyn, G. (2005). Voices of the terminally ill: uncovering the meaning of desire for euthanasia. *Palliative Medicine*, **19**, 343–350.

Monforte-Royo, C., Villavicencio-Chávez, C., Tomás-Sábado, J., and Balaguer, A. (2011). The wish to hasten death: a review of clinical studies. *Psycho-Oncology*, **20**, 795–804.

Monforte-Royo, C., Villavicencio-Chávez, C., Tomás-Sábado, J., Mahtani Chugani, V., and Balaguer, A. (2012). What lies behind the wish to hasten death? A systematic review and meta-ethnography from the perspective of the patients. *PLoS ONE*, **7**, e37117.

Morita, T., Kawa, M., Honke, Y., et al. (2004a). Existential concerns of terminally ill cancer patients receiving specialized palliative care in Japan. *Supportive Care in Cancer*, **12**, 137–140.

Morita, T., Sakaguchi, Y., Hirai, K., Tsuneto, S., and Shima, Y. (2004b). Desire for death and request to hasten death of Japanese terminally ill cancer patients receiving specialized inpatient palliative care. *Journal of Pain and Symptom Management*, **27**, 44–52.

Morita, T., Murata, H., Hirai, K., et al. (2007). Meaninglessness in terminally ill cancer patients: a validation study and nurse education intervention trial. *Journal of Pain and Symptom Management*, **34**, 160–170.

Morse, J. M. and Field, P. A. (1995). *Qualitative Research Methods for Health Professionals*. Thousand Oaks, CA: Sage.

Mystakidou, K., Rosenfeld, B., Parpa, E., et al. (2004). The schedule of attitudes toward hastened death: validation analysis in terminally ill cancer patients. *Palliative and Supportive Care*, **2**, 395–402.

Nissim, R., Gagliese, L., and Rodin, G. (2009). The desire for hastened death in individuals with advanced cancer: a longitudinal qualitative study. *Social Science and Medicine*, **69**, 165–171.

Noblit, G. and Hare, R. (1988). *Meta-Ethnography: Synthesizing Qualitative Studies*. Newbury Park, CA: Sage.

Olden, M., Rosenfeld, B., Pessin, H., and Breitbart, W. (2009). Measuring depression at the end of life: is the Hamilton Depression Rating Scale a valid instrument? *Assessment*, **16**, 43–54.

Pearlman, R. A., Hsu, C., Starks, H., et al. (2005). Motivations for physician-assisted suicide. *Journal of General Internal Medicine*, **20**, 234–239.

Rabkin, J. G., Wagner, G. J., and Del Bene, M. (2000). Resilience and distress among amyotrophic lateral sclerosis patients and caregivers. *Psychosomatic Medicine*, **62**, 271–279.

Ransom, S., Sacco, W. P., Weitzner, M. A., Azzarello, L. M., and McMillan, S. C. (2006). Interpersonal factors predict increased desire for hastened death in late-stage cancer patients. *Annals of Behavioral Medicine*, **31**, 63–69.

Rodin, G., Zimmermann, C., Rydall, A., et al. (2007). The desire for hastened death in patients with metastatic cancer. *Journal of Pain and Symptom Management*, **33**, 661–675.

Rosenfeld, B. (2000). Assisted suicide, depression and the right to die. *Psychology, Public Policy and Law*, **6**, 467–488.

Rosenfeld, B., Breitbart, W., Stein, K., et al. (1999). Measuring desire for death among patients with HIV/AIDS: The schedule of attitudes toward hastened death. *American Journal of Psychiatry*, **156**, 94–100.

Rosenfeld, B., Breitbart, W., Galietta, M., et al. (2000). The schedule of attitudes toward hastened death. Measuring desire for death in terminally ill cancer patients. *Cancer*, **88**, 2868–2875.

Schroepfer, T. A. (2006). Mind frames towards dying and factors motivating their adoption by terminally ill elders. *Journals of Gerontology*, **61**, S129–S139.

Tataryn, D. and Chochinov, H. M. (2002). Predicting the trajectory of will to live in terminally ill patients. *Psychosomatics*, **43**, 370–377.

Willems, D. L., Daniels, E. R., van der Wal, G., van der Maas, P. J., and Emanuel, E. J. (2000). Attitudes and practices concerning the end of life: a comparison between physicians from the United States and from The Netherlands. *Archives of Internal Medicine*, **160**, 63–68.

Wilson, K., Scott, J. F., Graham, I. D., et al. (2000). Attitudes of terminally ill patients toward euthanasia and physician-assisted suicide. *Archives of Internal Medicine*, **160**, 2454–2460.

Part V

Conclusion

Chapter 22

Concluding dialogue

KATHRIN OHNSORGE: Should patients be informed in advance about the possibility of palliative sedation until death, or do they not need to be informed if the decision for palliative sedation is reserved for physicians—as the ultima ratio measure, in situations of emergency or in the case of refractory symptoms? If patients must be informed in advance, should they then also have the possibility to choose palliative sedation if they feel that nothing else works?

SETTIMIO MONTEVERDE: The challenge of providing good medical care at the end of life consists in not intentionally hastening death, although death itself is unavoidable. In the case of refractory symptoms the doctrine of double effect is advocated to distinguish 'foreseen' from 'intended' consequences. The question of whether it is possible to clearly distinguish merely 'foreseen' from 'intended' consequences has led to an important debate within medical ethics that questioned the helpfulness of the doctrine for justifying clinical decisions at the end of life. Nevertheless, the doctrine is still considered to provide the ethico-legal ground for palliative sedation until death: triggered by physical or psychological symptoms, the escalation of drugs for symptom control is considered to be justified when no alternative is available, even if this hastens death. But this 'pragmatic' solution cannot hide two concomitant ethical tensions. The first stems from the temporal relatedness of allowing death and hastening dying. The second relates to the goals of care and the distinction of treating 'refractory' symptoms from treating 'suffering' from refractory symptoms by palliative sedation at the end of life. One important means of dealing with these normative tensions is to acknowledge that—although the level of normative safety should be as high as possible—a 'grey zone' of hastening death cannot be avoided as long as the patient's suffering triggers the therapeutic response. Another is to strengthen patients' and families' choices in the process of planning care in advance. If the doctor, by virtue of his or her knowledge about the illness trajectories, thinks it is possible that palliative sedation could be a realistic option for a given patient (due to the specific characteristics of the situation), the patient should be given the possibility of taking an active role in the decision. Withholding information from a conscious patient by advocating a kind of therapeutic privilege would be an act of inappropriate paternalism. Where the possibility of sedation can be foreseen (even for anticipated emergency cases), the consent of the patient or legal representative should also be foreseen.

    The doctrine of double effect is legitimately criticized for its justifiability. A 'shared ethical work' of doctors, patients, proxies, families, and co-workers is needed which removes the normative load of the situation exclusively from the doctor's shoulders and distributes it among the other actors. The patient's 'feeling that nothing else works' is a necessary but insufficient condition for palliative sedation. It should be assessed carefully in order to rule out that undertreated—but otherwise treatable—symptoms may trigger a premature use of sedatives.

H. CHRISTOF MÜLLER-BUSCH: Certainly patients should be informed in advance about palliative sedation as a therapeutic option that is widely accepted in palliative care. Early information about the indication, forms, possibilities, and goals of palliative sedation is an essential part of advance care planning, especially in patients at risk of developing refractory symptoms, emergency events, agitated anxiety, or intolerable suffering in the terminal or final phase. Prevention of suffering is one of the main intentions behind this early information about palliative sedation and effective communication about the possibilities and goals of palliative care. Information on palliative sedation as a therapeutic option to manage intolerable suffering by reducing consciousness or awareness should never be given with a negative connotation such as 'ultima ratio' or 'secret weapon'. It is a good therapeutic method in refractory suffering and not just an alternative possibility if patients and relatives ask for the hastening of death.

Like every treatment, the kind and depth of sedation must correspond to a medical indication. Offering palliative sedation on the basis of a medical indication lies within the responsibility of the physician, while the patient has the right to decide whether this form of therapy is adequate for his or her special situation. When deep sedation until death is indicated in certain circumstances this form of treatment should be performed after the patient has evaluated a trial period, during interruption of the sedative. In the communication process the potential side effects of palliative sedation, as well as its potential misuse as an alternative to euthanasia, should be discussed in a sensitive and respectful way.

LARS JOHAN MATERSTVEDT: In order to respect patient autonomy, physicians are required to inform competent patients about diagnosis, prognosis, and treatment options. It follows that all relevant aspects of palliative sedation must be 'put on the table', as they are. I very much agree with Christof that one should present palliative sedation as good treatment that we, fortunately, are able to provide—instead of some sort of desperate last resort, in case lighter and/or intermittent forms of palliative sedation prove inappropriate. If that is the case, the patient must be told that the sedation is going to be deep and is likely to be continuous until death. At the same time, it must be made absolutely clear to all involved that this is still proportionate medical treatment and not in any way a 'form of' euthanasia, which has nothing to do with treatment—that these are measures that are completely different in terms of intention (treatment versus deliberately ending life), procedure (drugs given to alleviate suffering versus drugs given to kill), and outcome (symptom relief versus immediate death).

I also believe we should not talk much about the doctrine of double effect in this context, if at all. Research suggests that life is not shortened when palliative sedation is provided in the last week or so of life, and if that is correct this doctrine will not apply under those circumstances. In any case, a randomized controlled trial to establish the fact of the matter is out of the question for clinical and ethical reasons, and so the evidence base is going to be poor. The concerns I have lie elsewhere: that deep and continuous palliative sedation turns one into a 'socially dead' person—or 'living dead'—and for that reason it is a radical intervention, and so one might legitimately ask in what sense it contributes to quality of life. And last but not least, the issue of the indications for deep and continuous palliative sedation is a difficult one; what if, for example, existential suffering appears as refractory where medical symptoms are being adequately controlled 'the normal way'? In any event, as a patient is not in a position to demand that particular treatments be given, it is at the discretion of the doctor to decide about this—a decision that may be hard indeed.

HEIKE GUDAT: There is another issue I would like to raise. In practice, some cancer patients are scarred by disease. After years of chemotherapy, operations, toxic drugs, and radiation, their body looks different and disease and treatments impair their cognition. They suffer from fatigue, lack of concentration, and difficulties in planning and acting. They live in the here and now; they themselves or their families tell us that they have become 'another person'. The narrative approach may be shaped by the actual situation. Maybe the patient has even lost the link to their former life or biography, 'how it felt'. How can we deal with such situations?

SETTIMIO MONTEVERDE: I think this is a very complex question, which refers to the issue of what constitutes a person and what role recognition by others (even significant others) plays. At first glance, I would say that it is still the one person (with 'experiential' and 'critical' interests) understood as a biopsychosocial and spiritual continuum at a moment where she or he experiences that this continuum is threatened by the illness and its repercussions on life. But I refrain from speaking of two people or personalities. Maybe I would help the relatives to articulate the threat of this perceived loss of continuity and what it means to them. But when speaking to the patient and the family I would rather invite them to seek 'disrupted *continuity*' in the way they communicate with the patient and experience the situation of the patient, instead of 'discontinuity'.

H. CHRISTOF MÜLLER-BUSCH: I would like to make only a very short comment on Heike's complex question, which raises important aspects of communication that respects the experience of illness and the burden of a long illness career. With respect to the changes in self-esteem and identity, we must acknowledge that there is no way back in chronic illness, but finding a purpose even in a scarred life can help to strengthen resilience. As Viktor Frankl said: 'meaning cannot be given, it must be found'. Even though we fail in empathic communication often enough, it is a good strategy not to try to give meaning in end-of-life care, but to have in mind resilience and the possibility that meaning can be found.

LARS JOHAN MATERSTVEDT: My own experience with cancer patients is through research on such patients who had a short life expectancy and were inpatients at a palliative medicine unit. Since Heike's question is clinical, I am accordingly in no position to make a qualified answer to it. That said, I have been seriously ill myself with a life-threatening disease, and came very close to dying. So in the capacity of a former patient I can at least relate to the issue of personal change. What struck me back then was how little autonomy I had in reality, and that clear thinking is difficult indeed when illness knocks you off your feet both physically and mentally. Furthermore, one doesn't know beforehand how one is going to respond to serious illness, so one might be surprised by oneself in this regard. I do believe that Heike's description fits nicely with the discussion in my chapter in this volume [Chapter 12] of what I call empirical, as opposed to ethical autonomy; that is to say, one's *ability* to act autonomously can in practice be severely impaired even though one has the *right* to choose for oneself—due to 'autonomy-reducing' factors of exactly the sort Heike mentions; I myself list clinical depression, hopelessness, pain, dyspnoea, nausea, delirium, fatigue, cachexia, the experience of meaninglessness, existential crisis/suffering, and dementia. So if a patient 'loses' himself or herself to the extent that Heike describes, it would seem you are indeed dealing with a 'new' or another person.

May I add that Heike's description also serves to show just how demanding the work of clinicians can be. Here the task before them is 'far away' from medicine; rather, it would appear to be existential in nature, in the sense of helping the patient find out who he or she actually is—or wants to be.

Author index

Subject index

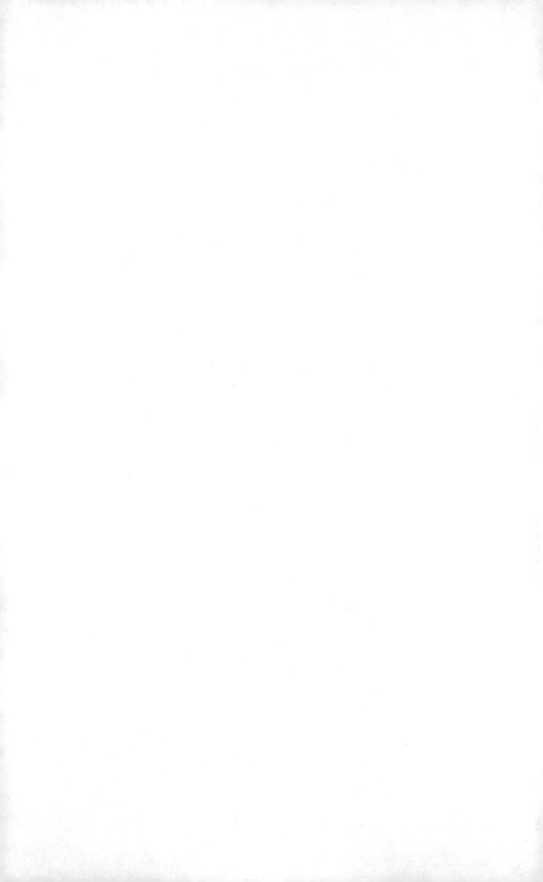